Study Guide

Lehne's Pharmacology for Nursing Care

Twelfth Edition

Jacqueline Rosenjack Burchum, DNSc, FNP-BC, CNE
Laura D. Rosenthal, DNP, RN, ACNP-BC, FAANP

Prepared by
Jennifer J. Yeager, PhD, MSN, RN
Associate Professor, School of Nursing
Tarleton State University
Stephenville, Texas

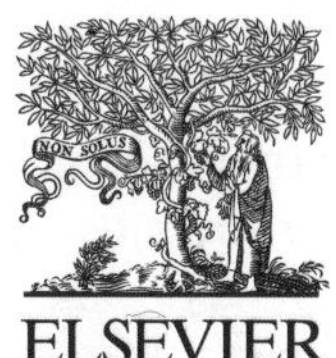

ELSEVIER

Elsevier
3251 Riverport Lane
St. Louis, Missouri 63043

STUDY GUIDE FOR LEHNE'S PHARMACOLOGY FOR NURSING CARE, TWELFTH EDITION **ISBN: 978-0-443-10619-4**

Previous editions copyrighted 2023, 2019, 2016

Executive Content Strategist: Lee Henderson
Sr. Content Development Manager: Lisa P. Newton
Publishing Services Manager: Deepthi Unni
Senior Project Manager: Kamatchi Madhavan
Design Direction: Gopal Venkatraman

Printed in India

Last digit is the print number: 9 8 7 6 5 4 3 2 1

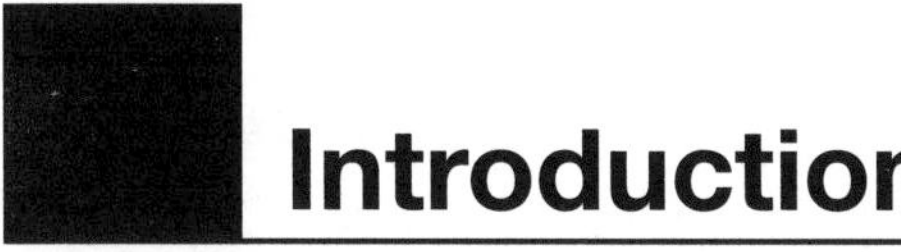

Introduction

The critical thinking, Next-Generation NCLEX® Examination (NGN) item types, and case study questions in this *Study Guide* include review of knowledge, application of knowledge to nursing care, analyses of nursing situations that require clinical judgment, and prioritization of nursing actions. When this book is used as a study guide, the questions that do not have a ▶ or ✳ before them are excellent tools to augment the initial reading of the textbook before attending class and to use for review after classroom activities. Knowledge of drug action, interactions, administration directives, and adverse effects is required before the nurse can engage in clinical decision-making.

The questions that have a ▶ or ✳ before them require more than repetition of the information in the textbook. Questions preceded by ▶ require application and analysis of information, whereas those preceded by ✳ require prioritization, including selecting the most important information or action. Identifying the correct answer to these questions requires careful examination of the data and reflection on the patient in a holistic manner. You will have to integrate other nursing knowledge, such as developmental consideration, pathophysiology, signs and symptoms, and laboratory values, as well as timing and prioritization of actions. These ▶ and ✳ critical thinking questions reflect the reasoning that students and new graduate nurses must be able to perform to safely administer pharmacotherapy. They are an excellent source of review when preparing for the NCLEX examination.

A useful strategy when presented with the case studies in this workbook is to read the last sentence first. Knowing the question that is being asked guides identification of pertinent information in the case. When reading the rest of the information in the case, identify key words and data. Identify assessment findings and laboratory values that are normal or abnormal. Think about the situation to identify whether it is a normal part of nursing care or if it requires collaboration with the provider.

Critical thinking by the nursing student requires assimilating classroom learning and clinical experience. No two experiences are the same. Be careful not to add information into the question based on your experience with patients when answering questions in this *Study Guide*. But *do* engage in discussion about similar patient experiences with faculty and peers. Be prepared to explain your thinking. It will enrich your learning experience.

The authors and Elsevier welcome any feedback you have about the content of the *Study Guide*.

Answers to the Case Studies can be reviewed online at http://evolve.elsevier.com/Lehne/.

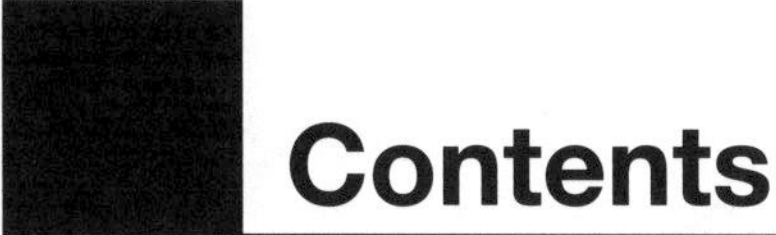

Contents

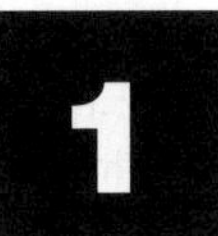

Orientation to Pharmacology

STUDY QUESTIONS

Matching

Match the term with its definition.

1. ___ Any chemical that can affect living processes.
2. ___ The medical use of drugs.
3. ___ The study of drugs and their interactions with living systems.
4. ___ The study of drugs in humans.
    a. Clinical pharmacology
    b. Drug
    c. Pharmacology
    d. Therapeutics

Completion

Fill in the blank with the property of an ideal drug that the nurse considers in the following situations.

5. The nurse teaches a patient to avoid engaging in hazardous activities when taking an antihistamine for allergy symptoms.

    ____

6. The nurse explains that a generic form of a newly prescribed drug is available to a patient who has limited insurance coverage for drugs.

    ____

7. The nurse researches if an antidote is available when administering drugs that have the potential to cause significant harm or death.

    ____

8. The nurse administers ciprofloxacin through a second intravenous line separate from all other drugs.

    ____

9. The nurse explains that quinapril and Accupril are names for the same drug.

    ____

10. The nurse reassesses the patient 20–30 minutes after administering an opiate analgesic.

    ____

11. During discharge teaching, the nurse assesses if the patient will be able to take a prescribed drug four times a day as ordered.

    ____

12. When a patient is, or could be, pregnant, the nurse researches the pregnancy and lactation information for every drug administered.

    ____

13. The nurse teaches patients that the medicine cabinet is a bad place to store medications because the heat and humidity can damage the drug.

    ____

14. The nurse is aware that African Americans often do not respond as well as Caucasians to angiotensin-converting enzyme inhibitors (ACEIs) prescribed for hypertension.

    ____

CRITICAL THINKING, PRIORITIZATION, AND DELEGATION QUESTIONS

✳15. Which patient would be **priority** when providing nursing care to multiple patients? A patient who:
    a. would like to know if a newly prescribed drug is available in generic form.
    b. has requested a laxative because they have not had a bowel movement in 2 days.
    c. received oral drugs 1 hour ago and now reports that they have raised, itchy, red bumps.
    d. is prescribed a drug, the name of which the nurse does not recognize.

▶16. Which *nursing* action would **best** meet the therapeutic objective of drug therapy?
   a. Assessing the patient for adverse effects of drug therapy for a newly prescribed drug
   b. Providing community education on how to read labels on over-the-counter drugs
   c. Checking a patient's blood pressure during their visit to the health center
   d. Recommending a patient talk to their prescriber before taking over-the-counter drugs

17. The nurse explains the importance of genetic testing prior to initiating drug therapy with clopidogrel. Which statement indicates the patient understands the importance of genetic testing:
   a. "By having genetic testing done, it will help determine the dosing of the drug."
   b. "This type of testing will determine if my age and weight affect how the drug works."
   c. "The testing may determine if I will have a reaction to the drug other people don't have."
   d. "If I don't get the testing done, I won't know if I have liver or kidney problems."

CLINICAL JUDGMENT CASE STUDY

The nurse is caring for a patient returning to the nursing unit following an esophagogastroduodenoscopy (EGD) under conscious sedation with midazolam for noncardiac chest pain. The patient returned to the unit at 1200. The patient did not take their 0900 oral drugs prior to the procedure because they were told to take nothing by mouth (NPO). The patient's medical history includes hypertension, heart failure, osteoarthritis, and depression. Prescribed drugs include carvedilol 12.5 mg twice daily, furosemide 40 mg daily, aspirin 81 mg daily, clopidogrel 75 mg daily, fluoxetine 80 mg daily, and Tylenol 8-Hour Arthritis Pain 650 mg three times per day. On exam, the patient is alert, responding to questions appropriately, and asking for a cup of coffee. Blood pressure is 145/85 mm Hg, pulse 68 bpm, respirations 14 bpm, temperature 97.3°F, and oxygen saturation 98% on 2 L of oxygen. The patient's adult child accompanied the patient today to drive them home; they are frequently asking when they can leave, as the adult child needs to get to work.

18. Which factors must the nurse consider when deciding which of the 0900 oral drugs should be administered at this time? **(Select all that apply; one, some or all may be correct.)**
   a. Mechanism of drug action
   b. Patient assessment findings
   c. Schedule of drug administration
   d. The ability to swallow the drugs
   e. Drugs given during the procedure
   f. Consequences if drug dosages are missed
   g. A responsible person is with the patient
   h. The patient can void

2 Application of Pharmacology in Nursing Practice

STUDY QUESTIONS

Matching

Match the nursing action with the eight aspects of drug therapy.

1. ___ Knowing the major adverse reactions of a drug, when they are likely to occur, early signs of development, and interventions to minimize discomfort and harm.
2. ___ The rights of drug administration coupled with the knowledge of pharmacology.
3. ___ Knowing the reason for drug use and being able to assess the patient's medication needs.
4. ___ Knowing the early signs of toxicity and the proper intervention when it occurs.
5. ___ Enhancing drug therapy through nonpharmacologic measures.
6. ___ Collecting baseline data, identifying high-risk patients, and determining the patient's capacity for self-care.
7. ___ Taking a thorough drug history, advising the patient to avoid drugs that may interact with prescribed medication, and monitoring for adverse interactions.
8. ___ The process to determine if a drug is beneficial or causes harm.
   a. Preadministration assessment
   b. Dosage and administration
   c. Promoting therapeutic effects
   d. Minimizing adverse effects
   e. Minimizing adverse interactions
   f. Making as-needed (PRN) decisions
   g. Evaluating responses to medication
   h. Managing toxicity

CRITICAL THINKING, PRIORITIZATION, AND DELEGATION QUESTIONS

9. The nurse is preparing to administer an antihypertensive drug. The nurse obtains a blood pressure reading of 110/70 mm Hg. Which action should the nurse take?
   a. Administer the medication because the antihypertensive medication is prescribed.
   b. Determine baseline blood pressure to determine if the medication should be administered.
   c. Call the prescriber and ask if the medication should be administered.
   d. Withhold the medication, as the blood pressure is below administration parameters.

►10. The nurse should withhold a drug and contact the prescriber if the patient reported an allergy to the drug with which symptom occurring shortly after the last time the drug was taken?
   a. Constipation
   b. Dry mouth
   c. New onset rash
   d. Diarrhea

11. Which postoperative patient assessment would warrant withholding an opiate analgesic that depresses the central nervous system (CNS)?
   a. Blood pressure 150/92 mm Hg
   b. Pulse 110 beats/min
   c. Respirations 9/min
   d. Temperature 102.2°F (39°C)

*12. Which patient problem would be most appropriate for a patient who is receiving an opiate analgesic that depresses the CNS?
   a. Fatigue
   b. Impaired physical mobility
   c. Risk for activity intolerance
   d. Risk for injury

*13. A patient who is admitted to the nursing unit from the postanesthesia care unit (PACU) is moaning in pain. The patient is due for another dose of pain medication. Which is the nursing priority?
   a. Administer prescribed pain-relieving drugs.
   b. Assess the patient's vital signs, tubes, and surgical site.
   c. Obtain the patient's pain rating on a scale of 1 to 10.
   d. Review the patient's allergy history.

14. The nurse is preparing to administer insulin based on the patient's bedside fingerstick blood glucose. Which action could be delegated to a licensed practical/vocational nurse (LPN/LVN)?
   a. Documenting the insulin that the RN administered
   b. Drawing up the insulin in the syringe
   c. Identifying the patient for medication administration
   d. Obtaining the bedside fingerstick blood glucose

CASE STUDY

A patient is admitted to the medical floor with uncontrolled hypertension.

<table>
<tr>
<td>
Military time: 1400 hrs
Patient states they live alone in a retirement apartment and have no children.
On admission, blood pressure is 185/104 mm Hg, pulse 112 beats per minute, respirations 14 breaths per minute, and temperature 99.0°F (37.2°C). Oxygen saturation on room air is 89%.
On exam, the patient's heart rhythm is irregular, lungs have fine bibasilar crackles bilaterally, and there is trace pitting edema in the lower extremities.
The patient denies headache or chest pain.
Medications:
Lisinopril/hydrochlorothiazide 20 mg/25 mg PO daily,
Metoprolol 100 mg PO daily,
Aspirin 81 mg PO daily,
Lovastatin 40 mg PO at bedtime,
Tylenol 8-Hour Arthritis Pain 650 mg PO 3 x day as needed for pain, and
Cetirizine, 10 mg PO daily.
The patient admits they split their pills to make them last longer, as they cannot afford them, and when taking drugs, the patient reports dizziness with standing and "just not feeling right."
</td>
<td>Highlight the assessment findings that require follow-up by the nurse.</td>
</tr>
</table>

3 Drug Regulation, Development, Names, and Information

STUDY QUESTIONS

Matching

Match the drug legislation with its action.

1. ___ Set standards for drug quality and purity in addition to strength.
2. ___ Requires drug companies to conduct pediatric clinical trials.
3. ___ Addressed drug safety.
4. ___ Implemented widespread changes in Food and Drug Administration (FDA) regulations.
5. ___ Required all drugs demonstrate effectiveness prior to marketing.
6. ___ Established rigorous oversight of drug safety after a drug has been approved.
7. ___ Allowed the FDA to regulate cigarettes.
8. ___ Purpose is to help combat a nationwide opioid epidemic.
   a. Federal Pure Food and Drug Act
   b. Family Smoking Prevention and Tobacco Control Act
   c. Food and Drug Administration Modernization Act
   d. Substance Use-Disorder Prevention that Promotes Opioid Recovery and Treatment (SUPPORT) for Patients and Communities Act
   e. Food, Drug, and Cosmetic Act
   f. FDA Amendments Act
   g. Harris-Kefauver Amendments
   h. Pediatric Research Equity Act

Completion

Fill in the blank with type of drug name.

9. The same ____________________________ name is never used for more than one medication.
10. The ____________________________ name tells the nurse the active ingredients of the drug.
11. The ____________________________ name of a drug will be the same, no matter which company produces the drug.
12. The ____________________________ name may suggest the action of the drug, such as PhosLo, which lowers phosphorus.
13. ____________________________ names of drugs in the same therapeutic class often have a similar suffix, making them easy to identify.
14. Drug Facts and Comparisons is organized by ____________________________ names.

NextGen Item Type: Matrix Multiple Choice

The nurse admits a patient with a history of hypertension, coronary artery disease, diabetes, and osteoporosis. While completing drug reconciliation, the nurse notes the patient's drug list has some drugs by generic name and others by brand name.

Click to specify which drug is listed by its generic name and which is listed by its brand name.

DRUG	GENERIC NAME	BRAND NAME
Diovan		
simvastatin		
hydrochlorothiazide		
Plavix		
aspirin		
Glucophage		
Aleve		

CRITICAL THINKING, PRIORITIZATION, AND DELEGATION QUESTIONS

15. Which should the nurse include when preparing discharge instructions?
   a. Ask the patient which name they use for the drug, and use only that name in discharge teaching.
   b. Explain generic names, and only use them so the patient does not become confused.
   c. Explain the brand names, and only use them because it is easier for the patient to remember.
   d. Review the prescriptions written for discharge, and include the brand name and generic name in discharge teaching.

16. A patient has been taking a brand-name drug for a chronic condition for several years. Recent changes in their insurance plan require the use of generic drugs whenever they are available. The patient asks the nurse if they should pay out of pocket to continue receiving the brand-name drug. The nurse's response should be based on which fact? **(Select all that apply.)**
    a. Continuing to use the brand-name drug will prevent confusion.
    b. Drugs requiring monitoring of blood levels should have levels checked when changing from brand-name to generic drugs.
    c. Generic drugs contain the same active ingredients as their brand-name counterparts.
    d. There is a difference in absorption between generic and brand-name drugs.
    e. Brand-name drugs contain different active ingredients than generic drugs.

17. The nurse is teaching a patient about tamsulosin (Flomax), which has been prescribed for difficulty voiding due to an enlarged prostate. Because the patient travels extensively and not all countries require prescriptions to get drugs, which is important for the nurse to teach the patient?
    a. Flomax may have different active ingredients in different countries.
    b. Drugs purchased in countries other than the United States and Canada are usually unsafe.
    c. Flomax is not available anywhere except in the United States and Canada.
    d. Doses of Flomax in countries that use the metric system are different than doses of drugs in the United States.

18. The nurse instructs the patient to inform their health care provider of all over-the-counter (OTC) drugs they take, explaining that just because a drug is available OTC does not mean it is without adverse effects. Which statement by the nurse conveys the risks associated with OTC drugs?
    a. "If you follow the instructions on the label, you shouldn't have any issues with side effects."
    b. "Serious health issues rarely occur with OTC drugs like acetaminophen and ibuprofen."
    c. "Taking OTC drugs along with prescription drugs may result in increased side effects such as nausea."
    d. "Self-medication with OTC drugs will reduce your need to visit a health care provider."

19. Which resource is most likely to provide current, complete positive and negative information about a drug? **(Select all that apply.)**
    a. Pharmaceutical sales representative
    b. Drug facts and comparisons
    c. Nurse's letter
    d. Prescriber's letter
    e. DailyMed

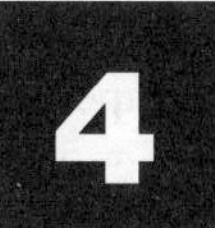

4 Pharmacokinetics

STUDY QUESTIONS

Matching

Match the terms and definitions relating to drug change and movement.

1. ___ Absorption
2. ___ Distribution
3. ___ Elimination
4. ___ Excretion
5. ___ Metabolism
6. ___ Pharmacokinetics
   a. Change in drug structure
   b. Change in drug structure and movement out of the body
   c. Movement from blood into tissue and cells
   d. Movement into and out of body
   e. Movement into the blood
   f. Movement out of the body

Match the method of movement with characteristics for that method of movement.

7. ___ May require expenditure of energy
8. ___ Requires small size
9. ___ Requires lipid solubility
   a. Passage through channels
   b. Direct penetration of the membrane
   c. Passage with the aid of a transport system

True or False

For each of the following statements, enter T for true or F for false.

10. ___ Cell membranes are composed of fat with phosphate.
11. ___ Most drugs enter cells through channels or pores.
12. ___ P-glycoprotein transports many drugs out of cells.
13. ___ A transport mechanism is needed for a water-soluble drug to enter a cell.
14. ___ Ionization is a process that allows a drug to enter a cell.
15. ___ If a quaternary ammonium compound drug is injected into a vein, it will produce effects, but it will not if taken orally.
16. ___ Polar drugs can enter fetal circulation and breast milk.
17. ___ Aspirin, like most drugs, is primarily absorbed in the small intestine.
18. ___ Enteric drugs should not be crushed because crushing these preparations can cause stomach distress or cause the acid in the stomach to alter the drug.
19. ___ A depot intramuscular (IM) injection of an antibiotic to treat syphilis will be completely effective within 24 hours after administration.
20. ___ The protein-bound portion of a drug in circulation is not able to exert its action.
21. ___ First-pass effect means most of the drug is activated by the liver, so it must be administered orally.
22. ___ A drug with extensive first-pass effect may be given sublingually to allow the drug to be absorbed directly into the systemic circulation.
23. ___ Adding a drug to a patient's drug regimen can cause the other drugs to be metabolized more slowly or more rapidly.
24. ___ Intestinal enzymes can release drugs from bile in the duodenum, causing the drug to be reabsorbed.
25. ___The nurse would expect that an intravenous (IV) antibiotic prescribed for bacterial meningitis would most likely get to the site of infection if the drug is water soluble.
26. ___ Chemotherapy is administered through a central IV line because chemotherapy is caustic to the vein and a large central vein has rapid blood flow, which dilutes and moves the medication quickly.

CRITICAL THINKING, PRIORITIZATION, AND DELEGATION QUESTIONS

✳27. The nurse is administering an IV push dose of an opiate analgesic. After administering half of the dose, the nurse notes that patient's respirations have decreased from 15/min to 11/min. Which is the priority nursing action?
   a. Assess the patient's current pain.
   b. Call the prescriber.
   c. Stimulate the patient.
   d. Stop administration of the rest of the drug.

✳28. The nurse inadvertently administers heparin 7500 units subcutaneously, instead of the heparin 5000 units that was prescribed to prevent postoperative deep vein thrombosis (DVT). Which is the priority nursing concern?
   a. Assessing the patient for DVT
   b. Consulting the prescriber for direction
   c. Completing an incident report
   d. Preventing excessive bleeding

▶29. The nurse realizes that when injecting insulin into the subcutaneous fat above the deltoid muscle in a very thin child, the drug may have been inadvertently administered into the muscle, leading to:
   a. the blood glucose levels drop too rapidly.
   b. Glucose levels do not drop rapidly enough.
   c. There will be change in blood sugar levels.
   d. adequate blood sugar control will be maintained.

▶30. Which laboratory test result suggests that a patient's excretion of a drug may be impaired?
   a. Aminotransferase (AST) 72 international units
   b. International normalized ratio (INR) 4.2
   c. Estimated glomerular filtration rate (eGFR) 30 mL/min
   d. White blood cell count (WBC) 13,000/mm^3

✳31. Which is a priority nursing action in postanesthesia care unit (PACU) to promote excretion of most anesthetics?
   a. Encourage deep breathing.
   b. Maintain a patient IV line.
   c. Monitor urine output.
   d. Prevent constipation.

32. Digoxin is a drug that has a narrow therapeutic range. When administering this drug, which action should the nurse take? **(Select all that apply.)**
   a. Administer the medication only on an as-needed (PRN) basis.
   b. Carefully monitor the patient for therapeutic and toxic effects.
   c. Be diligent about the timing of administering the medication.
   d. Monitor blood levels of the drug to assess if it is in the therapeutic range.
   e. Teach the patient that the drug takes several weeks to reach full effectiveness.

33. Grapefruit juice inhibits the cytochrome P450 CYP3A4 drug-metabolizing enzyme and inhibits P-glycoprotein in the intestines for days after ingestion. This especially affects calcium channel blockers, benzodiazepines, cyclosporine, and statin drugs. The nurse should teach a patient who is prescribed any of these drugs that drinking grapefruit juice can cause which problem?
   a. Excessive first-pass effect
   b. Excess levels of drug in the blood
   c. Lack of therapeutic effect of the drug
   d. Rapid excretion of the drug

34. A patient stopped taking levothyroxine 3 days ago. This drug has a half-life of 7 days. The patient tells the nurse that the drug must not have been necessary because they do not feel any different. Which is the basis of the nurse's explanation of why the patient has not noticed any change in how they feel?
   a. The patient's dose was probably too high, so the drug is still working.
   b. The patient could not have been taking the drug as prescribed.
   c. The drug probably was not needed if the patient has not experienced any symptoms.
   d. The drug's previous doses have not been completely eliminated from the body.

CASE STUDY

The nurse is caring for a hospitalized patient who has been prescribed the following medications: 0800, metformin 850 mg, and 0900, lisinopril 10 mg. Breakfast is served at 0810. Hospital policy states that medications may be administered 30 minutes before or after the designated time. To save time, the nurse plans to administer both medications at 0830.

1. Research the onset of these medications. Is this a good plan? Please explain why or why not.

5 Pharmacodynamics

STUDY QUESTIONS

True or False

For each of the following statements, enter T for true or F for false.

1. ___ Pharmacodynamics includes the study of how drugs work.
2. ___ In phase 2 of the dose-response relationship, the therapeutic effect does not increase with increasing the dose.
3. ___ *Maximal efficacy* is defined as the largest effect that a drug can produce.
4. ___ *Potency* is defined as the dose of drug needed to get the desired effect.
5. ___ Two drugs in the same therapeutic class with different recommended doses (2 mg versus 200 mg) can have equal effects.
6. ___ A drug that activates transcription factor may not reach a peak therapeutic effect until taken regularly for days to weeks.
7. ___ A drug that is selective for specific receptors will produce more unintended effects than a nonselective drug.
8. ___ If a drug is selective for specific receptors, it is safe.
9. ___ *Affinity* is the strength of attraction between a drug and its receptor.
10. ___ Drugs with high intrinsic activity cause an intense response.
11. ___ An agonist drug blocks the stimulation of a receptor.
12. ___ If a receptor is constantly bombarded by a drug, the cell can downregulate and decrease the response to the drug.
13. ___ A patient who suddenly stops taking an antagonist drug may experience hypersensitivity of the receptor and overstimulation.
14. ___ The 50% effective dose (ED_{50}) is usually the recommended dose for the drug.

CRITICAL THINKING, PRIORITIZATION, AND DELEGATION QUESTIONS

15. The nurse is reading research about a drug. The literature states that the drug is *potent.* Which describes the potency of a drug?
    a. The drug produces its effects at low doses.
    b. The drug produces strong effects at any dose.
    c. The drug requires high doses to produce its effects.
    d. The drug is very likely to cause adverse effects.
16. Which statement is true about drug-receptor interactions? (**Select all that apply**.)
    a. Drugs can mimic the actions of endogenous molecules.
    b. Receptors for drugs do not respond to hormones and neurotransmitters produced by the body.
    c. The binding of a drug to its receptor is usually irreversible.
    d. Drugs can block the actions of endogenous molecules.
    e. Drugs can give the cell new functions.

►17. The nurse is administering morphine sulfate to a hospice patient in severe pain. Knowing the drug's effects, which nursing interventions are indicated? (**Select all that apply**.)
    a. Assess respirations and hold the medication if adventitious breath sounds are present.
    b. Assess respiratory rate and hold the medication if respirations are weak or fewer than 12/minute.
    c. Maintain the patient on complete bed rest with all four side rails elevated to prevent injury.
    d. Assist the patient when ambulating to prevent injury.
    e. Encourage ambulation if not contraindicated to promote bowel motility.

18. A patient suddenly stops taking atenolol (Tenormin), a $beta_2$ receptor antagonist that slows the heart rate. Which assessment finding suggests hypersensitivity of $beta_2$ receptors?
    a. BP 80/56 mm Hg
    b. Pulse 118 beats/min
    c. Respirations 26/min
    d. Temperature 104°F (40°C)

19. When the therapeutic index of a drug is narrow, which should the nurse expect?
    a. Blood levels of the drug would be monitored throughout therapy.
    b. The drug would produce the desired effect at low doses.
    c. The drug would produce many adverse effects at low doses.
    d. The drug would only be used in an emergency.

NGN STAND ALONE ITEM TYPE: BOW-TIE

HEALTH HISTORY	NURSE'S NOTES	PHYSICIAN'S ORDERS	LABORATORY PROFILE
Time: 1040 hrs A patient comes to the emergency department with a decreased level of consciousness and severely depressed respirations. The person accompanying the patient reported finding an empty bottle of methadone HCL, an opiate, next to the patient. The patient has a history of heroin use disorder and is treated at a nearby rehabilitation center. They also have a history of alcohol use disorder and vaping. Vital signs: temperature 97.6°F; pulse 48; blood pressure 92/60; respirations 6 and shallow; oxygen saturation 80% on room air. Pupils are pinpointed. Skin is pale and clammy. Glucose level 154.			

After reviewing the EHR, complete the Bowtie chart, selecting the nursing actions to take, the potential condition, and the parameters to monitor.

Action to Take	Potential Condition	Parameter to Monitor
Action to Take		Parameter to Monitor

NURSING ACTIONS	POTENTIAL CONDITIONS	PARAMETERS TO MONITOR
Position on left side	Alcohol intoxication	Pain
Administer naloxone	Overdose	Blood pressure
Elevate the head of the bed	Hypoglycemia	Level of consciousness
Place on Oxygen at 2–4 L per NC	Hypoxia	Respirations
Perform CPR	Head injury	Heroin drug level

CASE STUDY

The nurse is caring for a patient taking digoxin, phenytoin, and theophylline.

1. What is the lab reference range for each drug? What is the therapeutic index of each drug (narrow or wide)?

2. If the patient's drug levels fall within each drug's reference range, can the nurse assume the patient will be free of toxicity? Why or why not?

6 Drug Interactions

STUDY QUESTIONS

True or False

For each of the following statements, enter T for true or F for false.

1. ___ A provider may prescribe a drug solely because of its interaction with another drug.
2. ___ Powdered drugs can be mixed once they are dissolved in a liquid.
3. ___ Alcohol, caffeine, tobacco, garlic, and orange and grapefruit juice can interact with drugs and cause adverse effects.
4. ___ Aluminum-containing antacids plus citrus beverages can result in excessive absorption of aluminum.
5. ___ The potassium-sparing effects of spironolactone tend to balance the potassium-wasting effects of hydrochlorothiazide.
6. ___ The nurse should consult with the provider regarding blood levels of oral drugs when a patient has gastrointestinal (GI) disturbances.

CRITICAL THINKING, PRIORITIZATION, AND DELEGATION QUESTIONS

✳7. The nurse is providing discharge teaching for a patient who will be taking metronidazole after discharge. The drug information states to caution the patient that a disulfiram-like reaction can occur. It is a priority to teach the patient to avoid which food or drink?
   a. Beer
   b. Chocolate
   c. High-fat food
   d. Sugar

▶8. The nurse is teaching a patient about their new drug. The instructions state to take it "with or without food". The patient asks how to tell if they should take it with or without food. Which is the appropriate nursing response?
   a. "When you are given the option always take your drugs on an empty stomach."
   b. "If upset stomach occurs after taking the drug on an empty stomach, then take it with food."
   c. "It would be best if you asked the pharmacist or the provider this question, not me."
   d. "Read the package insert, it will provide full instructions on how to take the drug."

9. Patients receiving certain drugs that are metabolized by the CYP3A4 enzyme should not drink grapefruit juice because grapefruit juice inhibits the CYP3A4 enzyme and the drug transporter P-glycoprotein. The patient asks what might happen if they drink grapefruit juice and take the medication. Which response should the nurse provide?
   a. "There will be impaired drug absorption."
   b. "The drug will not get to its site of action."
   c. "Impaired metabolism and excretion of the drug."
   d. "Liver damage due to drug toxicity."

✳10. A patient is prescribed clopidogrel to prevent blood clots after experiencing a myocardial infarction (MI). The patient self-prescribes omeprazole over the counter (OTC) for heartburn. Because omeprazole can inhibit the efficacy of clopidogrel, it is a priority for the nurse to teach the patient to report which effect?
   a. Dizziness
   b. Nausea and vomiting
   c. Joint pain
   d. Chest pain

11. A patient has been taking phenytoin, a drug with a narrow therapeutic index, to control seizures. If fluoxetine is prescribed to treat obsessive-compulsive disorder, drug interaction puts the patient at risk for which effect?
   a. Subtherapeutic effects of fluoxetine
   b. Phenytoin level becomes subtherapeutic
   c. Fluoxetine toxicity develops
   d. Toxicity from phenytoin

12. Tobacco induces the CYP1A2 liver enzyme. Methadone is metabolized by the CYP1A2 liver enzyme. If a patient with substance use disorder is treated with methadone and smokes cigarettes, which would be the expected effect?
   a. Diminish the effect of methadone
   b. Make the effect of methadone more intense
   c. Speed the elimination of methadone
   d. Slow the elimination of methadone

13. A patient has been prescribed sildenafil for erectile dysfunction. The nurse teaches the patient that metabolism of this drug may be increased, potentially decreasing the effect of sildenafil, if the patient uses which dietary supplement?
   a. Fish oil
   b. Iron
   c. Garlic
   d. Multivitamin

14. A patient who drinks grapefruit juice and does not inform the prescriber may experience muscle pain from the adverse effect of rhabdomyolysis, which is possible if the patient is prescribed which drug?
    a. Lovastatin for high cholesterol
    b. Nifedipine for hypertension
    c. Triazolam for insomnia
    d. Verapamil for atrial fibrillation

CLINICAL JUDGMENT CASE STUDY

The nurse has assumed care for a patient admitted 1 day ago with pneumonia. The patient's history includes hypertension, heart failure, osteoporosis, and Type 2 diabetes.

HEALTH HISTORY	NURSE'S NOTES	PHYSICIAN'S ORDERS	LABORATORY PROFILE

0700: Report received from night shift.

0730: Vital signs: blood pressure (BP) 112/68 mm Hg, heart rate 96 bpm, respirations 18 bpm, temperature 99.0°F (37.2°C), and oxygen saturation 90% on 2 L oxygen per nasal canula.

Orient to self only. When asked how they feel, the patient responded, "Dear, please give that cup of coffee to my visitor." The patient gestured to the chair in the room, but no one was there.

Lungs with bibasilar rhonchi posteriorly. Heart regular rate and rhythm, normal S_1S_2. No lower extremity edema. Abdomen with normoactive bowel sounds in all quadrants.

NURSE'S NOTES	LABORATORY PROFILE	PHYSICIAN'S ORDERS	HEALTH HISTORY
	Results	Reference Range	
Blood urea nitrogen	28 mg/dL	7–20 mg/dL	
Creatinine	1.6 mg/dL	0.7–1.3 mg/dL	
Sodium	145 mEq/L	135–145 mEq/L	
Potassium	5.2 mEq/L	3.7–5.2 mEq/L	
Hemoglobin	12 g/dL	12–15 g/dL	
Hematocrit	36%	36–48%	
White blood cells	11.0 × 10^9/L	4.5–10 × 10^9/L	
Lymphocytes	40%	20–40%	

MEDICATION ADMINISTRATION RECORD	0600	0700	0800	0900	1000	1100	1200
Cefazolin 500 mg IV every 8 hours Scheduled 0600, 1400, 2200							
Lisinopril 20 mg PO daily Scheduled 0900 BP __________							
Spironolactone 25 mg PO daily Scheduled 0900							
Metolazone 10 mg PO daily Scheduled 0900							
Aspirin 81 mg PO daily Scheduled 0900							
Lovastatin 20 mg PO every night Scheduled 2100							
Metformin 500 mg PO twice a day Scheduled 0800, 1700							
Empagliflozin 10 mg PO daily Scheduled 0800							
Tylenol 8-Hour Arthritis Pain 650 mg PO every 8 hours Scheduled 0600, 1400, 2200							

IV, Intravenous.

For each nursing action, check to specify whether the action is **Indicated, Contraindicated,** or **Nonessential** for the client's care.

NURSING ACTION	INDICATED	CONTRAINDICATED	NONESSENTIAL
Determine baseline mental status			
Review current list of drugs for interactions			
Administer drugs as ordered			
Continue to monitor patient without intervention			
Ask nursing assistant to double-check vital signs			
Determine if physical assessment has changed from previous			
Determine if any drugs are newly prescribed			

7 Adverse Drug Reactions and Medication Errors

STUDY QUESTIONS

Matching

Match the term with its description.

1. ___ Light-colored stool with nausea and vomiting.
2. ___ Estimated glomerular filtration rate (eGFR) 50 mL/minute and urinary output 750 mL/day; fluid intake 1500 mL/day.
3. ___ Fatigue and hemoglobin/hematocrit 28 mg/dL/9.2%, respectively.
4. ___ Frequent infections or infection with rare microbe and WBC count fewer than 5000/mm^3.
5. ___ Bronchospasm and laryngeal edema.
6. ___ Cardiac dysrhythmia and unexplained fainting.
   a. Anaphylaxis
   b. Hemolytic anemia
   c. Hepatotoxicity
   d. QT prolongation
   e. Nephrotoxicity
   f. Neutropenia

Completion

7. Withdrawal reactions occur when a drug is stopped when a person is ____________________ ____________________ on the drug.
8. A(n) ________________________ reaction is an immune response.
9. ________________________ means cancer causing.
10. Drugs that are ____________________________ can harm a fetus if the patient takes the drug while they are pregnant.
11. Effects that are nearly unavoidable secondary drug effects at therapeutic doses are called ________________ ____________________.
12. Genetic differences can cause uncommon drug responses. These are called __________________ reactions.
13. ____________________ disease is when a drug causes symptoms closely resembling a disease.
14. ____________________ is the detrimental physiologic effects caused by excessive drug dosing.

CRITICAL THINKING, PRIORITIZATION, AND DELEGATION QUESTIONS

15. Which is not an adverse effect of a drug as defined by the World Health Organization (WHO)?
    a. Constipation from codeine for pain
    b. Nausea and vomiting from chemotherapy
    c. Reflex tachycardia from calcium channel blocker
    d. Respiratory depression from an overdose of opioids
16. Adverse drug reactions occur more often when? (**Select all that apply**.)
    a. Patients take multiple drugs.
    b. Individuals take potent drugs.
    c. Medication errors occur.
    d. Children are less than 1 year.
    e. Multiple chronic conditions exist.

*17. The nurse has administered lisinopril. One hour after administration, the patient reports a tingling sensation of the lips. The nurse notes that the patient has perioral edema. Which action is of greatest **priority**?
    a. Document the finding.
    b. Hold the next dose.
    c. Notify the prescriber.
    d. Withhold food and water.

18. Which symptom suggests an ototoxic reaction to a drug?
    a. Dizziness
    b. Headache
    c. Nausea
    d. Tinnitus

▶19. Before administering lovastatin, the nurse reviews the patient's laboratory tests. Test results include alanine aminotransferase (ALT) 134 international units/L and aspartate aminotransferase (AST) 97 units/L. Which action is **most** appropriate at this time?
    a. Administer the drug.
    b. Obtain the vital signs.
    c. Call the prescriber.
    d. Hold the drug.

20. The nurse is mentoring a nursing student. The student states that it is unfair that the nursing program requires 100% proficiency on a dose calculation examination during the last semester because it is stressful for students. Which is the basis of the nurse's response to the student?
    a. Explain that students must be able to calculate drug doses under stress.
    b. Share with the student the policy that existed when the nurse was in school.
    c. Assist the student's efforts to overturn the policy because it is unrealistic.
    d. Tell the student 100% proficiency is required on the nursing board examination.

21. The nurse is caring for a patient who is experiencing severe pain. Morphine sulfate 10 mg intramuscularly (IM) is ordered every 4 hours as needed. The patient asks the nurse to administer the medication via an existing intravenous (IV) line because the patient dislikes the pain of an IM injection. Which action should the nurse take?
    a. Administer the medication IM as ordered.
    b. Use the IV line to give the drug as requested.
    c. Ask their supervisor what to do in this situation.
    d. Call the prescriber to request a change in route.

22. A nursing instructor is explaining changes that have taken place to reduce errors in drug administration. Which change has reduced errors that occur during transitions in care?
    a. Avoiding error-prone symbols
    b. Medication reconciliation
    c. Using barcode systems
    d. Computerized order entry

23. Which adverse effect should the nurse report to MedWatch?
    a. Itching with IV contrast administration
    b. Anaphylaxis with weekly allergy shots
    c. Hives after first dose of newly approved drug
    d. Hypoglycemia with administration of Levaquin

24. Which is **not** required on FD Aapproved medication guides for patients?
    a. Indications for taking the drug
    b. The safe dose range of the drug
    c. What to do if a dose is missed
    d. Who should not take the drug

25. Which is criterion for boxed warning in the drug literature?
    a. Risk for life-threatening risks
    b. Cause iatrogenic diseases
    c. Potential for anaphylaxis
    d. Patients must sign a consent

26. Which is the reason for isotretinoin to be part of the iPLEDGE program? The drug:
    a. can cause dysrhythmias.
    b. increases risk for suicide.
    c. interacts with 50% of all drugs.
    d. may cause major fetal harm.

CASE STUDY

Next-Generation NCLEX (NGN) Item Type: Bowtie

HEALTH HISTORY	NURSE'S NOTES	PHYSICIAN'S ORDERS	LABORATORY PROFILE

Time: 1100 hrs

Patient is a 20-year-old college student with a history of partial-onset seizures. They have been taking carbamazepine 600 mg extended release (ER) twice daily for some time. Since starting college, the drug has not been effective, with the patient experiencing two or more seizures a week. In addition to seizure disorder, the patient has a history of type I diabetes and anxiety.

Two days ago, the patient was started on brivaracetam 50 mg twice daily.

On rounds, the patient is drowsy and responds to questions with slurred speech. They answer questions appropriately, lungs are clear to auscultation, and the heart has a regular rate and rhythm. Abdomen with hyperactive bowel sounds.

Vital signs: temperature 97.8°F, blood pressure 121/64, pulse 77, respirations 18, oxygen saturation on room air 96%.

Intake/output last 24 hours: 1200 mL/395 mL.

After reviewing the electronic health record (EHR), complete the bowtie chart, selecting the nursing actions to take, the potential condition, and parameters to monitor.

Action to Take	Potential Condition	Parameter to Monitor
Action to Take		Parameter to Monitor

NURSING ACTIONS	POTENTIAL CONDITIONS	PARAMETERS TO MONITOR
Hold carbamazepine	Hypoglycemia	Intake/output
Check blood sugar	Postictal state	Percent meals eaten
Side rails x 2	Carbamazepine toxicity	Serum albumin level
Check liver function studies	Hypovolemia	Monitor serum drug levels
O_2 at 2 L per nasal canula		Seizures

8 Individual Variation to Drug Responses

STUDY QUESTIONS

Completion

1. Dose requirements for drugs with a narrow therapeutic range are more precisely calculated based on the patient's ______________________________ ______________________________ ________.

2. When a patient takes a drug for a long time and becomes tolerant, the nurse would expect the prescriber to ______________________ the dose to achieve the desired effect.

3. ______________________ is the ability of a drug to reach the systemic circulation from its site of administration.

4. ______________________ is a reduction in drug responsiveness brought on by repeated dosing over a short time.

5. If the nurse is administering warfarin to a malnourished patient with a serum protein level of 2.2 g/dL, the nurse would expect the patient to be at increased risk for ______________________.

6. Based on differences in the metabolism of alcohol, if both males and females consume the same amount of alcohol (on a weight-adjusted basis) and take the drug metronidazole, the disulfiram-like reaction between alcohol and the drug in the female should be more ______________________ and last ______________________ than for the male.

CRITICAL THINKING, PRIORITIZATION, AND DELEGATION QUESTIONS

► 7. A terminal cancer patient has been receiving narcotic analgesics for severe pain for more than 10 months. The prescriber has increased the dose of the long-acting opiate and added an "as-needed" opiate for breakthrough pain. Which action should the nurse take?
   a. Hold the higher dose of opiate until clarified.
   b. Discuss the new orders with the charge nurse.
   c. Refer the patient to counseling for drug misuse.
   d. Administer both of the drugs as ordered.

8. A nitroglycerin transdermal patch is ordered to be applied at 0900 and removed at 2100. The patch from the previous day is still in place when the nurse is preparing to administer the 0900 patch. Which action should the nurse take?
   a. Leave the old patch on and apply a new one.
   b. Apply the new patch and remove the old one.
   c. Hold the application of a new patch until tomorrow.
   d. Consult the healthcare provider for further directions.

► 9. A patient is ventilator dependent. Recent laboratory values include pH 7.48, pCO_2 32 mm Hg, and HCO_3 20 mEq/L, indicating respiratory alkalosis. Which effect could this imbalance have on acidic drugs?
   a. Ionization of the drug in blood
   b. Trapping of the drug in cells
   c. No impact on acidic drugs
   d. Binding of the acidic drug

10. Which symptom of an electrolyte imbalance would be of most concern to the nurse when a patient is prescribed digoxin?
   a. Fatigue
   b. Perioral tingling
   c. Dysrhythmia
   d. Muscle weakness

11. The nurse is caring for a female patient recently diagnosed with HIV. The nurse instructs the patient on the importance of follow-up liver function studies when taking which drug, as females develop hepatotoxicity more often than males?
   a. Zidovudines
   b. Stavudine
   c. Didanosine
   d. Nevirapine

12. The nurse is caring for a patient with Asian ancestry. The patient was admitted with new-onset seizures. Lab work prior to starting drug therapy indicates the patient has the HLA-B*1502 allele. The nurse knows which drug cannot be given to this patient, as this allele is linked to the increased risk of developing fatal skin conditions?
   a. Cannabidiol
   b. Carbamazepine
   c. Cenobamate
   d. Clonazepam

CASE STUDY

We know many of our patients do not adhere to their prescribed drug regimens.

1. What factors are known to negatively influence adherence?

2. How can nurses facilitate the removal of barriers to improve adherence?

9 Genetic and Genomic Considerations

STUDY QUESTIONS

True or False

For each of the following statements, enter T for true or F for false.

1. ___ Genomics is the examination of passing genetic traits from one generation to another through human genes.
2. ___ Genetics examines the effects of genes.
3. ___ Genetics takes into account a person's environment and lifestyle.
4. ___ Pharmacogenomics is the study of how genes affect a person's response to drugs.
5. ___ Precision medicine refers to a more general approach to finding effective strategies for treatment of similar groups of patients.
6. ___ The Food and Drug Administration (FDA) now requires genetic testing before using warfarin.
7. ___ A biomarker is a measurable substance that indicates the existence of genetic variation.
8. ___ Codeine cannot relieve pain in about 1 in 14 people of European heritage.

CRITICAL THINKING, PRIORITIZATION, AND DELEGATION QUESTIONS

9. The nurse preceptor is orienting the new RN to the clinic, stating that they gather specimens for genetic testing nearly every day. The new RN asks which can be used for genetic testing, depending on the test requirements. **(Select all that apply.)**
   a. Saliva
   b. Urine
   c. Stool
   d. Hair
   e. Tissue

10. The new RN asks their preceptor what has been done to remove barriers to genetic testing. Which response by the preceptor is the best?
    a. "The Genetic Information Nondiscrimination Act protects everyone from discrimination."
    b. "All insurance companies cover the testing."
    c. "The National Academy of Medicine states genomics education should be provided for all health professionals."
    d. "There are many guidelines to support clinical practice."

11. Which is the most common mechanism by which genetic variants modify drug responses?
    a. Absorption
    b. Distribution
    c. Metabolism
    d. Excretion

12. The nurse is caring for a patient who has undergone genetic testing to determine if they are thiopurine methyltransferase (TPMT) deficient. Which action would need to be taken if the patient is deficient?
    a. Make no change in drug dosage.
    b. Increase the drug dosage.
    c. Reduce the drug dosage.
    d. Do not give the drug.

13. The nurse knows that patients of European ancestry respond better to beta blockers than patients of African ancestry because blockade of hyperresponsive beta-1 adrenergic receptors (ADRB1) produces which response in blood pressure?
    a. Reduced
    b. Exaggerated
    c. Increased
    d. No change

14. The nurse is caring for a patient prescribed maraviroc. They understand that a patient prescribed this drug is infected with a specific strain of which virus?
    a. HPV
    b. HBV
    c. HCV
    d. HIV

15. The nurse is caring for a patient recently prescribed carbamazepine. The patient developed a severe skin reaction after starting the drug. The nurse knows patients of which origin develop this toxicity?
    a. African American
    b. Asian
    c. European
    d. Native American

CASE STUDY

The nurse is providing discharge instructions for a patient hospitalized with new-onset atrial fibrillation. The health care provider has recommended genetic testing prior to beginning warfarin. The patient asks the nurse to explain the benefits of genetic testing.

1. How should the nurse respond?

10 Introduction to Immunomodulators

STUDY QUESTIONS

True or False

For each of the following statements, enter T for true or F for false.

1. ___ A monoclonal antibody is a protein derived from a horse.
2. ___ Erenumab is approved for the prevention of migraine headache.
3. ___ Interleukin 5 is responsible for the functioning and survival of eosinophils.
4. ___ Bebtelovimab is approved for emergency use in patients with COVID-19 who do not require supplemental oxygen.
5. ___ Tyrosine kinase inhibitors block tyrosine kinases in cells that send growth signals.
6. ___ Teprotumumab-trbw reduces pain and swelling in patients with thyroid eye disease (TED), but it does not decrease proptosis.
7. ___ The degree of skin toxicity experienced by persons receiving erlotinib correlates positively to a therapeutic response to the drug.
8. ___ Proteasome inhibitors are used in the treatment of mantle cell lymphoma.
9. ___ It is recommended that patients receiving proteasome inhibitors have routine transthoracic echocardiograms due to the risk of cardiotoxicity.
10. ___ Proteasome inhibitors may cause more medication interactions than other immunotherapies.

Matching

Match the drug with its approved use.

11. ___ Teprotumumab
12. ___ Omalizumab
13. ___ Reslizumab
14. ___ Bezlotoxumab
15. ___ Erenumab

    a. *Clostridium difficile*
    b. Eosinophilic asthma
    c. Allergy-related asthma
    d. Prevention of migraine
    e. TED

CRITICAL THINKING, PRIORITIZATION, AND DELEGATION QUESTIONS

16. The nurse is caring for a patient with *C. difficile*. Despite treatment with oral vancomycin and metronidazole, the patient remains symptomatic and in distress. The nurse anticipates which drug will be ordered to treat this patient?
    a. Dupilumab
    b. Bezlotoxumab
    c. Mepolizumab
    d. Benralizumab

17. The nurse is caring for a patient with debilitating migraine headaches who has failed multiple treatment modalities. Understanding that migraines may result from vasodilation and release of inflammatory neuropeptides caused by calcitonin gene-related peptide (CGRP), which CGRP inhibitor does the nurse anticipate will be prescribed? (**Select all that apply**.)
    a. Erenumab
    b. Galcanezumab
    c. Benralizumab
    d. Mepolizumab
    e. Fremanezumab

18. The nurse is caring for a patient with TED. Orders have been received to begin teprotumumab 700 mg intravenously (IV) × 1. The nurse knows this drug is helpful in reducing which symptoms of TED? (**Select all that apply**.)
    a. Proptosis
    b. Blurred vision
    c. Light sensitivity
    d. Pain
    e. Dry eyes

19. The nurse is caring for a patient who began omalizumab 150 mg subcutaneously (SC) for allergy-related asthma last week. The patient is admitted with fever, nausea, tachypnea, and delirium. The patient is on seizure precautions. Which is the most likely cause of the patient's symptoms.
    a. Hepatotoxicity
    b. Anaphylaxis
    c. Cytokine release syndrome
    d. *Staphylococcus aureus* infection

20. The nurse is caring for a patient who is scheduled to begin carfilzomib, a proteasome inhibitor, as treatment for refractory multiple myeloma. The nurse conducts a thorough assessment of cardiac risk factors due to which potential serious adverse event(s). (**Select all that apply**.)
    a. Headache
    b. Heart failure
    c. Dysrrhythmias
    d. Hypotension
    e. Weakness

CASE STUDY

The patient arrives at the clinic to begin therapy with Galcanezumab 120 mg SC every month. Prior to administering the injection, the nurse educates the patient about the drug.

1. What is galcanezumab's mechanism of action?

2. What potential side effects should the nurse instruct the patient about?

11 Drug Therapy During Pregnancy and Breastfeeding

STUDY QUESTIONS

True or False

For each of the following statements, enter T for true or F for false.

1. ___ Drugs are not a common cause of birth defects.
2. ___ The health of the fetus supersedes the health of the mother when drugs are prescribed to pregnant patients.
3. ___ The health of the fetus depends on the health of the mother.
4. ___ Pregnant women should not take any drugs.
5. ___ The Birth Defects Study to Evaluate Pregnancy Exposures compared histories of women who gave birth to children with and without congenital anomalies.
6. ___ Hepatic metabolism decreases during pregnancy.
7. ___ Glomerular filtration increases during pregnancy.
8. ___ All drugs can cross the placenta to some extent.
9. ___ Drugs are most likely to pass into fetal circulation if they are water soluble.
10. ___ Angiotensin-converting enzyme inhibitor drugs for hypertension are prohibited during the second and third trimesters of pregnancy.

Matching

Match the drug with its potential teratogenic effect.

11. ___ Alcohol
12. ___ Ibuprofen
13. ___ Isotretinoin
14. ___ Lisinopril
15. ___ Methotrexate
16. ___ Phenytoin
17. ___ Tetracycline
18. ___ Valproic acid
    a. Cardiovascular defects
    b. Limb malformations
    c. Growth delay
    d. Low birth weight
    e. Neural tube defects
    f. Premature closure of the ductus arteriosus
    g. Renal failure
    h. Tooth anomalies

CRITICAL THINKING, PRIORITIZATION, AND DELEGATION QUESTIONS

19. Based on pharmacokinetics, drugs are most likely to pass into fetal circulation if they are
    a. highly polar.
    b. ionized.
    c. protein bound.
    d. lipid soluble.
20. A patient with a history of heroin use disorder has delivered a full-term infant. Which signs and symptoms suggest the infant is experiencing withdrawal symptoms? **(Select all that apply.)**
    a. Shrill cry
    b. Irritability
    c. Lethargy
    d. Hypotension
    e. Low Apgar score
21. A patient who is pregnant with a history of controlled hypertension asks the nurse why the provider changed their high blood pressure medication from amlodipine to nifedipine. The nurse's response is based on which knowledge?
    a. Nifedipine is more effective for treating hypertension during pregnancy.
    b. There is no known risk of fetal harm with use of nifedipine during pregnancy.
    c. The dose of amlodipine is more potent than the dose of nifedipine.
    d. Amlodipine crosses the placenta, but nifedipine does not.

22. Which is an important role of the nurse when a patient who is pregnant has a known exposure to a teratogen during week 4 of pregnancy?
    a. Ordering an ultrasound
    b. Calling test results to the parents
    c. Providing emotional support
    d. Recommending abortion
23. Which instruction should be included in patient teaching regarding breastfeeding and drug therapy?
    a. Do not take any drugs.
    b. Avoid drugs that have a long half-life.
    c. Take needed drugs just after breastfeeding.
    d. Use sustained-release formulas of drugs.

CASE STUDY

A patient with a history of heroin use disorder has delivered a full-term infant.

1. What should be included in the nursing care to address possible drug withdrawal in the neonate?

2. Exposure to teratogens during the embryonic period can produce gross malformation in the fetus. What nursing actions can help decrease teratogenesis during this period?

12 Drug Therapy in Pediatric Patients

STUDY QUESTIONS

True or False

For each of the following statements, enter T for true or F for false.

1. ___ All drugs that are considered safe to administer to adults are safe for administration to pediatric patients if the dose is adjusted appropriately for size.
2. ___ For drug purposes, infancy is defined as from the end of 4 weeks to 1 year of age.
3. ___ The majority of drugs used in pediatrics have never been tested on children.
4. ___ Intramuscular absorption of drugs is slower in the infant than in the adult.
5. ___ Toddlers often need higher doses per body weight than preschool children.
6. ___ Approximating safe doses of drugs for children is most accurate when calculated based on weight.

Matching

Match the pediatric group with the proper age range:

7. ____ Infants
8. ____ Adolescents
9. ____ Premature infants
10. ____ Neonates
11. ____ Full-term infants
12. ____ Children

a. Less than 36 weeks gestational age
b. 36 to 40 weeks gestational age
c. First 4 postnatal weeks
d. Weeks 5 to 52 postnatal
e. 1 to 12 years
f. 12 to 16 years

CRITICAL THINKING, PRIORITIZATION, AND DELEGATION QUESTIONS

13. Which drug is considered inappropriate for use in children due to the increased risk of adverse effects? **(Select all that apply.)**
    a. Aspirin
    b. Famotidine
    c. Tetracycline
    d. Mineral oil
    e. Loratadine

*14. A pregnant patient received morphine sulfate late in labor. The neonate was born 22 minutes later. Because the drug crosses the placenta and the characteristics of the blood-brain barrier of the neonate, which neonatal assessment finding would be of most concern to the nurse?
    a. Blood pressure 90/45 mm Hg
    b. Heart rate 160 beats/min
    c. Respirations 22/min
    d. Temperature 98.1°F (36.7°C)

15. The nurse is teaching the parents of a 5-year-old strategies to promote adherence. Which strategy will the nurse include in teaching?
    a. Set up a reward system when taking medications.
    b. Administer all medications on an empty stomach.
    c. Use warm water to rinse the taste out of the mouth.
    d. Always use tablets as they are easier to swallow.

16. Which drug is potentially safe to administer to children?
    a. Acetaminophen
    b. Dextromethorphan
    c. Pseudoephedrine
    d. Phenylephrine

17. The immaturity of which pharmacokinetic process in infants may result in drug sensitivity?
    a. Area under the curve
    b. Protein binding
    c. Drug levels
    d. Receptor sites

18. The safe dose of a liquid drug for a 6-month-old is 0.75 mL. Which would be the best option to accurately measure and administer the drug?
    a. A 1mL syringe
    b. Household spoon
    c. Measuring spoon
    d. Medicine cup

DOSE CALCULATION QUESTIONS

19. The prescriber has prescribed 225 mg of a drug twice a day for a 7-year-old child who is 43 inches tall and weighs 45 lb. The recommended adult dose of this drug is 500 mg twice a day. Based on body surface area, is this dose safe?

20. The drug is available in an elixir of 250 mg/5 mL. How much medication will the nurse administer?

CASE STUDY

New parents tell the nurse that getting their infant to take an oral suspension of an antibiotic impossible is. They tell the nurse they have been putting the medicine into the baby's formula.

1. Are there problems with the parent's method of drug administration? Please explain your answer.

2. What can the nurse do to increase adherence to the drug regimen?

13 Drug Therapy in Older Adult Patients

STUDY QUESTIONS

True or False

For each of the following statements, enter T for true or F for false.

1. ___ The goal of therapy for the older adult is to cure the disease.
2. ___ There is a wider individual variation in drug response in the older adult.
3. ___ Older adults are less sensitive to drugs.
4. ___ Older adults absorb less of the dose of medication than young adults.
5. ___ Absorption of many drugs slows with aging.
6. ___ Changes in body fat and lean body mass that occur with aging can cause lipid-soluble drugs to have a decrease in effect and water-soluble drugs to have a more intense effect.
7. ___ Liver enzyme activity often is increased in the older adult.
8. ___ Drug accumulation secondary to decreased renal excretion is the most common cause of adverse reactions in older adults.
9. ___ A reduction in the number of receptors and/or decreased affinity for receptors in the older adult may decrease the response to drugs that work by receptor interactions.

CRITICAL THINKING, PRIORITIZATION, AND DELEGATION QUESTIONS

*10. When evaluating kidney function in the frail older adult, it is a **priority** for the nurse to review the results of which test?
a. Serum blood urea nitrogen (BUN)
b. Serum creatinine
c. Creatinine clearance
d. Renal ultrasound

11. An older adult with liver disease is receiving several drugs that are normally highly protein bound. The patient's serum albumin is 2.4 mg/dL (normal 3.5–5 mg/dL). Drug effects in this patient may be
a. increased.
b. decreased.
c. unchanged.
d. unknown.

►12. The nurse is preparing to administer ketorolac to a frail 83-year-old who has joint pain. Which of the following symptoms would warrant withholding the drug and contacting the prescriber?
a. Constipation
b. Difficulty waking up
c. Dizziness from position change
d. Tarry stools

*13. Which assessment is a priority before administering prazosin to a geriatric patient?
a. Alertness and orientation
b. Blood pressure (BP) and pulse
c. Bowel and bladder elimination
d. Intake and output

*14. The nurse is aware that anticholinergic adverse effects of drugs commonly cause more problems in older adults than in younger adults. Which anticholinergic effect would be a **priority** to report to the prescriber?
a. Blurred vision upon waking
b. Dry mouth at night
c. Has not voided in 16 hours
d. No bowel movement for 48 hours

15. The nurse is aware that an older adult patient is at risk for which problem when prescribed tolterodine?
a. Altered bowel pattern
b. Disturbed cognition
c. Fluid volume deficit
d. Impaired skin integrity

16. Which factor increases the risk of poor adherence in the older adult? **(Select all that apply.)**
a. Multiple comorbidities
b. Cost of medications
c. Presence of side effects
d. Living with family
e. Few visits to providers

17. An older adult is prescribed labetalol for new-onset atrial fibrillation. The nurse knows that this drug may be less effective in the older adult than younger adults due to which factor?
a. Increased receptor affinity
b. Reduction in beta receptors
c. Idiosyncratic drug response
d. Drug accumulation

CASE STUDY

1. A 76-year-old male is placed on hospice with end-stage chronic obstructive pulmonary disease (COPD). He has a history of coronary artery disease and diabetes.
   a. What changes in medications might be expected?

   b. Why?

14 Basic Principles of Neuropharmacology

STUDY QUESTIONS

Matching

Match the term with its definition.

1. ___ Areas on the axon where neurotransmitters are stored.
2. ___ Areas on the postsynaptic cells that can be stimulated or blocked by drugs.
3. ___ Drugs that activate receptor activity.
4. ___ Drugs that prevent receptor activity.
5. ___Moving the axon potential down the neuron.
6. ___ Arrival of this at an axon terminal triggers release of a transmitter.
7. ___ Molecules from the axon terminal that bind to receptors on the postsynaptic cell.
8. ___ The process by which information is carried across the synaptic gap.
9. ___ The process by which the parts of neurotransmitters are recycled back to the neuron from which they were released.
   a. Action potential
   b. Agonist
   c. Antagonist
   d. Axonal conduction
   e. Neurotransmitter
   f. Receptor
   g. Reuptake
   h. Synaptic transmission
   i. Vesicle

True or False

For each of the following statements, enter T for true or F for false.

10. ___ The impact of a drug on a neuronally regulated process is dependent on the ability of that drug to influence receptor activity.
11. ___ Activation of a receptor always results in speeding up a physiologic process.
12. ___ Drugs can cause an increase in the formation of neurotransmitters.
13. ___ Drugs can promote, but cannot prevent, transmitter release.
14. ___ Selective serotonin reuptake inhibitors increase the release of serotonin from the vesicles into the synapse.
15. ___ Selectivity is one of the most desirable qualities that a drug can have.

CRITICAL THINKING, PRIORITIZATION, AND DELEGATION QUESTIONS

16. Selective serotonin reuptake inhibitors are a class of antidepressant drugs. Which is their mechanism of action?
   a. The synthesis of serotonin is decreased in the axon.
   b. Decrease the return of serotonin to the axon from which it was released.
   c. Increase the release of serotonin from the vesicles into the synapse.
   d. The number of receptors for serotonin is increased.
17. A cholinergic drug that mimics the action of acetylcholine causes the heart rate to slow because of which mechanism?
   a. Blocks receptors for acetylcholine
   b. Causes an increased release of acetylcholine
   c. Release of acetylcholine is decreased
   d. Stimulates cardiac receptors for acetylcholine
18. Which characteristic allows naloxone to reverse respiratory depression caused by an opiate? **(Select all that apply.)**
   a. Binding to opiate receptors is reversible.
   b. Opiates have a shorter half-life than naloxone.
   c. The affinity of naloxone to the receptor is stronger.
   d. Naloxone is selective for opiate receptors.
   e. The dose of naloxone is larger than the dose of the opiate.

19. Drugs that block transmitter reuptake have which effect on receptor activation?
    a. Decrease receptor activation.
    b. Increase receptor activation.
    c. There is no effect on receptor activation.
    d. The effect on receptor activation is unknown.

CASE STUDY

Why must the nurse be cautious when administering nonselective blockers of α_1, β_1, and β_2 receptors to patients with the following chronic disorders?

1. Asthma
2. Benign prostatic hyperplasia
3. Diabetes mellitus

15 Physiology of the Peripheral Nervous System

STUDY QUESTIONS

Matching

Match the divisions of the nervous system to functions that can be influenced by drugs.

1. ___ Regulation of smooth muscle
2. ___ Thinking, emotion, and processing data
3. ___ The somatic and autonomic nervous systems
4. ___ Heart, secretory glands, and smooth muscle
5. ___ Has three principle functions
   a. Autonomic
   b. Central
   c. Parasympathetic
   d. Peripheral
   e. Somatic

Completion

6. Stimulation of the somatic nervous system causes contraction of ________________.
7. Parasympathetic stimulation of the eye causes __________ __________ and __________ __________.
8. Sympathetic stimulation of the lungs causes __________ and increased __________ __________.
9. Parasympathetic stimulation of the heart causes __________ of the heart rate.
10. Sympathetic stimulation of the gastrointestinal tract causes slowing of gastrointestinal __________ and __________.
11. Parasympathetic stimulation of the urinary bladder causes urinary __________.
12. Sympathetic stimulation shunts blood from organs to __________ __________.
13. The __________ __________ is the most important feedback loop of the autonomic nervous system.
14. The __________ __________ __________ provides the predominant tone in most organs.

CRITICAL THINKING, PRIORITIZATION, AND DELEGATION QUESTIONS

►15. A patient with a blood pressure (BP) of 188/104 mm Hg takes a potent vasodilating drug to lower the BP. One hour after administration, the BP has dropped to 135/78 mm Hg in response to the drug. Which additional assessment finding is an expected response to this rapid change in BP?
   a. Capillary refill of 2 seconds
   b. Rubor when legs dangling
   c. Pulse increase of 20–30 beats/min
   d. Increased urine output by 15 mL/h

16. Most drugs that affect muscarinic receptors of the parasympathetic nervous system produce adverse effects by which mechanism?
   a. High doses are needed to achieve therapeutic effects.
   b. Most drugs that affect muscarinic receptors are nonselective.
   c. Most muscarinic receptors are stimulated by epinephrine.
   d. Muscarinic receptors are present on all postganglionic neurons.

17. A military nurse receives a soldier from a combat zone who may have been exposed to an aerosolized nerve gas. Because nerve gas inhibits the enzyme cholinesterase, the nurse should assess for which signs and symptoms?
   a. Wheezing
   b. Mydriasis
   c. Headache
   d. Constipation

►18. The nurse would consult with the provider if an anticholinergic drug was prescribed for a patient with which health issue?
   a. Diarrhea
   b. Salivation
   c. Hypotension
   d. Urinary retention

✳19. Doxazosin, an α_1 adrenergic blocking drug, is prescribed for a patient with benign prostatic hyperplasia (BPH). A priority nursing concern for this patient is assessing for which signs and symptoms?
   a. Sweating
   b. Dizziness
   c. Heartburn
   d. Weakness

20. Which is the only neurotransmitter that activates β_2 adrenergic receptors?
    a. Acetylcholine
    b. Dopamine
    c. Epinephrine
    d. Norepinephrine

21. Tamsulosin is a drug that selectively blocks α_{1A} receptors in the bladder, neck, and iris. It would be a priority to report current or past use of this drug to a surgeon who is planning to do which type of surgery?
    a. Cataract removal
    b. Colon resection
    c. Herniorrhaphy
    d. Valvuloplasty

►22. A decrease in the inactivation of norepinephrine occurs with the administration of a monoamine oxidase (MAO) inhibitor. Which is a priority assessment when administering an MAO?
    a. Glucose level
    b. BP
    c. Kidney function
    d. Liver function

CASE STUDY

A patient receives a nonselective drug administered to slow the heart rate, and it acts by blocking stimulation of β_1 and β_2 sympathetic nervous system receptors. What would be the possible related adverse effects on the following organs or processes? What are the appropriate nursing actions for these adverse effects?

1. Eyes

2. Respiratory rate

3. Airway

4. Gastrointestinal motility

5. Production of glucose by the liver and release into the blood

6. Heart

16 Muscarinic Agonists

STUDY QUESTIONS

Administration and Consultation

1. The nurse is preparing to administer a muscarinic agonist. If the following preadministration assessment findings were present, indicate if it would it be safe to administer the drug (administer) or if consultation with the provider would be indicated (consult).
   a. Pulse 110 beats/min ________________
   b. Blood pressure (BP) 100/60 mm Hg __________
   c. Wheezing ________________
   d. Drooling ________________
   e. Postoperative abdominal distention __________
   f. Recent bowel resection ________________
   g. Recent vaginal delivery of a 7-lb neonate _____________
   h. Postvoid residual of 350 mL of urine, without obstruction ________________
   i. Positive hemoccult of stool ________________
   j. TSH 0.2 microunits/mL, T_4 18 mcg/dL ________________

CRITICAL THINKING, PRIORITIZATION, AND DELEGATION QUESTIONS

2. A young camper finds some wild mushrooms and eats them. Which symptom suggests to the camp nurse that the camper is experiencing muscarinic poisoning? **(Select all that apply.)**
   a. Tachycardia
   b. Hypertension
   c. Profuse salivation
   d. Dilated pupils
   e. Wheezing

*3. The emergency department nurse receives a patient by ambulance with suspected poisoning from exposure to muscarinic insecticide. The priority nursing action is to prepare for which?
   a. Relieve the pain of muscle spasms
   b. Possible cardiorespiratory collapse
   c. Place the patient in a side-lying position
   d. Administer intravenous fluids

4. The nurse is caring for a patient with type 1 diabetes, peripheral neuropathy, and neurogenic bladder. The patient is prescribed bethanechol 10 three times per day. The nurse knows that the drug is prescribed for which physiologic response to activation of muscarinic receptors?
   a. Change in distance vision
   b. Contraction of detrusor muscle
   c. Increased watering of mouth
   d. Increased gastrointestinal motility

5. The nurse is preparing to administer a patient's morning medications, which include bethanechol. After reviewing the diagnosis accompanying the patient's medications, the nurse prepares to call the provider, as bethanechol is contraindicated in patients with which diagnosis? **(Select all that apply.)**
   a. Hypertension
   b. Constipation
   c. Hypotension
   d. Hyperthyroid
   e. Bradycardia

6. A patient is seen in the emergency department with severe headache, changes in vision, difficulty breathing, bradycardia, abdominal pain and cramping, and uncontrolled shaking. Upon questioning, the patient states they were just started on pilocarpine four times per day for Sjogren syndrome. The nurse caring for the patient prepares to administer which drug to treat the patient's symptoms?
   a. Neostigmine
   b. Physostigmine
   c. Atropine
   d. Mecamylamine

DOSE CALCULATION QUESTION

The patient is prescribed pilocarpine 30 mg per day to treat xerostomia following treatment of laryngeal cancer. Pilocarpine 7.5-mg tablets are available.

1. How many tablets should the nurse administer?

CASE STUDY

Y. L. has a long-standing history of type 1 diabetes. As a result, the patient has developed urinary retention secondary to neurogenic bladder. To treat the issue, bethanechol is prescribed. Muscarinic agonists, such as bethanechol, mimic acetylcholine at muscarinic receptors.

1. What effects does activation of muscarinic receptors produce?

2. What other name are muscarinic agonists known by?

3. How does bethanechol relieve urinary retention?

17 Muscarinic Antagonists

STUDY QUESTIONS

Administration and Consultation

1. The nurse is preparing to administer a muscarinic antagonist. If the following preadministration assessment findings are present, then indicate if it would it be safe to administer the drug (administer) or if consultation with the prescriber would be indicated (consult).
   a. Pulse 118 beats/min ________________
   b. Mild wheezing in patient with maintenance IV________________
   c. Drooling ________________
   d. Postoperative abdominal distention ___________
   e. Recent bowel resection ________________
   f. Postvoid residual of 350 mL of urine, obstruction unknown ________________
   g. Postoperative delirium ________________

CRITICAL THINKING, PRIORITIZATION, AND DELEGATION QUESTIONS

✳ 2. The emergency department nurse receives a patient brought in by ambulance with suspected poisoning from exposure to scopolamine. Which is the priority nursing action?
   a. Administer activated charcoal.
   b. Prepare for possible respiratory arrest.
   c. Place the patient in a side-lying position.
   d. Initiate intravenous fluid infusion.

3. Which signs would the nurse use to differentiate between psychosis and excessive muscarinic blockade? (**Select all that apply**.)
   a. Hallucinations
   b. Dry mouth
   c. Delirium
   d. Dry skin
   e. Hyperthermia

4. Which form of antidote would the nurse expect to be prescribed for a person who is at risk of exposure to toxic levels of insecticide or nerve gas?
   a. Extended-release tablet
   b. Enteric-coated tablet
   c. Subcutaneous injection
   d. Self-injectable pen

5. Oxybutynin is a prescribed anticholinergic drug that is available in five formulations. A patient has experienced many adverse effects when taking oxybutynin immediate-release (IR) tablets for overactive bladder (OAB). The patient asks the nurse how the transdermal patch could cause fewer adverse effects if it is essentially the same drug. The nurse's response is based on which factor?
   a. Absorption bypasses intestinal metabolism.
   b. It is water soluble and poorly absorbed.
   c. The oral IR form is chemically different.
   d. Transdermal is less effective than the IR oral form.

✳ 6. The nurse is administering trospium to a 78-year-old patient who has a history of OAB, diabetes, osteoarthritis, and osteoporosis. As the nurse explains the drug action, the patient asks how this drug is different from oxybutynin, which is less expensive. The nurse should explain that the priority reason for the provider choosing trospium instead of oxybutynin, based on age and chronic conditions, is the prevention of which side effect?
   a. Blood sugar spikes
   b. Constipation
   c. Dry mouth
   d. Central nervous system effects

► 7. The emergency department provider orders clarithromycin 500 mg orally twice a day and continuation of all home medications for a patient with advanced HIV admitted with a mycobacterium infection. The patient's home regimen includes darifenacin extended release (ER) 15 mg once a day, delavirdine 400 mg three times daily, nevirapine 200 mg twice a day, and ritonavir 600 mg twice a day. Based on possible drug interactions with darifenacin, which action should the nurse take?
   a. Give the medications with food to prevent gastrointestinal distress.
   b. Administer clarithromycin 1 hour after home medications.
   c. Review the home medications and the medication order with the prescriber.
   d. Ask the provider to discontinue the darifenacin ER 15 mg daily.

8. The nurse should review the patient's history for unexplained fainting or long-QT syndrome before administering which medication? (**Select all that apply**.)
   a. Darifenacin
   b. Fesoterodine
   c. Solifenacin
   d. Tolterodine
   e. Trospium

9. Which response to tolterodine would the nurse expect if a patient were also prescribed ketoconazole? (**Select all that apply**.)
   a. Adverse effects are increased.
   b. Adverse effects are reduced.
   c. Beneficial effects are enhanced.
   d. Beneficial effects are decreased.
   e. QT interval is prolonged.

10. Trospium 20 mg once a day is prescribed for an older adult patient with OAB. The nurse instructs the patient to take the medication at what time of day?
   a. One hour before breakfast
   b. One hour after breakfast
   c. With the first bite of breakfast
   d. Anytime during the day

11. The nurse is caring for a patient who has taken an overdose of amitriptyline. Which action should the nurse implement? (**Select all that apply**.)
   a. Support breathing.
   b. Administer atropine.
   c. Initiate IV hydration.
   d. Ice-water submersion.
   e. Give physostigmine.

12. Which intervention for dry mouth caused by anticholinergic drugs would be least likely to produce adverse effects?
   a. Cough drops
   b. Mouthwash
   c. Sipping fluid
   d. Hard candy

*13. A patient is prescribed oxybutynin topical. The nurse should teach the patient which action to avoid inadvertent, excessive dosing of this drug?
   a. Drink a full glass of water with the drug.
   b. Wash hands after administering the drug.
   c. Take the drug at the same each day.
   d. Administer the drug on an empty stomach.

DOSE CALCULATION QUESTIONS

14. A patient is prescribed 5 mg of oxybutynin syrup every 12 hours. Oxybutynin syrup is available as 5 mg/5 mL. How much syrup should the nurse administer per dose?

15. The recommended subcutaneous dose of atropine for a child is 0.01 mg/kg, not to exceed 0.4 mg.
   a. What is the recommended dose for a child who is 32 inches long and weighs 24 lb?
   b. Based on the recommended dose, what amount of drug should the nurse draw into the syringe if atropine is available as 0.5 mg/mL?

CLINICAL JUDGMENT CASE STUDY

The nurse is caring for a patient with a history of type 2 diabetes, hypertension, depression, and overactive bladder who is admitted to a medical unit with the diagnosis of altered mental status.

HEALTH HISTORY	NURSE'S NOTES	PHYSICIAN'S ORDERS	LABORATORY PROFILE
1400: Vital statistics (VS) on admission: BP 182/110 mm Hg, pulse 118 bpm, respirations 12 bpm, and temperature 102.4°F. The patient is unable to identify the surroundings and cries out that there are spiders coming out of the walls. The patient resists efforts to open their eyes for pupil assessment. Skin is flushed and warm; mucous membranes are dry. Bowel sounds are hypoactive, and there are multiple areas of dullness when percussing the abdomen. The bladder is palpable above the pubic symphysis, with bladder scan reading 650 mL. Admission laboratory test results include blood urea nitrogen (BUN) 32 mg/dL, creatinine 2.3 mg/dL, glucose 178 mg/dL, and white blood cell (WBC) 12,400 mm^3. Creatinine clearance is 24 mL/min. Medications include metformin, lisinopril, sertraline, and tolterodine.			

1. **Use a highlighter to identify the assessment findings that suggest muscarinic toxicity in the case study**.

18 Cholinesterase Inhibitors and Their Use in Myasthenia Gravis

STUDY QUESTIONS

Matching

Match the medication to its use.

1. ___ Used to reverse inhibition of cholinesterase in organophosphate poisoning
2. ___ Used to treat drug-induced muscarinic blockade
3. ___ Irreversible cholinesterase inhibitor used to treat glaucoma
4. ___ Irreversible cholinesterase inhibitor nerve agent that can be used in bioterrorism
5. ___ Antidote for cholinergic crisis
6. ___ Short-acting reversible cholinesterase inhibitor that does not cross the blood-brain barrier
7. ___ For dementia secondary to Alzheimer disease
8. ___ Drug used to treat myasthenic crisis
   a. Atropine
   b. Echothiophate
   c. Rivastigmine
   d. Pyridostigmine
   e. Physostigmine
   f. Pralidoxime
   g. Tabun
   h. Neostigmine

CRITICAL THINKING, PRIORITIZATION, AND DELEGATION QUESTIONS

9. Which are effects of cholinesterase inhibitors?
   a. Increase transmission only at neuromuscular junctions
   b. Intensify transmission at all cholinergic junctions
   c. Decrease transmission only at neuromuscular junctions
   d. Reduce transmission at all cholinergic junctions

10. Therapeutic doses of cholinesterase inhibitors have which effect? (**Select all that apply**.)
    a. Pupils constrict
    b. Tachycardia
    c. Hypertension
    d. Slow respirations
    e. Excessive salivation

11. Toxic levels of cholinesterase inhibitors result in which symptoms? (**Select all that apply.**)
    a. Diaphoresis
    b. Bronchospasm
    c. Mydriasis
    d. Constipation
    e. Tachycardia

✳12. Which is a priority concern when neostigmine is used to reverse neuromuscular blockade in postoperative patients?
    a. Respiration
    b. Diaphoresis
    c. Nausesa
    d. Incontinence

13. A 66-year-old male with myasthenia gravis has been taking pyridostigmine for 18 months. He is admitted to the hospital for a prostate biopsy. The pyridostigmine is scheduled to be administered. Which action should the nurse take?
    a. Administer the drug.
    b. Hold pyridostigmine.
    c. Assess for urine retention.
    d. Consult with the urologist.

14. The nurse is caring for a patient with myasthenia gravis who is prescribed pyridostigmine 240 mg three times daily. The patient states that they are experiencing an extreme increase in muscle weakness and that they need the nurse to administer 300-mg doses. Which action should the nurse take?
    a. Administer 240-mg dose as ordered.
    b. Give 300 mg as requested by the patient.
    c. Call the provider for directions on what to do.
    d. Assess for signs of myasthenic/cholinergic crisis.

DOSE CALCULATION QUESTIONS

15. Pyridostigmine 210 mg is ordered by mouth three times a day. The pharmacy stocks 60-mg scored tablets. How many tablets should the nurse administer for one dose?

16. Neostigmine is administered to reverse nondepolarizing neuromuscular blockade in an initial dose of 0.03 mg/kg. The patient weighs 154 lb. Neostigmine is available as an injectable solution of 0.5 mg/mL. How many milliliters of neostigmine should be administered?

CASE STUDIES

Case Study 1

A patient who is receiving a reversible cholinesterase inhibitor for myasthenia gravis is brought into the emergency department by their family because of extreme muscle weakness and difficulty breathing.

1. In this situation, why is it important to determine if the cause of the weakness is myasthenic crisis versus cholinergic crisis?

2. What assessments should the nurse perform? What questions should the nurse ask the patient and family? Why?

3. The provider is unsure, by history, if the patient is experiencing myasthenic crisis or cholinergic crisis. They order administration of edrophonium to differentiate. What should the nurse do, along with preparing to administer the edrophonium?

4. The nurse is completing discharge teaching for this patient. What teaching should the nurse provide to help the patient monitor the response to medication for his myasthenia gravis?

Case Study 2

The nurse has been asked to speak to a 4-H group in a farming community on preventing poisoning by organophosphate insecticides. The nurse has stressed the importance of following all directions provided on the insecticide label and seeking clarification from an adult if any directions are unclear.

5. What information should the nurse include to prevent:
   a. exposure through the skin or eyes when using insecticides?

   b. exposure through the respiratory tract when using insecticides?

   c. oral exposure?

6. What would the nurse include in an explanation of why insecticides have such potential for poisoning humans?

7. What information would the nurse include when explaining which symptoms warrant seeking immediate medical attention when using pesticides?

8. What information should be provided regarding the treatment for pesticide poisoning?

19 Drugs That Block Nicotinic Cholinergic Transmission

STUDY QUESTIONS

Matching

Match the term with its definition.

1. ___ Muscle twitching
2. ___ Process that leads to muscle contraction
3. ___ Pumping positively charged ions from inside to outside the cell membrane
4. ___ Uneven distribution of electrical charges across the inner and the outer cell membrane
5. ___ Positive charges move inward, making the inside of a membrane more positively charged than the outside of the membrane
   a. Depolarization
   b. Excitation-contraction coupling
   c. Fasciculations
   d. Polarization
   e. Repolarization

CRITICAL THINKING, PRIORITIZATION, AND DELEGATION QUESTIONS

6. A patient who is 8 weeks pregnant must have surgery. The anesthesiologist administers vecuronium to achieve muscle relaxation. Which is the most likely effect of this medication on the developing fetus?
   a. Very little effect
   b. Respiratory depression
   c. Bradycardia
   d. Teratogenesis
7. A patient is scheduled to have a nondepolarizing neuromuscular blocking agent administered. Which preoperative laboratory test result should be reported to the anesthesiologist, as it could affect paralysis?
   a. Alanine aminotransferase (ALT) 30 IU/L
   b. Blood urea nitrogen (BUN) 14 mg/dL
   c. Fasting blood glucose 175 mg/dL
   d. Potassium 3.1 mEq/L
8. The patient is at greater risk for enhanced neuromuscular blockade when which of the following antibiotics are used? (**Select all that apply**.)
   a. Amoxicillin
   b. Doxycycline
   c. Levofloxacin
   d. Gentamicin
   e. Polymyxin B
9. Which drug decreases the risk of hypotension when atracurium is administered?
   a. Acetaminophen
   b. Hydromorphone
   c. Diphenhydramine
   d. Indomethacin
10. The nurse should assess for and plan interventions to relieve muscle pain 12–24 hours after surgery for patients who have received which of the following drugs?
    a. Atracurium
    b. Pancuronium
    c. Succinylcholine
    d. Tubocurarine
11. An anesthesia resident is supervising the reversal of the neuromuscular blockade for an adult patient who has received succinylcholine. The resident directs the nurse to administer 0.5 mg of neostigmine intravenously (IV). Which action should the nurse take?
    a. Administer the medication slowly and monitor respirations.
    b. Question the order because the drug intensifies neuromuscular blockade.
    c. Ensure mechanical ventilation is available and then administer the drug.
    d. Ask the resident to order atropine, as it should also be administered.

*12. A patient will be receiving succinylcholine before electroconvulsive therapy. Which is the priority nursing action?
    a. Have diphenhydramine oral available.
    b. Teach the patient that they may have muscle pain.
    c. Moisten the mouth periodically.
    d. Ensure mechanical ventilation is available.

DOSE CALCULATION QUESTION

13. Dantrolene 2.5 mg/kg is prescribed STAT by rapid IV infusion for a 220-lb patient who is experiencing malignant hyperthermia after anesthesia with succinylcholine. How many milligrams should the nurse administer?

CASE STUDIES

Case Study 1

The postanesthesia care unit (PACU) nurse is caring for a patient who received a competitive neuromuscular blocking agent during surgery to remove a cancerous section of the bowel. The patient is admitted to the PACU with mechanical ventilation and a nasogastric (NG) tube for low-intermittent suction.

1. What are the priority assessments that the PACU nurse must monitor while the patient is still under the effects of the competitive neuromuscular blocking agent?

2. The nasogastric tube is draining a large amount of bile-colored liquid. How does this affect potassium levels and nursing care?

3. As the patient regains neuromuscular functioning, the nurse instructs the patient to take deep breaths. How does deep breathing counteract the adverse effects of histamine release stimulated by the competitive neuromuscular blocking agent?

Case Study 2

A patient is receiving a neuromuscular blocker for prolonged paralysis during mechanical ventilation.

4. Describe measures that should be included in nursing care and their rationale.

5. The patient spikes a temperature of 102°F within an hour after the neuromuscular agent infusion is begun. The infusion of the neuromuscular blocking agent is stopped, the patient receives a dose of dantrolene, and the patient's temperature begins to drop. Why was dantrolene administered to lower this patient's temperature instead of an antipyretic such as acetaminophen?

20 Adrenergic Agonists

STUDY QUESTIONS

Matching

Match the receptor with the main therapeutic uses of receptor stimulation.

1. ___ Dilation of renal vasculature
2. ___ Vasoconstriction
3. ___ Increased force of myocardial contraction
4. ___ Relief of severe pain
5. ___ Promotes bronchodilation
   a. α_1
   b. α_2
   c. β_1
   d. β_2
   e. Dopamine

True or False

For each of the following statements, enter T for true or F for false.

6. ___ Catecholamines are inactivated before reaching systemic circulation if administered orally.
7. ___ Catecholamines cross the blood-brain barrier, activating the central nervous system.
8. ___ Catecholamines include the drugs epinephrine, norepinephrine, isoproterenol, dopamine, and dobutamine.
9. ___ Catecholamines are effective when administered by any parenteral route.
10. ___ Catecholamine solutions should be discarded as soon as discoloration develops.
11. ___ Catecholamines are destroyed by monoamine oxidase (MAO) and catechol-*O*-methyltransferase (COMT) enzymes in the liver and intestinal wall.

CRITICAL THINKING, PRIORITIZATION, AND DELEGATION QUESTIONS

12. Direct-acting adrenergic drugs mimic the action of which neurotransmitters? (**Select all that apply**.)
   a. Acetylcholine
   b. Dopamine
   c. Epinephrine
   d. Norepinephrine
   e. Serotonin

✳13. The nurse is caring for a patient who is receiving an intravenous (IV) dopamine drip. The nurse has been assessing their patient's vital signs every 15 minutes. The nurse notes that since the last assessment, the IV has extravasated. Which is the priority nursing intervention?
   a. Stop the IV infusion.
   b. Administer phentolamine.
   c. Notify the provider.
   d. Restart the IV line.

14. The nurse is caring for a patient receiving IV epinephrine and knows they must monitor the patient for excessive cardiovascular activation. Which is an indication of excessive activation? (**Select all that apply**.)
   a. Oral temperature 102.5°F
   b. Respirations 16 per minute
   c. Blood pressure 175/98 mm Hg
   d. Pulse 130 beats per minute
   e. Oxygen saturation 96%

15. The nurse is working in the emergency department. A local anesthetic combined with epinephrine is often used when suturing wounds that need a small area of anesthesia and are likely to bleed. Assessment findings that would warrant consultation with the prescriber before administering a drug containing epinephrine include what? (**Select all that apply**.)
   a. Hypotension
   b. Peripheral edema
   c. Chest pain
   d. Poor capillary refill
   e. Bradycardia

*16. The nurse has administered epinephrine intramuscularly (IM) to a patient with a history of asthma and type 1 diabetes mellitus. It is a priority to assess for which effect?
   a. Hyperglycemia
   b. Hypotension
   c. Photophobia
   d. Fasciculations

17. A patient has a history of depression. Treatment with which antidepressant is most likely to decrease the inactivation of dopamine and increase the risk of toxicity? (**Select all that apply**.)
   a. Bupropion
   b. Nortriptyline
   c. Sertraline
   d. Phenelzine
   e. Duloxetine

18. Phenylephrine is available over the counter (OTC) as a nasal decongestant. A patient states that they understand why the label says it should not be used if they have high blood pressure, but they do not understand why it should not be used by patients with diabetes. The nurse's response is based on knowledge that phenylephrine can cause which effect?
   a. Anorexia
   b. Diaphoresis
   c. Hypoglycemia
   d. Hyperglycemia

19. The nurse is administering an IV dobutamine infusion. Eight hours after the infusion began, the nurse notes that the solution has become discolored. Which action should the nurse take?
   a. Continue the IV infusion.
   b. Administer phentolamine.
   c. Notify the provider.
   d. Hang a new IV bag.

DOSE CALCULATION QUESTIONS

20. A patient in cardiogenic shock is ordered an IV infusion of dopamine at a rate of 300 mcg/kg/min. The patient weighs 154 lb. The dopamine infusion is available in a dilution of 200 mg/250 mL. The infusion pump is calculated in mL/hour. What is the flow rate the nurse will program into the infusion pump?

21. Dobutamine HCl is available in a vial of 250 mg/20 mL. The prescribed dose for a patient weighing 110 lb is 250 mcg/kg/min. What is the recommended dilution and administration rate?

CASE STUDY

A 4-year-old child comes to the emergency department with angioedema, wheezing, and hypotension after eating a peanut butter cookie. Epinephrine is administered.

1. Describe how epinephrine treats the symptoms of anaphylactic shock.

2. The child is prescribed an epinephrine autoinjector. What should the nurse teach the parents and the child about administering the medication?

3. How can the parents ensure that their young child has the epinephrine autoinjector available at all times?

21 Adrenergic Antagonists

STUDY QUESTIONS

Matching

Match the physiologic action with the desired therapeutic response following alpha-blockade

1. ___ Blood pressure (BP) 90/60 mm Hg to 120/80 mm Hg
2. ___ Brisk capillary refill
3. ___ Postvoid residual less than 75 mL
   a. Reduced contraction of smooth muscle in trigone and sphincter
   b. Direct dilation of arterioles and indirect dilation of veins
   c. Prevent alpha-mediated vasoconstriction

True or False

For each of the following statements, enter T for true or F for false.

The nurse would consult the provider before administering alfuzosin if the nurse just learned the patient has a history of

4. ___ Q-T prolongation
5. ___ Advanced HIV infection
6. ___ Diabetes mellitus type 2
7. ___ Erectile dysfunction
8. ___ Frequent urinary tract infections
9. ___ Hepatitis B
10. ___ Hypertension
11. ___ Ventricular dysrhythmia

CRITICAL THINKING, PRIORITIZATION, AND DELEGATION QUESTIONS

12. Which are adverse effects of alpha blockade? (**Select all that apply.**)
    a. Orthostatic hypotension
    b. Decreased blood volume
    c. Inhibition of ejaculation
    d. Reflex tachycardia
    e. Nasal congestion

13. Alfuzosin is contraindicated in patients with which condition? (**Select all that apply.**)
    a. History of QT prolongation
    b. Moderate hepatic impairment
    c. Sexual dysfunction
    d. Hypertension
    e. Kidney dysfunction

14. A patient has just been prescribed prazosin. Which statement from the patient would indicate a need for further teaching?
    a. "I should avoid driving and other hazardous activities for 12–24 hours after taking this drug."
    b. "I should take the medication first thing in the morning, along with my breakfast."
    c. "I should sit on the edge of the bed for a few minutes before standing up when I get up in the morning."
    d. "I should be sitting or lying 30–60 minutes after I take the first dose of this drug."

*15. A patient with coronary artery disease is receiving terazosin for hypertension. It would be a priority for the nurse to report to the prescriber which effect of the drug?
    a. Drop of 15 mm Hg in systolic BP with position changes
    b. Headache
    c. Increase in pulse of 20 beats/min
    d. Nasal congestion

16. When administering tamsulosin, which assessment would indicate that therapy has achieved the desired effect?
    a. Voiding 250 mL every 2–3 hours while awake
    b. Position changes without dizziness
    c. Absence of dysuria when voiding
    d. Postvoid residual less than 300 mL

17. Which is the proper way to administer tamsulosin?
    a. Take with food
    b. On an empty stomach
    c. 30 minutes after eating
    d. Sit up for 30 minutes after administration

▶18. In addition to teaching a patient with a new prescription for prazosin actions to reduce orthostatic hypotension, the nurse must also teach the patient to take their first dose at bedtime to prevent which side effect?
   a. Nasal congestion
   b. Reflex tachycardia
   c. First-dose hypotension
   d. Nausea and vomiting

19. The generic names of β_1 and β_2 receptor antagonists share what common suffix?
   a. -azole
   b. -lol
   c. -osin
   d. -sartan

▶20. Which assessment finding would warrant withholding a β-blocker and consulting the provider?
   a. Apical pulse 48 beats/min
   b. BP 110/70 mm Hg
   c. 2+ ankle edema
   d. Capillary blood glucose 90 mg/dL

▶21. The nurse is caring for a full-term neonate whose mother took the drug betaxolol throughout pregnancy. Which assessment finding would be a priority to report to the pediatrician?
   a. Apical pulse 80 beats/min
   b. BP 65/45 mm Hg
   c. Plasma glucose 48 mg/dL
   d. Respirations 35/min

✳22. Which of these new assessment findings, if identified 1 hour after administering metoprolol, would be a priority to report to the prescriber?
   a. Drop in apical pulse from 80 to 65 beats/min
   b. Warm, flushed, dry skin
   c. Crackles throughout lung fields
   d. Migraine headache

23. Which of these conditions, if identified on admission assessment, would be a concern to the nurse if the provider ordered propranolol? **(Select all that apply.)**
   a. Atrioventricular (AV) block
   b. Preexisting heart failure
   c. Prostatic hypertrophy
   d. Diabetes mellitus
   e. Rhinitis due to ragweed

24. The nurse should report which findings in a patient who is prescribed metoprolol to the prescriber?
   a. Creatinine 1.2 mg/dL
   b. Dyspnea with exertion
   c. Capillary blood glucose 85 mg/dL
   d. Sinus rhythm on electrocardiogram

✳25. Which would be of most concern to the nurse if a patient is prescribed propranolol?
   a. Apical pulse 94 beats/min
   b. BP 157/88 mm Hg
   c. Urinary urgency
   d. Wheezing

26. Esmolol is approved to treat which condition?
   a. Ventricular dysrhythmia
   b. Supraventricular tachycardia
   c. Hypertension
   d. Heart failure

✳27. It is a priority for the nurse to monitor for excessive cardiosuppression when a patient is prescribed metoprolol and which other drug?
   a. Rizatriptan
   b. Amiloride
   c. Terazosin
   d. Verapamil

DOSE CALCULATION QUESTIONS

28. Phentolamine 1 mg intravenous (IV) is ordered as prophylaxis of hypertension 1 hour prior to surgery for a child with pheochromocytoma. The drug is available in a vial of 5 mg/2 mL. How many milliliters will be administered?

29. Labetalol is prescribed by continuous intravenous infusion at 2 mg/min, to be adjusted by patient response. It is supplied as 200 mg/250 mL. The intravenous pump is calibrated in milliliters per hour. What rate will the nurse initially program into the pump?

CASE STUDIES

Case Study 1

A 58-year-old male has just been prescribed prazosin for hypertension.

1. Explain the common adverse effects and nursing teaching needed to provide both comfort and safety for this patient.

2. What assessments should be performed before the nurse administers an α_1-adrenergic antagonist for hypertension, and what assessment findings would warrant not administering the medication and notifying the prescriber?

3. The patient's BP is not controlled by his prescribed α_1 antagonist. The prescriber has added a loop diuretic and a β_1 blocker. The patient asks, "Why do I have to take three different medications for my BP? Can't I just have a higher dose of one medication?" How should the nurse explain the rationale for this drug regimen?

4. Why is it very important to address ejaculation problems and other adverse effects with this patient?

Case Study 2

A 45-year-old male is being treated for hypertension. Several antihypertensive medications have been tried without success. They also have been taking glargine insulin 22 units every morning and aspart insulin on a sliding scale according to blood sugar for diabetes. Their prescriber orders metoprolol 50 mg once a day. When the patient tries to fill the prescription using their insurance, the pharmacist notifies them that their insurance covers only the less expensive β-blocker, propranolol, unless the patient experiences adverse effects or has an absolute contraindication for the use of propranolol. The prescriber can appeal to the insurance company and justify the use of the more expensive decision. The prescriber asks the office nurse to initiate the insurance appeal form.

5. Describe and explain the adverse effects that this patient might experience relating to their diabetes diagnosis and propranolol.

6. The insurance appeal is approved, and the patient receives metoprolol, a β_1-selective adrenergic antagonist. The patient states, "I'm glad I do not have to take propranolol. I have had frequent episodes of hypoglycemia because, with my job, I cannot always eat when I should." What should the nurse do and why?

7. The nurse discovers that this patient has a history of poor adherence to medication regimens. Why are β-adrenergic blockers poor choices for this patient?

22 Indirect-Acting Antiadrenergic Agents

STUDY QUESTIONS

Completion

1. Indirect-acting antiadrenergic drugs' net effect is to reduce activation of ________________ ________________ receptors.
2. ________________ is the primary use for centrally acting α_2 agonists.
3. The effect of centrally acting α_2 agonists is like that of ____ ____ ________________.
4. The most common adverse effects of clonidine are ____, ____, and ________________________.
5. The principal mechanism of blood pressure (BP) reduction with methyldopa is ____________________.

CRITICAL THINKING, PRIORITIZATION, AND DELEGATION QUESTIONS

6. Clonidine is used off-label to treat which condition? (**Select all that apply**.)
   a. Bradycardia
   b. Opioid withdrawal
   c. Smoking cessation
   d. Insomnia
   e. Tourette syndrome
7. The nurse is teaching a 56-year-old truck driver about taking clonidine. Which information should be included in the teaching about drug administration?
   a. Administer twice daily.
   b. Take at bedtime.
   c. Eat before taking.
   d. Take on an empty stomach.

*8. It would be a priority to withhold clonidine and report which laboratory test result?
   a. Alanine aminotransferase (ALT) 55 IU/L
   b. Creatinine 1.4 mg/dL
   c. Human chorionic gonadotropin (hCG) 900 IU/mL
   d. White blood cell (WBC) count 10,500 mm^3

9. The nurse is teaching a patient who has been prescribed clonidine for hypertension. Which of the following statements suggests a need for additional teaching?
   a. "Effects like drowsiness should get better after I take the drug for several weeks."
   b. "Nightmares are a sign of drug toxicity, and I need to call my provider."
   c. "I should inform all of my health care providers that I am taking this drug."
   d. "Increasing fiber and fluid in my diet can decrease the risk of constipation."
10. A patient has been taking methyldopa for 12 months. Which laboratory test should be monitored throughout therapy? (**Select all that apply**.)
   a. Coombs
   b. Red cell count
   c. Potassium
   d. Blood glucose
   e. Troponin T

▶11. A patient has been taking methyldopa 250 mg twice a day for 8 months. Vital signs are blood pressure (BP) 170/90 mm Hg, pulse 104, and respiratory 20. The nurse is reviewing new laboratory test results, which include ALT 40 international units/L, creatinine 0.8 mg/dL, blood urea nitrogen (BUN) 20 mg/dL, Coombs test positive, sodium 145 mEq/L, and potassium 4.8 mEq/L. Which action should the nurse take?
   a. Administer the medication as ordered.
   b. Notify the prescriber of the lab results.
   c. Recheck all of the patient's vital signs.
   d. Hold the medication until after rounds.

12. Which indirect-acting antiadrenergic agent may be used inappropriately by persons with substance use disorder?
   a. Methyldopa
   b. Clonidine
   c. Guanfacine
   d. Tizanidine

DOSE CALCULATION QUESTIONS

13. Clonidine 0.4 mg twice daily is prescribed. Available are 0.2-mg tablets. How many tablets should be administered for each dose?

14. Methyldopa for intravenous infusion 10 mg/mL is prepared in 5% dextrose in water. The 100-mL bag is to be infused in 30 minutes. What rate should the nurse program into the intravenous pump if it is calibrated in milliliters per hour?

CASE STUDY

A 50-year-old female who plays tennis regularly has been prescribed guanfacine 10 mg once a day for hypertension not controlled by other agents. The prescriber asks the office nurse to provide teaching regarding this medication.

1. What should the nurse teach about side effects?

2. What should the nurse teach about drug-herb supplement interactions and drug-food interactions?

3. What serious reactions can occur if this drug is stopped abruptly?

23 Introduction to Central Nervous System Pharmacology

CRITICAL THINKING, PRIORITIZATION, AND DELEGATION QUESTIONS

1. Which are medical applications of central nervous system (CNS) drugs? (**Select all that apply.**)
   a. Anesthesia
   b. Heart failure
   c. Constipation
   d. Pain relief
   e. Seizure suppression
2. Which drugs can cross the blood-brain barrier?
   a. Lipid soluble
   b. Protein bound
   c. Highly ionized
   d. Water soluble
3. Alterations in drug therapeutic and side effects over time are a result of which ability of the brain?
   a. Tolerance
   b. Dependence
   c. Adaptability
   d. Metabolism
4. A patient who has been taking an opiate analgesic for chronic pain due to terminal cancer needs higher doses to produce the same pain relief as when originally prescribed. This may be an example of what?
   a. Misuse
   b. Dependence
   c. Tolerance
   d. Withdrawal

CASE STUDY

A patient has recently been diagnosed with major depression. Medication has just been prescribed that alters CNS neurotransmission. The patient verbalizes concerns to the nurse because the medication is "not working." They are also experiencing some daytime sedation.

1. How should the nurse respond?
2. The patient asks why drug companies have not been able to develop new psychotherapeutic drugs that do not have adverse effects. What would be the basis of the nurse's response?
3. There are many psychotherapeutic drugs that are effective in treating patients' symptoms. What factors decrease patient adherence with these medications?

24 Drugs for Parkinson Disease

STUDY QUESTIONS

Completion

Name the class of drugs by action.

1. ________________ ________________ activate dopamine receptors in the striatum.
2. ________________________________ inhibit metabolism of levodopa in the periphery.
3. ________________ ________________ block muscarinic receptors in the striatum.
4. ________________ ________________ inhibit inactivation of dopamine in the striatum.
5. ________________ promotes dopamine synthesis.
6. ________________ promotes dopamine release and may block dopamine reuptake.

CRITICAL THINKING, PRIORITIZATION, AND DELEGATION QUESTIONS

7. Which is a realistic outcome for a patient receiving drug therapy for Parkinson disease (PD)?
   a. Absence of tremor
   b. A normal gait
   c. Improved ability for self-care
   d. Reversal of neurodegeneration

8. How do selegiline and rasagiline improve mild PD symptoms?
   a. Stimulation of γ-aminobutyric acid release
   b. Prevention of dopamine breakdown
   c. Blocking of muscarinic receptors
   d. Increasing dopamine secretion

9. A PD patient who is receiving levodopa displays slow, involuntary writhing movements of the extremities. The nurse holds the medications and notifies the prescriber. Which terminology should the nurse use when documenting this movement?
   a. Ballismus
   b. Choreoathetosis
   c. Fasciculation
   d. Myoclonus

10. Which finding would be of most concern if the nurse is preparing to administer levodopa?
    a. Ataxia
    b. Amber urine
    c. Dizziness
    d. Tics

11. Which drug would **NOT** be a concern if prescribed for the psychological effects of PD and the adverse effects of treatment with levodopa/carbidopa?
    a. Chlorpromazine
    b. Clozapine
    c. Haloperidol
    d. Risperidone

*12. Which is the most appropriate nursing action when the nurse notes an asymmetric, irregular, darkly pigmented mole on the back of a patient who is receiving levodopa and rasagiline for PD?
    a. Notify the provider.
    b. Assess vital signs.
    c. Consult a dermatologist.
    d. Stop both drugs.

13. Which is the effect of adding carbidopa to levodopa?
    a. Has a synergistic therapeutic effect with levodopa
    b. Allows for an increase in levodopa dosage
    c. Decreases the risk of nausea and vomiting
    d. Increases the conversion of levodopa to dopamine

*14. The nurse is caring for a patient who has just begun therapy with ropinirole. It is priority for the nurse to include which information when teaching the patient about side effect?
    a. Nausea is common with this drug
    b. This drug can cause sleep attacks
    c. Get up slowly to avoid fainting
    d. Dizziness is common with this drug

15. The medication administration record (MAR) for a patient with PD lists apomorphine 1 mg subcutaneous with trimethobenzamide 300 mg, up to three doses per day as needed. The drug is an acute *rescue* treatment for which episode?
    a. A sleep attack
    b. An off episode
    c. Lack of impulse control
    d. Psychotic reaction

✳16. It would be of greatest priority to consult the provider if which new finding in a patient who is prescribed bromocriptine?
   a. Dyskinesias
   b. Confusion
   c. Erythromelalgia
   d. Valvular disease

✳17. A patient who is receiving tolcapone complains of nausea and abdominal pain. His urine is dark amber. Which laboratory test results would be most significant when the nurse reports these symptoms to the prescriber?
   a. ALT 175 IU/L
   b. Creatinine 1.1 mg/dL
   c. Hgb 12 g/dL
   d. Na^+ 142 mEq/L

18. The nurse notes an orange color in the urine of a PD patient who is scheduled to receive a dose of entacapone. Which action should the nurse take?
   a. Assess for symptoms of liver failure.
   b. Consult with the provider.
   c. Continue nursing care.
   d. Hold the medication.

19. Which drug should **NOT** be prescribed when a patient is prescribed selegiline? **(Select all that apply.)**
   a. Butorphanol
   b. Fluoxetine
   c. Hydromorphone
   d. Meperidine
   e. Sertraline

DOSE CALCULATION QUESTIONS

20. Pramipexole 1.5 mg by mouth is prescribed. The hospital pharmacy stocks pramipexole 0.25 mg. How many tablets should the nurse administer?

21. Orally disintegrating selegiline 2.5 mg once a day is prescribed. Available is selegiline 1.25 mg. How many tablets will the nurse administer?

CLINICAL JUDGMENT CASE STUDY

The nurse admits a patient who has recently been diagnosed with PD.

HEALTH HISTORY	NURSE'S NOTES	PHYSICIAN'S ORDERS	LABORATORY PROFILE

1400:

Admission note:

The patient is a welder, married, with two adult children and one college-aged child. The patient has a 40-pack-a-year history of smoking; the patient quit smoking 2 years ago.

Patient reports the tremor is starting to interfere with the precision of their work, and they have noticed some unsteadiness when working on scaffolding. These symptoms are causing anxiety and concern about the ability to continue working, as the welding job provides insurance for the family.

Medical history includes hypertension, type 2 diabetes, and chronic obstructive pulmonary disease.

On exam, the patient has resting tremor bilateral upper extremities; voice is soft without slurring. Although the patient's stance has widened and steps do not always clear the floor, there is no shuffling and near-normal arm movement with ambulation. The patient can complete all activities of daily living without assistance.

Medication reconciliation: metformin 500 mg twice a day, lisinopril/hydrochlorothiazide 10 mg/12.5 mg, and budesonide/formoterol 80 mcg/4.5 mcg 2 puffs twice a day.

Orders received to start the patient on selegiline.

Which teaching should the nurse provide about possible adverse effects of selegiline? **(One, some, or all may apply.)**
   a. Take the drug no later than noon to decrease the risk of insomnia.
   b. Avoid stimulating television before bedtime.
   c. Change positions slowly to avoid orthostatic hypotension.
   d. Avoid foods high in tyramine.
   e. Avoid taking the drug with food.
   f. Reduce the dosage of drug if dyskinesias occur.
   g. Twenty percent of patients taking the drug have nightmares.

25 Drugs for Alzheimer Disease

STUDY QUESTIONS

True or False

For each of the following statements, enter T for true or F for false.

1. ___ A blood test can confirm the diagnosis of Alzheimer disease (AD).
2. ___ An early symptom of AD is loss of appetite.
3. ___ There is no effective therapy for the core symptoms of AD.
4. ___ Effects of drugs for AD are long lasting.
5. ___ High levels of the neurotransmitter acetylcholine are found in patients with AD.
6. ___ Neuritic plaques are found in the hippocampus and cerebral cortex of patients with AD.
7. ___ Production of an abnormal form of a protein (τ) results in neurofibrillary tangles of AD.
8. ___ Apolipoprotein E4 (apoE4) is protective for AD.
9. ___ Research suggests that many AD patients experience more intense symptoms on waking up in the morning.
10. ___ Research suggests cholinesterase inhibitors enhance transmission by central cholinergic neurons.
11. ___ The American College of Physicians recommends trying a cholinesterase inhibitor in all patients with mild to moderate AD.
12. ___ The neuronal damage that occurs with AD is irreversible.
13. ___ Olanzapine may reduce the neuropsychiatric symptoms of AD.

CRITICAL THINKING, PRIORITIZATION, AND DELEGATION QUESTIONS

14. Neuronal degeneration in the hippocampus results in which symptom of AD?
    a. Language difficulties
    b. Urinary incontinence
    c. Inability for self-care
    d. Short-term memory

*15. The nurse is caring for a patient who is receiving rivastigmine for AD. Which is the nursing priority related to the most common adverse effect of the drug?
    a. Ensure adequate nutrition.
    b. Monitor serum electrolytes.
    c. Assess for skin reactions.
    d. Resolve drug-drug interactions.

16. Adverse effects of cholinesterase inhibitors come from parasympathetic stimulation. Which nursing intervention prevents a common adverse effect?
    a. Encourage hydration.
    b. Moisturize the skin.
    c. Provide adequate fiber.
    d. Provide lip moisturizers.

17. The nurse should be particularly cautious when administering a cholinesterase inhibitor drug to any patient with a history of which condition? (**Select all that apply**.)
    a. Asthma
    b. Chronic obstructive pulmonary disease (COPD)
    c. Bradycardia
    d. Hypertension
    e. Headaches

18. Which treatment for dyspepsia could potentially decrease the renal excretion of memantine and cause toxicity?
    a. Calcium carbonate
    b. Dexlansoprazole
    c. Nizatidine capsules
    d. Sodium bicarbonate

19. Which result would warrant withholding administration of memantine and notifying the provider?
    a. Alanine aminotransferase (ALT) 112 international units/L
    b. Blood urea nitrogen (BUN) 18 mg/dL
    c. Estimated glomerular filtration rate (eGFR) 45 mL/min
    d. Brain natriuretic peptide (BNP) 75 pg/mL

20. Prior to beginning therapy with aducanumab, which actions are required? (**Select all that apply.**)
    a. Obtain echocardiogram imaging.
    b. Conduct a cognitive assessment.
    c. Perform magnetic resonance imaging (MRI).
    d. Screen for taking anticoagulants.
    e. Assess for amyloid-related imaging abnormalities.

21. The home caregiver of a patient with AD tells the nurse that the patient has become increasingly agitated, has become aggressive, and is paranoid. They ask if there are any medications to help. Which is the appropriate response from the nurse?
    a. "I will talk to the provider and see if we can do a trial of lorazepam."
    b. "There is nothing to try; start looking for long-term care placement."
    c. "Diphenhydramine has been shown to help, and it is over the counter (OTC)."
    d. "Olanzapine may help; talk to the provider about the risks and benefits."

DOSE CALCULATION QUESTIONS

22. Galantamine extended-release (ER) 16 mg orally once a day is prescribed. Available is galantamine ER 8 mg. How many capsules should the nurse administer?

23. Memantine is prescribed as 5 mg by mouth in the morning (0800) and 10 mg by mouth in the evening (1800). The nurse is preparing to administer the 0800 dose. Available is memantine 2-mg/mL oral solution. How much memantine should the nurse administer, and how should the nurse measure this dose?

CASE STUDY

A patient with a history of AD, diabetes mellitus (DM), hypertension, and seasonal allergies has been admitted with a hip fracture following a fall while wandering around the house at night. They are scheduled for an open reduction and internal fixation of the fracture in the morning. On admission, the nurse discovers that the patient's spouse had been administering ginkgo biloba for the past 8 months in the hope that it would improve memory.

1. Why is it important for the nurse to report the use of ginkgo to the orthopedic surgeon?

2. The patient's spouse is concerned that the patient's confusion, memory loss, and wandering have not improved much and that they seem to have gotten worse since the weather got warm and the flowers started to bloom. The patient's spouse has provided a list of all the patient's prescribed medications, which include hydrochlorothiazide, metformin, and galantamine. Based on the patient's history, what class of OTC medication does the nurse need to report to the prescriber because it could be contributing to the patient's sudden decline in functioning?

3. What assessments (including reviewing laboratory tests) should the nurse perform before administering galantamine, and what findings would warrant consulting the prescriber?

4. The patient's ALT is 178 international units/L, and bilirubin is 3.2 mg/mL. The prescriber instructs the patient's spouse and the patient to discontinue the galantamine, not take any OTC antihistamines, and start taking rivastigmine. The patient's spouse asks the nurse why the prescriber changed the medication to one in the same class if the galantamine is not working well and is hurting the patient's liver.

5. The nurse should teach the patient's spouse what information regarding the adverse effects of rivastigmine?

6. The patient's spouse heard from friends of something sold in the health food store to cure AD. The friend said that the store provided results of research that state that the supplement is effective in improving memory in AD patients. The patient's spouse is on a limited budget and asks the opinion of the nurse. How should the nurse respond?

26 Drugs for Multiple Sclerosis

STUDY QUESTIONS

True or False

For each of the following statements, enter T for true or F for false.

1. ___ Initiation of the disease process is thought to be linked to genetics, environmental factors, and microbial pathogens.
2. ___ Current drug therapy repairs the myelin sheath on peripheral nerves.
3. ___ Although MS causes more disability than other neurologic diseases, life expectancy is only slightly reduced.
4. ___ Most clinicians employ the Katz Index of Independence in Activities of Daily Living to quantify the impact of MS symptoms.
5. ___ Drug therapy for MS can decrease the severity of relapses.
6. ___ Current drug therapy for MS can maintain quality of life.
7. ___ Persons with MS may experience visual impairment, emotional lability, and cognitive impairment.
8. ___ Interferon Beta can slow disease progression in relapsing MS.
9. ___ All patients with relapsing-remitting MS should receive an immunomodulator.
10. ___ Interferon β, glatiramer, and fingolimod are more effective than natalizumab in the treatment of relapsing forms of MS.
11. ___ Primary progressive MS is characterized by recurrent, clearly defined episodes of neurologic dysfunction (relapses) separated by periods of partial or full recovery.

CRITICAL THINKING, PRIORITIZATION, AND DELEGATION QUESTIONS

12. A 26-year-old patient seeks medical care for blurred vision and severe muscle weakness. Which information from their history suggests possible risk factors for MS? (**Select all that apply**.)
    a. Ten-pack-year history of smoking
    b. Has a part-time job in fast food
    c. Missed classes due to mononucleosis
    d. Parent with cerebrovascular disease
    e. Grandparents were Norwegian immigrants

13. Which of the following best describes treatment of relapsing-remitting MS with immunomodulators?
    a. Always administer orally
    b. Used only during relapses
    c. Continue use indefinitely
    d. Only be used during recovery

14. The nurse is administering high-dose intravenous (IV) methylprednisolone to a patient who is experiencing an acute relapse of MS. Which chronic condition could be adversely affected by this treatment?
    a. Asthma
    b. Diabetes
    c. Hypertension
    d. Osteoarthritis

15. A patient with MS hospitalized with pneumonia is receiving interferon β-1a intramuscular (IM) 30 mcg once a week. It would be of greatest priority for the nurse to report which laboratory result to the prescriber?
    a. C-reactive protein 8 mg/L
    b. Hemoglobin A1c 5.2%
    c. Platelets 50 × 10^9/L
    d. Hemoglobin 13 g/dL

16. The nurse is administering mitoxantrone to a patient who did not respond to other immunomodulating drugs. The nurse should hold the medication and contact the provider if the patient exhibits which of the following?
    a. Low blood glucose
    b. Orthostatic hypotension
    c. Elevated blood pressure
    d. Shortness of breath

17. A patient is scheduled to receive mitoxantrone. Which would be a reason to withhold the medication and contact the provider? (**Select all that apply**.)
    a. Platelets 400 × 10^9/L
    b. Direct bilirubin 0.1 mg/dL
    c. Ejection fraction of 60%
    d. hCG 350 IU/L
    e. Neutrophils 250 cells/mm^3

18. Which immunizations are contraindicated in a patient receiving mitoxantrone? (**Select all that apply**.)
    a. Hepatitis B vaccine
    b. Influenza vaccine
    c. Measles, mumps, and rubella
    d. Tetanus toxoids
    e. Varicella virus vaccine

19. A patient with MS experiences nausea, vomiting, tea-colored urine, clay-colored stools, and right upper quadrant (RUQ) tenderness. Alanine transaminase (ALT) is 200 international units/L, and aspartate aminotransferase (AST) is 190 units/L (U/L). The nurse would consult with the provider if the patient was prescribed which drug? (**Select all that apply**.)
    a. Interferon β-1b
    b. Mitoxantrone
    c. Interferon β-1a
    d. Cladribine
    e. Alemtuzumab

20. Which symptom suggests a complication of detrusor-sphincter dyssynergia in an MS patient?
    a. Dysuria
    b. Urinary retention
    c. Nocturia
    d. Urinary urgency

21. Which teaching is appropriate regarding the administration of bulk-forming products used for fecal incontinence?
    a. Give after meals
    b. Administer before meals
    c. Take fiber at night
    d. With 240 mL of fluid

22. An MS patient reports they are still depressed and fatigued despite being prescribed fluoxetine for 4 months. Which is the most appropriate nursing intervention?
    a. Encourage increased caffeine consumption.
    b. Explain the drugs take many months to help.
    c. Discuss this problem with the provider.
    d. Implement 1:1 suicide precautions.

DOSE CALCULATION QUESTIONS

23. A patient is prescribed an initial subcutaneous dose of 8.8 mcg of interferon 1a for the first 2 weeks of therapy. The drug is supplied as 8.8-mcg/0.2-mL prefilled, single-use syringes. How much drug should the patient administer with each dose?

24. The nurse prepares natalizumab 300 mg/15 mL in 100 mL of normal saline solution for IV infusion. The drug is to be administered over 1 hour. The tubing has a drop factor of 10 gtt/mL. How many drops per minute will be infused?

CASE STUDY

A 36-year-old college professor has been diagnosed with relapsing-remitting MS after the birth of her first child.

1. What assessments are important for the nurse to include when caring for this patient?

2. Her symptoms have significantly improved. What are the primary factors of the pathophysiologic process of MS that explain how the symptoms can abate but the disease is still present?

3. Identify current and potential nursing problems for this patient.

4. When the nurse is administering medications, the patient refuses the drug, stating, "What's the use? My mom had MS, and the drugs didn't help. She died in 1990. She was only 57 years old." What should be the basis of the nurse's response?

5. The patient with MS is started on the immunomodulator interferon β-1a IM 30 mcg once a week. What should the nurse include in teaching regarding this drug?

6. The patient and the prescriber have tried treatment with the immunomodulators without success. They have agreed to try the immunosuppressant mitoxantrone. What teaching should the nurse provide to this patient?

7. What steps does the nurse need to take before administering the mitoxantrone by IV infusion?

8. The patient is experiencing urinary incontinence. What pharmacologic and nonpharmacologic measures can be employed to prevent this problem?

27 Drugs for Seizure Disorders

STUDY QUESTIONS

Matching

Match the term with its definition.

1. ___ Abnormal motor phenomena.
2. ___ Any seizure activity that lasts 15–30 minutes or longer.
3. ___ Brief loss of consciousness with or without mild, symmetric motor activity.
4. ___ General term that applies to all types of epileptic events.
5. ___ Group of hyperexcitable neurons that start seizure activity.
6. ___ Muscle rigidity followed by muscle jerks and then a period of central nervous system (CNS) depression.
7. ___ Partial seizure that evolves into generalized seizure activity.
8. ___ Repetitive movements that lack purpose, such as lip smacking.
9. ___ Seizure activity in young children associated with an elevated temperature.
10. ___ Severe form of epilepsy with developmental delay and a mixture of partial and generalized seizures.
11. ___ Sudden, very brief, local, *or* generalized muscle contraction.
12. ___ Sudden loss of muscle tone.
13. ___ Discrete symptoms determined by the brain region involved; there is no loss of consciousness.
14. ___ Trance-like state for 45–90 seconds followed by automatism.
    a. Absence seizure
    b. Atonic seizure
    c. Automatism
    d. Focal impaired awareness
    e. Convulsions
    f. Febrile seizure
    g. Focus
    h. Lennox-Gastaut syndrome
    i. Myoclonic seizure
    j. Focal to bilateral tonic-clonic seizures
    k. Seizure
    l. Focal aware
    m. Status epilepticus
    n. Tonic-clonic seizure

CRITICAL THINKING, PRIORITIZATION, AND DELEGATION QUESTIONS

15. Antiseizure drugs act through which mechanisms? (**Select all that apply**.)
    a. Prolong sodium channel inactivation
    b. Calcium channel blockade
    c. Facilitate potassium influx
    d. Block actions of glutamate
    e. Potentiate the actions of γ-aminobutyric acid (GABA)
16. Developmentally, which would be the most likely reason an 18-year-old male patient may refuse to seek treatment for possible seizure activity?
    a. Concern about loss of driver's license
    b. Feels drugs are not likely to be helpful
    c. Fear of injury when playing sports
    d. Concern about addiction to antiseizure drugs
17. Which should be included when teaching when a patient about withdrawing them from antiseizure drugs?
    a. Drug should be gradually decreased over a year.
    b. The drug should be withdrawn over several months.
    c. Antiseizure drugs should be stopped all at once.
    d. Withdrawal is done by trial and error.
18. Research suggests that there is a statistically significant increased risk of thoughts of suicide when a patient is prescribed which antiseizure drug? (**Select all that apply**.)
    a. Carbamazepine
    b. Depakene
    c. Lamotrigine
    d. Phenytoin
    e. Topiramate

19. Which is true regarding new-generation antiseizure drugs versus first-generation antiseizure drugs?
    a. Birth defects are more common with new-generation drugs.
    b. New-generation drugs do not induce drug-metabolizing enzymes.
    c. Research suggests newer antiseizure drugs are more effective.
    d. There is less clinical experience with newer antiseizure drugs.

✳20. Which action is priority concerning phenytoin's narrow therapeutic index?
    a. Check plasma levels of the drug.
    b. Increase intake of dairy products.
    c. Have regular dental checkups.
    d. Use two reliable forms of birth control.

✳21. Which laboratory test result would be of most concern to the nurse when a 27-year-old patient is admitted after injuries sustained in a motor vehicle accident is prescribed phenytoin, omeprazole, diazepam, and heparin?
    a. Alanine aminotransferase (ALT) 35 IU/L
    b. Human chorionic gonadotropin (hCG) 3270 mIU/mL
    c. Partial thromboplastin time (PTT) 60 seconds
    d. Phenytoin 15 mcg/mL

✳22. When caring for a patient receiving phenytoin, which assessment finding is a priority to report to the prescriber?
    a. Morbilliform-like rash
    b. Nystagumus
    c. Hyperplasia of gum tissue
    d. Mild hypotention

23. Parents have received instructions regarding the administration of phenytoin suspension 5 mL (250 mg) twice daily to their child. Which statement made by the parents suggests a need for further teaching?
    a. "We must be sure to shake the medication thoroughly."
    b. "We should give our baby a teaspoonful of the drug at each dose."
    c. "We should give the medication with breakfast and bedtime."
    d. "It is important that we space the drug doses as instructed."

24. Which side-effect is likely to occur with carbamazepine therapy, but not phenytoin?
    a. Sedation
    b. Hyponatremia
    c. Neuralgia
    d. Gingival overgrowth

✳25. Which nursing action is priority when the patient prescribed carbamazepine has an absolute neutrophil count (ANC) of 500/mm^3?
    a. Handwashing
    b. Limited visitors
    c. No fresh fruit or vegetables
    d. Protective isolation

✳26. Which is the priority nursing action when a patient who is prescribed carbamazepine reports vertigo?
    a. Ensuring patient safety
    b. Paging the provider
    c. Reviewing most recent lab results
    d. Withholding the medication

27. The nurse is teaching a patient about the adverse effects of carbamazepine. Which instructions should be included in this teaching? (**Select all that apply**.)
    a. Call your provider if you develop a fever.
    b. Plan your day to allow for rest periods.
    c. Stop taking the drug if you experience double vision.
    d. Do not take the medication with grapefruit juice.
    e. Report new onset peripheral edema to the provider.

✳28. To prevent a life-threatening skin reaction, it would be a priority to review which laboratory results if administering carbamazepine to a patient of Asian descent?
    a. Aspartate aminotransferase (AST)
    b. Blood urea nitrogen (BUN)
    c. Complete blood cell count (CBC)
    d. Human leukocyte antigen (HLA)-B*1502

29. The nurse instructs patients who have just received a prescription for carbamazepine to avoid consuming grapefruit juice for which time period?
    a. 4 hours after taking the drug
    b. No more than twice a week
    c. Never when taking the drug
    d. 2 hours before taking the drug

✳30. It would be priority for the patient to report which adverse effect of valproic acid?
    a. Abdominal pain
    b. Belching
    c. Hair loss
    d. Weight gain

31. A female who is of childbearing age must take valproic acid to control seizures. Which statement suggests a need for further teaching?
    a. "Folic acid supplements are a good idea in case of pregnancy."
    b. "I should stop taking the drug if I find out that I am pregnant."
    c. "I need to inform my provider that I am taking valproic acid."
    d. "To be safe, I need to use two reliable forms of birth control."

32. Which is the best goal for a child who is prescribed ethosuximide for absence seizures?
    a. Normal participation in school activities
    b. No adverse effects from the drug
    c. Plasma levels within the therapeutic range
    d. Suppression of neurons in the thalamus

33. A patient is admitted with a phenobarbital overdose. Which nursing action is priority?
    a. Assess respiratory status.
    b. Initiate intravenous (IV) fluids.
    c. Obtain drug level.
    d. Initiate seizure precautions.

34. A patient with a history of hypertension and focal impaired awareness seizures has been prescribed oxcarbazepine 100 mg twice a day and hydrochlorothiazide. It is important for the nurse to assess for which condition? (**Select all that apply**.)
    a. Dry mucous membranes
    b. Hyperactive bowel sounds
    c. Muscle spasms
    d. Headache
    e. Brittle hair

35. If a patient receiving lamotrigine develops a rash, which action should the nurse take?
    a. Assess vital signs.
    b. Continue nursing care.
    c. Consult with the provider.
    d. Review laboratory test results.

36. Pregabalin can cause angioedema. Which information should the nurse teach the patient to do if they experience symptoms of angioedema?
    a. Prevent injury during the seizure.
    b. Elevate the extremities.
    c. Seek emergency medical care.
    d. Take the drug with food.

37. Which is true about levetiracetam?
    a. Can cause muscle weakness.
    b. Decreases effectiveness of warfarin.
    c. Causes blockade of sodium channels.
    d. Should be administered with food.

►38. A ketogenic diet is especially dangerous when a patient with epilepsy is prescribed which drug?
    a. Levetiracetam
    b. Pregabalin
    c. Tiagabine
    d. Topiramate

39. Which laboratory test result would be of most concern to the nurse when a patient is prescribed topiramate?
    a. Creatinine 1.5 mg/dL
    b. Bicarbonate (HCO_3) 20 mEq/L
    c. Hematocrit (Hct) 32%
    d. White blood cell (WBC) 4600/mm^3

40. Which symptom suggests a serious adverse effect when a patient is prescribed topiramate for tonic-clonic seizures?
    a. Ataxia
    b. Reduced sweating
    c. Sudden eye pain
    d. Weight loss

41. Which is the most appropriate action if the nurse notes that tiagabine is ordered but no other antiseizure drugs are prescribed?
    a. Administer the medication.
    b. Ask the charge nurse what to do.
    c. Withhold the medication.
    d. Consult with the provider.

►42. The nurse would consult the provider before administering zonisamide if the nurse notes that the patient had a known anaphylactic reaction to which drug?
    a. Acarbose
    b. Insulin aspart
    c. Glipizide
    d. Metformin

DOSE CALCULATION QUESTIONS

43. A 5-year-old patient who weighs 35 lb is newly prescribed phenytoin 20 mg every 12 hours. The suggested initial dose is 2.5 mg/kg/day in divided doses. Is this a safe and effective dose for this child?

44. Phenytoin mg is available as a suspension of 125 mg/mL. How much drug should be administered if the prescribed dose is 20 mg twice a day?

CASE STUDY

A 26-year-old patient who is 8 months pregnant is admitted to the neurologic intensive care unit with the diagnosis of head injury. An automobile accident has left the patient unconscious. On admission, an IV line of dextrose 5% in half-normal saline ($D_5{}^{1/2}$ NS) at 50 mL/h is started. Within the first 24 hours on the unit, the patient has several tonic-clonic seizures. Standing orders on the unit allow the nurse to administer diazepam 5 mg IV push. The provider is notified of the seizure and orders an IV loading dose of phenytoin 800 mg followed by 100 mg every 6 hours, a phenytoin level the next day, and IV cimetidine 300 mg twice a day.

1. What nursing precautions are needed when administering phenytoin and cimetidine IV?

2. Phenytoin is available for IV infusion in a concentration of 50 mg/mL. How long should the nurse take when administering the 800-mg loading dose?

3. What symptoms should the nurse be alert for because of the possible interaction of phenytoin and cimetidine?

4. The next day, the phenytoin level is 14 mcg/mL. Why is it critical for the nurse to closely monitor plasma drug levels of phenytoin?

5. One week later, the patient goes into labor. Based on initiation of phenytoin near the end of the pregnancy, what fetal effects are most likely to occur?

6. What precautions might be taken to protect the fetus during drug therapy, during delivery, and after delivery?

7. Two weeks later, the patient is stabilized and has been transferred to the neurologic progressive unit. On admission, the nurse notes a fine maculopapular rash on the patient's trunk. What should the nurse do and why?

8. Phenytoin is discontinued. Carbamazepine is substituted as the patient's antiseizure drug. The patient is concerned about taking seizure medication because she wants to have more children. She has been advised about possible adverse effects to the fetus. In addition to referring concerns to the provider, what information could the nurse provide about seizures, antiseizure drugs, and pregnancy?

28 Drugs for Muscle Spasm and Spasticity

STUDY QUESTIONS

True or False

For each of the following statements, enter T for true or F for false.

1. ___ Most drugs used to treat spasticity do not relieve acute muscle spasm.
2. ___ Muscle-relaxant drugs shorten the time of rehabilitation from traumatic injuries that cause muscle spasm.
3. ___ The therapeutic effects of muscle relaxants are similar to the effect of taking aspirin.
4. ___ Diazepam is the most effective muscle relaxant.
5. ___ Most centrally acting muscle relaxants are not effective in treating spasticity associated with cerebral palsy.
6. ___ The nurse should assess all patients who are prescribed a centrally acting muscle relaxant for feelings associated with depression.
7. ___ Dark brown or black urine should be reported to the prescriber of methocarbamol.
8. ___ It is important for the nurse to review the blood urea nitrogen (BUN) lab results when a patient is prescribed tizanidine, metaxalone, or dantrolene.
9. ___ Blocking the neurotransmitter γ-aminobutyric acid (GABA) reduces spasticity.
10. ___ Baclofen decreases spasticity.

CRITICAL THINKING, PRIORITIZATION, AND DELEGATION QUESTIONS

*11. The priority nursing interventions and teaching for a patient receiving a centrally acting muscle relaxant are related to:
   a. elimination.
   b. emotional support.
   c. nutrition.
   d. safety.

12. Which teaching point must be included when talking to patients prescribed methocarbamol or chlorzoxazone?
   a. "To avoid rebound hypertension, taper the drug off."
   b. "Patients taking this drug may experience photophobia."
   c. "This drug may change the color of your urine; it's harmless."
   d. "You will only receive 5 days of pills due to the risk of dependence."

13. A patient prescribed a centrally acting muscle relaxant must be taught to avoid which drug?
   a. Diphenhydramine
   b. Acetaminophen
   c. Ferrous gluconate
   d. Polyethylene glycol

14. The nurse would consult the provider if baclofen was prescribed to relieve muscle spasms for a patient with which condition? (**Select all that apply**.)
   a. Cerebral palsy
   b. Cerebrovascular accident
   c. Multiple sclerosis
   d. Spinal cord injury
   e. Electrolyte depletion

DOSE CALCULATION QUESTIONS

15. Diazepam 2 mg orally every 8 hours is prescribed for muscle spasms. The drug is available as 5 mg/mL. How much should the nurse administer at each dose?

16. Dantrolene 250 mg by rapid intravenous (IV) infusion is prescribed. The recommended dose to treat malignant hyperthermia is initially 2 mg/kg. The patient weighs 185 lb. Is this a safe dose?

CASE STUDIES

Case Study 1

A 19-year-old is admitted to the neurologic intensive care unit after a motorcycle accident. They are paraplegic with severe lower extremity muscle spasms, receiving intrathecal baclofen. A pump is being used to infuse the drug, because abrupt discontinuation can cause rhabdomyolysis and multiple organ system failure.

1. What is rhabdomyolysis, what organ is particularly sensitive to its effects, and what assessment findings would suggest that this is occurring?

2. The patient is transferred to a rehabilitation unit. Baclofen 20 mg is prescribed four times a day. What assessments should be included in the nurse's plan of care for this patient relating to drug therapy?

3. Developmentally, this patient is at risk for nonadherence to therapy. Why should the patient be discouraged from abrupt discontinuation of baclofen?

4. Dantrolene would be more convenient for this patient because it only needs to be taken once a day. Why is it not a good choice for this patient?

Case Study 2

A patient with multiple sclerosis is admitted with pneumonia. They are receiving cyclobenzaprine to relieve muscle spasms.

5. What are the common anticholinergic adverse effects associated with this drug and nursing interventions related to these effects?

6. What nonpharmacologic interventions and teaching could the nurse provide to help relieve the patient's discomfort and prevent complications?

Case Study 3

A patient returns to the postanesthesia care unit after general anesthesia. Vital signs have increased from normal to a temperature of 103.6°F, pulse 116 beats/min, respirations 22 breaths/min, and BP 145/99 mm Hg. The patient is developing muscular rigidity.

7. Why are antipyretics not appropriate to treat this fever?

8. The patient is prescribed dantrolene 150 mg IV push. Why is it important to position the patient on their side with the side rails up?

29 Local Anesthetics

STUDY QUESTIONS

True or False

For each of the following statements, enter T for true or F for false.
Using a vasoconstrictor, such as epinephrine, with a local anesthetic,

1. ___ Allows for the use of less anesthetic.
2. ___ Causes local vasoconstriction.
3. ___ Can cause adverse effects from systemic absorption of the vasoconstrictor.
4. ___ Causes local vasodilation.
5. ___ Delays onset of anesthesia.
6. ___ Delays systemic absorption.
7. ___ Improves blood flow to the affected area.
8. ___ Increases the risk of toxicity.
9. ___ Reduces blood flow to the affected area.
10. ___ Reduces the risk of toxicity.
11. ___ Requires the use of a larger dose of anesthetic.

CRITICAL THINKING, PRIORITIZATION, AND DELEGATION QUESTIONS

►12. The nurse is assisting the emergency department provider with anesthetizing and suturing multiple wounds on the extremities of a patient who was attacked by a dog. Which of these new developments would be of most concern to the nurse?
a. Perioral numbness
b. Morbilliform rash
c. Respirations 24/min
d. Restlessness

►13. A pregnant patient received an epidural anesthetic 10 minutes before delivering at 39 weeks of gestation. The neonate is brought to the nursery from the delivery room. Which finding would be a concern to the nursery nurse?
a. Apical pulse 160 beats/min
b. Positive Babinski sign
c. Respirations 22/min
d. Temperature 36.8°C (98.2°F)

✳14. A patient is admitted to a surgical floor at 1000 hours post–total abdominal hysterectomy performed with spinal anesthetic. During assessment at 1400 hours, the nurse notes that the patient has not voided. The patient denies a need to void. Which nursing action should be implemented?
a. Administer bethanechol 5 mg subcut.
b. Assist patient to the bathroom to void.
c. Sit the patient upright on a bedpan.
d. Use portable ultrasound to scan bladder.

15. Topical local anesthetic should be applied in which way to minimize risk?
a. Followed by heat to increase absorption
b. Using the smallest amount needed
c. Gently to areas of skin that are abraded
d. Applied as a thick film over affected area

✳16. Which symptom is a priority to report to the provider following administration of a local anesthetic?
a. Pulse 120 beats/min
b. Blood pressure 100/60 mm Hg
c. Respirations 24/min
d. Temperature 38°C (100.4°F)

17. The nurse must notify the provider if the patient has a known allergy to chloroprocaine and is to receive which medication?
a. Bupivacaine
b. Lidocaine
c. Mepivacaine
d. Tetracaine

18. Which are potentially severe cardiovascular effects when cocaine is used as a local anesthetic? (**Select all that apply**.)
a. Respiratory arrest
b. Fatal dysrhythmias
c. CNS depression
d. Hypertension
e. Talkativeness

✳19. A patient received intravenous regional anesthetic containing lidocaine without epinephrine for ankle surgery. It is a priority to assess for bradycardia, hypotension, and respiratory depression from the lidocaine at which time?
   a. Immediately after injection
   b. At the time of incision
   c. In postanesthesia care unit
   d. When back on the med-surg unit

20. A parent brings their 5-year-old to the emergency department with dyspnea and cyanosis. During questioning, it is revealed that the parent had applied topical benzocaine to areas of eczema to keep the child from scratching it. The nurse suspects which reaction?
   a. Anaphylaxis
   b. Psychogenic reaction
   c. Methemoglobinemia
   d. Hyperventilation

CASE STUDIES

Case Study 1

An 8-year-old child, accompanied by their parents, comes to the emergency department with a scalp laceration sustained when falling off their bicycle. The plan includes administration of lidocaine with epinephrine to close the wound with six to eight interrupted sutures. The child is tearful but cooperative.

1. What are the nursing responsibilities for this procedure?

2. The patient asks if they can use over-the-counter topical lidocaine anesthetic on their toe when sensation returns to relieve discomfort. What teaching should the nurse provide?

30 General Anesthetics

STUDY QUESTIONS

Matching

Match the anesthetic drug or adjunctive drug to the adverse effect.

1. ___ High risk of bacterial infection.
2. ___ Hypotension can occur from peripheral vasodilation.
3. ___ Can delay awakening after surgery.
4. ___ Delirium and unpleasant psychologic reactions can occur postoperatively.
5. ___ Can cause dangerous cardiorespiratory effects, including respiratory and cardiac arrest.
6. ___ Nausea and vomiting occur more often than with other inhaled anesthetics.
7. ___ Can obscure depth of anesthesia.

a. Neuromuscular blocking agents
b. Opioids
c. Nitrous oxide
d. Isoflurane
e. Ketamine
f. Propofol
g. Midazolam

CRITICAL THINKING, PRIORITIZATION, AND DELEGATION QUESTIONS

8. Which is the primary goal of using multiple agents to achieve balanced anesthesia?
   a. Rapid induction of anesthesia
   b. Ensuring adequate blood flow to kidneys
   c. Adequate analgesia and muscle relaxation
   d. Reduction of nausea and vomiting

9. Which statement is true concerning nitrous oxide?
   a. The drug can be administered at low doses to achieve anesthesia.
   b. Surgical anesthesia cannot be obtained with nitrous oxide alone.
   c. It achieves safe anesthesia if administered in a high-enough dose.
   d. The drug will make the patient unresponsive to painful stimuli.

✳10. The nurse is caring for a patient in the postanesthesia care unit (PACU). Which is the priority nursing assessment?
   a. Respiratory status
   b. Level of consciousness
   c. Determining level of pain
   d. Measuring urinary output

11. The nurse should assess all postoperative patients who have received inhaled anesthesia for which condition?
   a. Diarrhea
   b. Excessive salivation
   c. Urinary urgency
   d. Wheezing

►12. The nurse is completing the preoperative checklist for a same-day surgery patient who has been called to the operating room (OR). The patient makes a comment to the nurse that they hope they "really knock me out" because they need a lot of a drug to get a good effect. On further discussion, the patient reveals that they have a 2 year history of illicit oxycodone use and that their last dose was 6 hours ago. Which action should the nurse take?
   a. Call the OR and cancel the surgery.
   b. Note the medication on the patient's chart.
   c. Notify anesthesiologist of the finding.
   d. Complete the preoperative checklist.

►13. A male patient who has received midazolam has just been admitted to the recovery area. He tells the nurse that he needs to urinate. Which action should the nurse take?
   a. Assist the patient to the bathroom and stay with them.
   b. Provide the patient with a urinal to use while still in bed.
   c. Help the patient to stand to use the urinal.
   d. Use a bedpan, assisting the patient with positioning.

►14. Which assessment finding would warrant the nurse withholding morphine from a postoperative patient?
   a. Blood pressure 160/92 mm Hg
   b. Pain 9 on a scale of 1–10
   c. Respirations 8/min
   d. Temperature 103.6ºF (38.2°C)

✳15. A 14-month-old patient received isoflurane and succinylcholine during surgery. Which immediate postoperative assessment finding would be a priority concern?
   a. Blood pressure 86/54 mm Hg
   b. Pulse 68 beats/min
   c. Respirations 30/min
   d. Temperature 103.6°F (39.8°C)

*16. The emergency department has sent a patient for emergency surgery, including general anesthetic with isoflurane. The family has just arrived, and the nurse has learned that the patient has been taking amlodipine. Which is the priority nursing assessment?
   a. Blood pressure for hypotension
   b. Apical heart rate for bradycardia
   c. Respirations for hypopnea or apnea
   d. Temperature for malignant hyperthermia

17. Which is the reason nitrous oxide is widely used in surgery?
   a. Balanced anesthesia can be achieved with nitrous oxide alone.
   b. It does not have significant cardiac or respiratory depression.
   c. Unconsciousness is achieved at very low doses.
   d. Postoperative nausea and vomiting are uncommon.

18. Which is the purpose of administering methohexital in the OR?
   a. Decrease respiratory secretions
   b. Prevent muscle contraction
   c. Reduce sensation of pain
   d. Produce unconsciousness

19. A cataract surgery patient receives midazolam and fentanyl. The nurse would expect these medications to produce which effects? (**Select all that apply.**)
   a. Amnesia
   b. Analgesia
   c. Flaccid paralysis
   d. Sedation
   e. Unconsciousness

CASE STUDIES

Case Study 1

A patient with a history of lung cancer has been admitted the evening before surgery and is scheduled for a thoracotomy at 8 a.m. under balanced general anesthetic. They are 5 feet 6 inches tall and weigh 210 lb. The patient has a productive cough and admits to tobacco use for the last 40 years, smoking one pack of cigarettes per day. They have hypertension and take hydrochlorothiazide, which has been effective in keeping their blood pressure under control.

1. Describe the ideal anesthetic for this patient.

2. What would be priority concerns of the PACU nurse for this patient relating to general anesthetic?

3. What actions should the PACU nurse employ relating to this concern?

Case Study 2

The nurse is admitting a patient with a history of type 2 diabetes mellitus and hypertension to the same-day surgery unit. The patient is scheduled for an inguinal herniorrhaphy.

4. What type of agents would be included if this patient is to receive balanced anesthesia?

5. What data are important for the nurse to collect relating to scheduled general anesthesia?

6. The patient is in the PACU and has just awakened but is very drowsy. Describe nursing interventions relating to the effects of inhalation anesthetic that are needed when a patient first awakens.

7. The postoperative patient reports having awakened during surgery and being in pain but being unable to tell the surgeon. What should the nurse do?

31 Opioid Analgesics, Opioid Antagonists, and Nonopioid Centrally Acting Analgesics

STUDY QUESTIONS

True or False

For each of the following statements, enter T for true or F for false.

1. ___ An opiate is a drug that contains compounds found in opium, while an opioid may be a laboratory-created compound.
2. ___ Activation of delta receptors is responsible for the delusions and delirium that are seen with certain opioids.
3. ___ Enkephalins, endorphins, and dynorphins are body substances with opioid-like properties.
4. ___ The respiratory depression and euphoria that occur with opioid analgesics are related to activation of mu opioid receptors.
5. ___ Buprenorphine has less constipation and sedative effects than morphine.
6. ___ An agonist-antagonist blocks pain when taken alone but improves the pain-relieving effect of another opioid if in the blood at the same time.
7. ___ The dose of oral morphine is higher than the intravenous (IV) dose because hepatic first pass metabolizes some of the drug before it reaches the central nervous system.

CRITICAL THINKING, PRIORITIZATION, AND DELEGATION QUESTIONS

8. Which effect is produced by pure opioid agonists? (**Select all that apply**.)
   a. Euphoria
   b. Constipation
   c. Analgesia
   d. Cyanosis
   e. Mydriasis

9. The nurse is caring for a patient receiving an opioid analgesic for pain. The patient reports a history of severe nausea with previous administrations of opioids. Which is the priority nursing action?
   a. Pretreat with promethazine.
   b. Administer antiemetics as needed.
   c. Have the patient be still when nauseated.
   d. Ensure an emesis basin is available.

▶10. A nurse is caring for a patient receiving opioid analgesics. Which are important for the nurse to monitor? (**Select all that apply**.)
   a. Level of consciousness
   b. Withdrawal syndrome
   c. Respiratory status
   d. Oxygen saturation
   e. Dysrhythmias

*11. A neonate is born to a known heroin addict. The infant is exhibiting symptoms of opioid withdrawal. Which is the priority as the nurse cares for the neonate in the nursery?
   a. Altered nutrition
   b. Disturbed sleep
   c. Fluid deficit
   d. Parenting

12. A cancer patient who is receiving oxycodone for pain relief develops a rash after being prescribed an antibiotic. The prescriber discontinues the antibiotic and prescribes diphenhydramine. Which is a possible effect of the combination of oxycodone and diphenhydramine?
   a. Delirium
   b. Fever
   c. Hypotension
   d. Urinary retention

*13. Which is the reason the dosage of naloxone must be carefully titrated in a person with opioid addiction?
   a. Effects of the drug persist for an hour
   b. The drug may precipitate acute withdrawal
   c. A large dose can cause respiratory arrest
   d. Naloxone is not effective in opioid addicts

14. A patient has been prescribed a fentanyl patch. Which is the reason patients should be taught not to apply heat in the area of the patch?
   a. It inactivates the drug.
   b. It loosen the drug patch.
   c. It prolongs the drug's effect.
   d. It causes respiratory depression.

15. A patient with which condition is at increased risk for severe hypotension when administered morphine? (**Select all that apply**.)
   a. Liver impairment
   b. Hypotension
   c. Crohn disease
   d. Kidney dysfunction
   e. Prostatic hyperplasia

16. Which drug is used to treat opioid-induced constipation when other measures are inadequate?
    a. Sodium phosphate
    b. Polyethylene glycol
    c. Methylnaltrexone
    d. Pentazocine

*17. The nurse answers a call to the ED from a female who is prescribed fentanyl lozenge on a stick. She states that she found her 2-year-old grandson with the medication in his mouth. She took it away from him, and he is standing next to her crying. Which nursing action is greatest priority?
    a. Call 911 immediately.
    b. Assess amount of drug consumed.
    c. Contact the poison hotline.
    d. Rinse out the child's mouth.

18. Transmucosal fentanyl is **NOT** to be used for which source of pain? (**Select all that apply**.)
    a. Acute pain
    b. Postoperative pain
    c. Headache
    d. Athletic injury
    e. Cancer pain

*19. An aphasic patient who has been receiving meperidine 75 mg every 4 hours for pain for the past 36 hours has suddenly become restless and irritable. The last dose of meperidine was 4 hours ago. Why is it important for the nurse to withhold the meperidine, complete assessment, and contact the provider with the findings?
    a. Respiratory depression is imminent.
    b. Physical dependence may occur.
    c. Tolerance to the meperidine has developed.
    d. Toxicity from a metabolite may be occurring.

20. Which diagnostic test is a priority to review when a patient is prescribed methadone?
    a. Alanine aminotransferase (ALT)
    b. Electrocardiogram (ECG)
    c. Estimated glomerular filtration rate (eGFR)
    d. Brain natriuretic peptide (BNP)

*21. A cancer patient has been taking increasing doses of oxycodone for pain relief. Which teaching can prevent the adverse effect that is most likely to persist with long-term use of this drug?
    a. Consume adequate fluid.
    b. Change positions slowly.
    c. Exercise as tolerated.
    d. Take deep breaths every hour.

22. A cancer patient has received instructions regarding the administration of controlled-release oxycodone. Which of these statements made by the patient would indicate a need for further teaching?
    a. "I need to inform my doctor if I have pain between doses."
    b. "It is okay to crush the pills and take them with applesauce."
    c. "All of my health care providers should know I am taking this drug regularly."
    d. "If I am allergic to acetaminophen, it is still okay to take this drug."

23. The nurse would consult the provider if they identified that a patient had a history of which chronic condition and was prescribed tramadol for pain relief?
    a. Heart failure
    b. Asthma
    c. Dementia
    d. Seizure disorder

DOSE CALCULATION QUESTIONS

24. A patient is prescribed 3 mg of morphine by IV route every 3 hours as needed for postoperative pain. Available are vials containing 5 mg/mL. How many milliliters of morphine will the nurse administer at each dose? The drug handbook recommends that morphine be diluted in 5 mL of sterile water and administered slowly over 5 minutes. The 10-mL syringe is marked in 0.2-mL increments. How many seconds should elapse between each push of 0.2 mL of the diluted morphine?

25. Naloxone 10 mcg/kg is prescribed to treat respiratory depression for a 7-lb neonate. The drug is available as 0.4 mg/mL. What is the amount of naloxone that should be administered?

CASE STUDY

The nurse is providing preoperative teaching to a patient who has been admitted for an abdominal hysterectomy. Patient-controlled analgesia (PCA) is anticipated as the mechanism of postoperative pain relief.

1. What preoperative teaching should the nurse provide this patient to enhance pain relief and prevent adverse effects, including respiratory depression?

2. Postoperatively, the patient is ordered morphine IV via a PCA pump for her postoperative pain. The pump is set to deliver 1 mg of morphine per injection and up to a maximum of 5 mg/h. What are the advantages and disadvantages of PCA?

3. The patient appears to be sleeping. Their skin is pale, and respiratory rate is 8/min and shallow. What should the nurse do, in order of priority?

4. What measures, other than drug therapy, can the nurse employ to reduce this patient's pain?

32 Pain Management in Patients with Cancer

STUDY QUESTIONS

Matching

Match the types of pain to their origin.

1. ___ Injury to bone, joint, muscle.
2. ___ Injury to peripheral nerves.
3. ___ Injury to organs.
4. ___ Injury to tissue.
   a. Neuropathic
   b. Nociceptive
   c. Somatic
   d. Visceral

CRITICAL THINKING, PRIORITIZATION, AND DELEGATION QUESTIONS

5. Which are potential outcomes for patients with unrelieved pain? (**Select all that apply**.)
   a. Risk for suicide increases.
   b. Death is accelerated.
   c. Increased health system cost.
   d. Recovery is delayed.
   e. Provider burden increased.

6. Which is the most reliable indicator of the need for pain relief in the oncology patient?
   a. Changes in vital signs
   b. Invasiveness of the cancer
   c. Patient reluctance to move
   d. Request for pain relief

✳7. When developing plan for pain management, which is the desired outcome?
   a. Pain at ≤3 out of 10
   b. Able to perform ADLs
   c. Relief at patient's desired goal
   d. Total relief of cancer pain

8. A patient with cancer whose history includes type 2 diabetes mellitus informs the nurse that they are experiencing constant burning pain in their feet. Based on the type of foot pain commonly experienced by patients with diabetes, the nurse would consult the prescriber regarding possibly ordering which drug?
   a. Acetaminophen
   b. Carbamazepine
   c. Naproxen
   d. Morphine

✳9. Which laboratory test results would be a priority to report to the provider when a patient with cancer receiving chemotherapy is taking a pain reliever that contains ibuprofen?
   a. Total bilirubin 1.2 mg/dL
   b. Creatinine 1.3 mg/dL
   c. Platelet count 60,000/mm^3
   d. White blood cell 5500/mm^3

10. Following surgery, a patient with cancer is receiving morphine sulfate IV 10 mg every 4 hours for pain. The provider has discontinued the IV morphine and ordered morphine sulfate 20-mg tablets every 4 hours. Which is the appropriate action when switching opioids?
   a. Taper the current opioid before starting the equianalgisic.
   b. Stop the current opioid and replace it with an equianalgesic.
   c. Slowly increase the dose of equianalgesic before stopping the current opioid.
   d. Taper the current opioid while slowly increasing the dose of the equianalgesic.

▶11. The nurse knows that respiratory depression is most likely to occur with which pain regimen?
   a. A loading dose of 10 mg of morphine before starting patient-controlled analgesia (PCA)
   b. Increased IV dosage of morphine from 5 to 7 mg
   c. PCA morphine of 1 mg/dose up to a maximum of 5 mg/hr
   d. 60 mg of IV morphine every hour in a patient morphine tolerant.

12. A patient has been taking oral opioids for moderate pain associated with prostate cancer that has metastasized to the spine. Surgery is performed, and the patient is experiencing moderate to severe postoperative pain. Which analgesic is most appropriate?
   a. Buprenorphine IV
   b. Fentanyl transdermal patch
   c. Intermittent intramuscular (IM) dosing of meperidine
   d. Morphine sulfate via a PCA pump

✳13. Which is most concerning to the nurse when a patient is prescribed an NSAID analgesic on a regular basis?
   a. Lack of adequate pain relief
   b. Heartburn
   c. Rigid abdomen
   d. Swollen ankles

14. Celecoxib 200 mg twice a day is prescribed for a patient with cancer that has metastasized to the bone. Which adverse effect is more likely to occur with celecoxib than with other NSAIDs?
    a. Blood pressure elevation
    b. Cerebrovascular accident
    c. Gastrointestinal bleed
    d. Physical dependence

*15. Which laboratory test result would be of greatest priority to report to the prescriber in a patient with cancer taking carbamazepine?
    a. Blood urea nitrogen (BUN) 23 mg/dL
    b. Fasting blood glucose (FBG) 233 mg/dL
    c. Platelets 149,000/mm^3
    d. White blood cell count (WBC) 3000/mm^3

*16. What is of greatest priority when naloxone is administered to combat respiratory depression associated with opioid use for patients with cancer?
    a. Hydration
    b. Level of consciousness
    c. Presence of gag reflex
    d. Return of pain

17. The nurse is preparing to administer metoclopramide to a patient with cancer experiencing nausea associated with opioid use. The patient states their friend had a prescription for ondansetron and asks why they aren't receiving it too. Which is the best response concerning ondansetron?
    a. "Causes more constipation."
    b. "Increased urinary retention."
    c. "Has been known to cause anxiety."
    d. "It is a prokinetic drug, not an antiemetic."

*18. Which is the priority concern when a patient combines prescribed opioids with alcohol?
    a. Loss of consciousness
    b. Orthostatic hypotension
    c. Physical dependence
    d. Respiratory depression

DOSE CALCULATION QUESTION

19. Morphine 10 mg is prescribed via IV push. The drug book recommends administering at a rate of 4–5 mg/min. The drug is available as 10 mg/mL and has been further diluted in 10 mL normal saline. The nurse prepares to administer the drug. How much should the nurse administer every 15 seconds?

CASE STUDY

A cancer patient is being discharged on oxycodone and acetaminophen in a fixed-dose combination formulation.

1. What teaching should the nurse provide regarding the opioid and nonopioid components of this drug?

The patient's pain is not relieved by two tablets of oxycodone 10 mg and acetaminophen 325 mg, taken every 4 hours. The provider has discontinued the drug and ordered oxycodone CR 40 mg twice a day, oxycodone IR 5 mg every 6 hours as needed, and Tylenol 8-hour arthritis pain 650 mg every 8 hours. The patient is overwhelmed by the multiple medications and asks why they cannot just take three of the combination oxycodone and acetaminophen tablets every 4 hours.

2. How should the nurse respond?

3. What interventions can the nurse offer to help the patient understand their analgesic regimen?

4. What teaching should the nurse provide regarding the adverse effects of constipation?

5. What teaching can the nurse provide to enable the patient to assist the provider with decisions regarding analgesic prescription?

33 Drugs for Headache

STUDY QUESTIONS

Matching

Match the drug, or class of drug, for prevention of migraines to their side effect.

1. ___ Pancreatitis
2. ___ May exacerbate asthma
3. ___ Metabolic acidosis
4. ___ Formation of antibodies to treatment
5. ___ Dysrhythmias
6. ___ Coronary vasospasm
7. ___ Somnolence

   a. Tricyclic antidepressants
   b. Sumitriptan
   c. Divalproex
   d. Erenumab
   e. β-Blockers
   f. Topiramate
   g. Ubrogepant

CRITICAL THINKING, PRIORITIZATION, AND DELEGATION QUESTIONS

8. Which is true concerning migraines? (**Select all that apply**.)
   a. Cannot be treated effectively after the pain starts.
   b. Involve inflammation of intracranial blood vessels.
   c. Vasoconstriction of intracranial blood vessels is a cause.
   d. Usually develop in the morning after arising.
   e. Should implement therapy at the earliest sign of attack.

9. Which is the primary reason why abortive medication for migraine headaches should not be used more than 1 or 2 days a week?
   a. Abuse potential
   b. Coronary vasospasm
   c. Tolerance to drug
   d. Overuse headache

10. Which triptan is available as a nasal spray? (**Select all that apply.**)
    a. Rizatriptan
    b. Sumatriptan
    c. Zolmitriptan
    d. Almotriptan
    e. Naratriptan

11. Which is priority when a patient is prescribed meperidine for migraine headaches?
    a. Abuse potential
    b. Respiratory distress
    c. Constipation
    d. Relief of headache

*12. Which is priority to report to the provider if the nurse was preparing to administer ergotamine to a patient who is experiencing the start of a migraine headache?
    a. Oxygen saturation 96%
    b. Blood pressure 90/58 mm Hg
    c. Capillary refill of 12 seconds
    d. Flashes of light in visual fields

13. Which is the rationale for administering both ergotamine and metoclopramide to abort a migraine headache?
    a. Decreases vomiting
    b. Minimizes sensitivity to light
    c. Prevents myalgia
    d. Reduces cranial vasodilation

14. The nurse would consult the provider before administering ergotamine or triptan drugs for migraine headache to a patient with which condition? (**Select all that apply**.)
    a. Cardiovascular disease
    b. Diabetes mellitus
    c. Hypertension
    d. Infection
    e. Peptic ulcer disease

15. Which is true about triptan therapy for migraine headaches?
    a. It prevents recurrence of the headache.
    b. Combination therapy increases relief.
    c. Primary adverse effect is vasoconstriction.
    d. Therapy relieves sensitivity to light.

✳16. The nurse administered sumatriptan subcutaneously at 2100 hrs to a patient with a history of smoking. One hour after administration, the patient reports heavy arms and chest pressure. Which is the priority nursing action?
   a. Apply oxygen at 2 L per nasal canula.
   b. Evaluate the chest pain.
   c. Continue nursing care.
   d. Notify the provider.

17. A patient does not inform their primary care provider (PCP) that they are prescribed duloxetine by their rheumatologist. The PCP prescribes a triptan for migraines. Which symptom is possible with this combination?
   a. Confusion
   b. Fainting
   c. Hypotension
   d. Vomiting

18. For which patient would botulinum toxin A be appropriate for prevention?
   a. Headache days a month
   b. Cluster headaches
   c. 19 headache days a month
   d. Good results using a triptan

✳19. A patient is prescribed propranolol for migraine prevention. Which assessment would be priority to report to the provider?
   a. BP 130/80 mm Hg
   b. Expiratory wheezing
   c. Excessive thirst
   d. Pulse 98 beats/min

20. A patient is receiving lithium carbonate for prevention of cluster headaches. This drug has a narrow therapeutic index. Which drug level would fall into the safe and effective range?
   a. 0.1 mEq/L
   b. 0.3 mEq/L
   c. 0.7 mEq/L
   d. 1.1 mEq/L

21. Ubrogepant provides relief of which symptoms in 38% of patients? (**Select all that apply**.)
   a. Somnolence
   b. Nausea
   c. Phonophobia
   d. Photophobia
   e. Dysarthria

22. Which drug is a safe alternative for the treatment of acute migraine in persons with cardiovascular disease?
   a. Ergotamine
   b. Lasmiditan
   c. Sumatriptan
   d. Ubrogepant

DOSE CALCULATION QUESTIONS

23. Dihydroergotamine mesylate is available in solution (1 mg/mL). Prescribed is 1000 μg intramuscular (IM). How much drug should the nurse administer?

24. Naratriptan 5 mg is prescribed. Available are 2.5-mg tablets. How many should the nurse administer?

CASE STUDY

A patient is seen in the emergency department (ED) with a chief complaint of severe, frequent headaches that begin midmorning and grow progressively worse throughout the day. The patient reports occasional nausea and vomiting. Advil has been minimally successful in treating the headaches. The headaches are pulsatile and usually unilateral. All of the patient's laboratory findings are within normal limits. Sumatriptan 6 mg subcutaneously is prescribed to be administered now, along with a prescription for Imitrex STATdose Pen 6 mg to be taken as directed.

1. Describe what the nurse should include in teaching this patient about administering the self-injecting pen.

2. The patient attempts to fill the prescription at the hospital outpatient pharmacy, but insurance does not cover sumatriptan. Dihydroergotamine is prescribed in place of the sumatriptan. What teaching needs to be provided by the ED nurse regarding the administration of dihydroergotamine?

3. What teaching regarding preventing toxicity from dihydroergotamine should be provided to this patient?

4. The patient tells the nurse that a friend takes ergotamine and "got hooked" and had to go to the hospital to "get off of it." What would the nurse include when comparing ergotamine and dihydroergotamine?

5. The patient is instructed to seek follow-up with their PCP. The PCP discusses the use of prophylactic drugs to prevent the migraine headaches. What drugs might be considered?

34 Antipsychotic Agents and Their Use in Schizophrenia

STUDY QUESTIONS

True or False

For each of the following statements, enter T for true or F for false.

1. ___ High-potency antipsychotic drugs are more likely to be effective than low-potency drugs.
2. ___ When administered in therapeutically equivalent doses, both high-otency and low-potency drugs elicit an equivalent antipsychotic response.
3. ___ High-potency antipsychotic drugs treat both positive and negative symptoms more effectively than low-potency drugs.
4. ___ Second-generation antipsychotic (SGA) and first-generation antipsychotic (FGA) drugs are equally effective.
5. ___ Risk of extrapyramidal symptoms (EPS) is higher in FGAs.
6. ___ Antipsychotic drugs promote weight gain through blockade of H1 receptors in the brain.
7. ___ SGA drugs only cause minor adverse effects.
8. ___ Antipsychotic drugs can cure schizophrenia if taken as prescribed.

CRITICAL THINKING, PRIORITIZATION, AND DELEGATION QUESTIONS

9. A patient who is receiving chemotherapy for breast cancer is prescribed chlorpromazine. There is no mention of other medical or psychiatric disorders in the patient's history. Which is the most likely reason why this patient is receiving the drug?
   a. Constipation
   b. Insomnia
   c. Vomiting
   d. Hypotension

10. Which extrapyramidal adverse effect of antipsychotic drugs would the nurse expect to occur only after an extended period of drug therapy?
    a. Repetitive, slow, twisting movements of the tongue and face
    b. Severe spasms of the mouth, face, neck, or back
    c. Slow movement, tremor, and rigidity
    d. Uncontrollable need to be in motion

*11. Which is the priority when a patient is experiencing acute laryngeal dystonia?
    a. Airway clearance
    b. Anxiety treatment
    c. Control of pain
    d. Ensuring patient safety

*12. Which of these findings, in a patient who has been receiving a neuroleptic, should be reported to the provider immediately?
    a. Hypotension
    b. Difficulty speaking
    c. Involuntary movements
    d. Laryngeal dystonia

*13. Which would be the priority nursing action to reduce hyperthermia caused by neuroleptic malignant syndrome?
    a. Acetaminophen 500 mg orally
    b. Dantrolene as prescribed, STAT
    c. Increase fluid intake to 1500 mL/day
    d. Place ice bags under the patient's arms

►14. In a patient taking an FGA, which apical pulse obtained upon standing, when assessing orthostatic vital signs, would be a reason to withhold the drug and consult the provider?
    a. 90 beats/min
    b. 62 beats/min
    c. 122 beats/min
    d. 78 beats/min

*15. A 68-year-old patient who is prescribed an FGA is diagnosed with benign prostatic hyperplasia. Which assessment would be of greatest priority related to the drug and this condition?
    a. Abdominal pain
    b. Blood pressure
    c. Dizziness
    d. Intake and output

16. Which symptom would be of greatest concern when administering an FGA that causes QT prolongation?
    a. Elevated blood glucose
    b. Worsening fatigue
    c. Sudden fainting
    d. Increased thirst

17. Which statements suggest that a family member needs additional teaching regarding the administration of an oral liquid FGA? (**Select all that apply**.)
    a. "Chilling the drug for an hour after diluting it in juice makes it tastes better."
    b. "I need to be careful not to dilute it too much, so I am sure that they take all of it."
    c. "If I spill the drug on me, I need to rinse my skin with warm, soapy water."
    d. "The drug should be kept in the bottle that it comes in and put it in a dark cabinet."
    e. "They should take the drug themself so that they don't think I am poisoning them."

18. Thioridazine should be avoided in patients with which risk factors? (**Select all that apply**.)
    a. Bradycardia
    b. Hypomagnesemia
    c. Cerebrovascular disease
    d. Hyperkalemia
    e. Severe heart failure

19. Which is another name for SGAs?
    a. Atypical antipsychotics
    b. High-potency antipsychotics
    c. Low-potency antipsychotics
    d. Typical antipsychotics

20. It is important for the nurse to teach patients who are prescribed any neuroleptic to avoid taking which over-the-counter medication?
    a. Acetaminophen
    b. Acetylsalicylic acid
    c. Diphenhydramine
    d. Pseudoephedrine

21. A patient is prescribed haloperidol decanoate 2 mg intramuscular (IM) every 4 weeks. Which injection site is recommended for depot preparations?
    a. Deltoid muscle
    b. 2 inches from umbilicus
    c. Vastus lateralis muscle
    d. Subcutaneous fat of upper arm

✳22. In a patient taking haloperidol, which laboratory test result would be a priority to report to the provider?
    a. Creatinine 1.2 mg/dL
    b. Blood glucose 286 mg/dL
    c. Potassium 3.2 mg/dL
    d. Triglycerides 97 mg/dL

23. It is important for the nurse to assess for excessive hunger, thirst, and urination if a patient is prescribed which drug? (**Select all that apply**.)
    a. Chlorpromazine
    b. Clozapine
    c. Haloperidol
    d. Olanzapine
    e. Risperidone

✳24. It would be a priority to report which assessment finding in a patient receiving clozapine?
    a. Orthostasis
    b. Urine residual of 150 mL
    c. Temperature 104°F (40°C)
    d. Weight gain of 2 lb in 1 month

►25. Which laboratory tests are important for the nurse to monitor when caring for a patient prescribed risperidone? (**Select all that apply**.)
    a. Liver function tests
    b. Lipid panel
    c. Creatinine
    d. Hemoglobin A1c
    e. Thyroid panel

DOSE CALCULATION QUESTIONS

26. Chlorpromazine 100 mg IM three times a day is ordered. The drug is available as 25 mg/mL. How many milliliters should be injected? Will the drug be administered in one or two injections?

CASE STUDY

An 82-year-old patient who resides in a nursing facility is admitted to the hospital with pneumonia. They become agitated and are not oriented to the place. The on-call hospitalist is consulted.

1. Why is it important to inform the hospitalist about the presence or absence of a history of dementia?

   Haloperidol 0.5 mg every 4 hours is prescribed as needed when nonpharmacologic measures cannot control agitation, and there is concern they may harm herself. Two hours after administering the drug orally, the nurse notes that the patient is moaning. Their eyes are rolled upward, and their back is arched.

2. What action should the nurse take first?

3. What other assessment data are important for the nurse to collect and communicate to the provider?

35 Antidepressants

STUDY QUESTIONS

Completion

1. The most common symptom of depression in addition to depressed mood is __________ __________ or __________ in usual activities and pastimes.
2. Due to the risk of suicide, close observation is important during the first few months of antidepressant therapy and __________ __________.
3. Initial response to antidepressant drug therapy occurs in _____ to _____ weeks.
4. Relapse is more likely if a patient discontinues pharmacotherapy sooner than _____ to _____ months after symptom remission.
5. Tricyclic antidepressants (TCAs) are reserved for patients who have not responded to first-line drugs because they have __________ __________ __________.
6. Selective serotonin reuptake inhibitors (SSRIs) should be administered in the morning because they are __________ and can cause __________.
7. Overdose of TCAs can cause death because of effects on the __________.
8. When taken at doses and times as prescribed, __________ antidepressants can still cause hypertensive crisis and death.
9. Patients who are prescribed amitriptyline hydrochloride for depression should consult the provider or pharmacist before taking any over-the-counter __________ or __________ __________.
10. Fluoxetine causes __________, delayed __________, or absent __________ and decreased __________ __________ in 70% of men and women.
11. Patients who are prescribed a monoamine oxidase inhibitor (MAOI) should not eat foods containing __________.

CRITICAL THINKING, PRIORITIZATION, AND DELEGATION QUESTIONS

✳12. When assessing a patient receiving an antidepressant, which question would be priority?
   a. "Does weight gain from the medications concern you?"
   b. "Are you having thoughts about harming yourself?"
   c. "Do you experience dizziness when you stand up?"
   d. "Have you had any difficulty voiding?"

13. Which is the reason for administering tricyclic antidepressants at bedtime? (**Select all that apply**.)
   a. Facilitates adherence due to ease of dosing
   b. Ensures energizing effects of drug occur in the daytime
   c. Promotes sleep by causing nighttime sedation
   d. Reduces the side effect of anorexia
   e. Reduces intensity of daytime side effects

14. When a patient who is receiving an antidepressant verbalizes suicidal ideation, which is the priority nursing action?
   a. Administer the antidepressant.
   b. Ask the patient for more information.
   c. Notify the provider immediately.
   d. Provide a safe environment.

15. Which common side effects occur with administration of fluoxetine? (**Select all that apply**.)
   a. Headache
   b. Dry mouth
   c. Insomnia
   d. Weight gain
   e. Photophobia

✳16. Which laboratory test result, if identified in a patient receiving fluoxetine and warfarin, would be a priority to report to the provider?
   a. Aspartate aminotransferase (AST) 30 IU/L
   b. Creatinine 0.8 mg/dL
   c. International normalized ratio 4.5
   d. Platelets 250,000/mm^3

17. The nurse should consult the provider regarding which order?
   a. Fluoxetine 20 mg per oral (PO) each bedtime
   b. Mirtazapine 15 mg PO each bedtime
   c. Bupropion 100 mg twice daily
   d. Imipramine 75 mg PO daily

18. The nurse would assess the patient for unexplained bleeding when a patient is prescribed fluoxetine and:
   a. cetirizine.
   b. lithium.
   c. aspirin.
   d. torsemide.

*19. The nursery nurse sees that a neonate, whose mother has been taking sertraline for major depression throughout pregnancy, is tremulous and very irritable. Which assessment finding would be of most concern to the nurse?
   a. Difficulty calming
   b. Flexed extremities
   c. Pulse 148 beats/min
   d. Flaring nostrils, grunting

*20. The nurse is reviewing laboratory test results for a patient whose drug regimen includes desvenlafaxine. Which result would be priority to report to the provider?
   a. Estimated glomerular filtration rate (eGFR) 75 mL/min
   b. Human chorionic gonadotropin (hCG) 900 mIU/mL
   c. AST 30 U/L
   d. Alanine transaminase (ALT) 75 IU/L

21. In a patient prescribed duloxetine, which condition would concern the nurse?
   a. Rheumatoid arthritis
   b. Autoimmune hepatitis
   c. Diabetic neuropathy
   d. Stress urinary incontinence

22. A patient tells the nurse that they have been experiencing erectile dysfunction since they were prescribed paroxetine. Which is an appropriate response?
   a. Encourage the patient to share this concern with the provider.
   b. Instruct the patient not to take the antidepressant on weekends.
   c. Ask the provider to change his prescription to bupropion.
   d. Withhold the drug until the issue is resolved.

*23. Which is the priority assessment when a patient is switched from a TCA antidepressant to an MAOI?
   a. Blood glucose
   b. Temperature
   c. Oxygen saturation
   d. Apical pulse rate

24. Which is a property of SSRIs? (**Select all that apply**.)
   a. Blockage of transmitter reuptake occurs quickly.
   b. Therapeutic effects take weeks to develop.
   c. Causes central nervous system excitation.
   d. Long-term treatments result in weight loss.
   e. Most common side effect is sexual dysfunction.

25. Which data would be of greatest concern when a patient is prescribed desipramine?
   a. Dry mouth
   b. Racing heart
   c. Sunburns easily
   d. Constipation

*26. The nurse has received a hand-off report at shift change. Which patient is priority for the nurse to assess?
   a. Amitriptyline—sleepiness and constipation
   b. Fluoxetine—nausea and diarrhea
   c. Tranylcypromine—headache and vomiting
   d. Venlafaxine—anorexia and sweating

27. Which foods can cause a hypertensive crisis when a patient is prescribed an MAOI? (**Select all that apply**.)
   a. Apples
   b. Yeast bread
   c. Bologna
   d. Cottage cheese
   e. Soy sauce

28. A nurse providing teaching for a patient newly prescribed selegiline. Which should be included concerning orthostatic hypotension?
   a. Avoid certain foods.
   b. Change positions slowly.
   c. Drink coffee daily.
   d. Monitor pulse daily.

29. The nurse should closely monitor the temperature in a postoperative patient who is prescribed phenelzine and is receiving which drug for postoperative pain?
   a. Butorphanol
   b. Hydrocodone
   c. Hydromorphone
   d. Meperidine

*30. It would be priority to report the development of which new condition in a patient taking bupropion?
   a. Anemia
   b. Diabetes mellitus
   c. Epilepsy
   d. Glaucoma

*31. Which laboratory result would be of greatest concern to the nurse in a patient receiving mirtazapine?
   a. Absolute neutrophil count (ANC) 95 cells/mcL
   b. Blood urea nitrogen (BUN) 22 mg/dL
   c. ALT 75 IU/L
   d. White blood cell (WBC) 11,000/mm^3

32. Which is most important for the nurse to include in patient teaching for a patient who has been prescribed trazodone?
   a. Drink at least 2500 mL of fluid each day.
   b. Increase fluid and fiber in the diet.
   c. Report symptoms of a urinary tract infection.
   d. Seek medical care if erection does not subside after 4 hours.

33. Which should be included in teaching the patient who reveals that they self-medicate with St. John wort?
    a. Inform all providers that they are using this drug.
    b. The herb is effective when to treating major depression.
    c. St. John wort has not been shown to be effective.
    d. This herb is safe because it is natural and not a drug.

DOSE CALCULATION QUESTIONS

34. Paroxetine controlled release (CR) 50 mg is prescribed once a day. Available are 25-mg and 62.5-mg CR tablets. What should the nurse administer?

35. Venlafaxine ER 150 mg is prescribed. The hospital pharmacy stocks 75-mg ER capsules. How many capsules should the nurse administer?

CASE STUDIES

Case Study 1

A 28-year-old patient, who is a high school science teacher with two children, comes to the community mental health center at their family's urging because of lack of interest in usual activities, difficulty concentrating, excessive sleepiness, and feeling "down" every day for the past 3 months. Desipramine 50 mg at bedtime is prescribed.

1. Developmentally, what are the advantages of this particular TCA for this patient?

2. The patient is hopeful that the medication will help. They ask, "If the drugs work, why do I have to meet with the doctor every week?" What is the basis of the response to this question?

3. What symptoms should the patient, family members, and/or caregivers be told to report?

4. The patient asks why the drug is supposed to be taken at bedtime. How should the nurse respond?

5. What teaching should the nurse provide regarding these common adverse effects of TCAs? (1) Sedation, (2) orthostatic hypotension, and (3) anticholinergic effects.

6. The patient is concerned about cost because the provider has prescribed only 1 week's supply at a time. What would be the rationale for such a small prescription amount?

7. The patient is admitted for an inguinal herniorrhaphy. When providing history information, the patient states that they have been taking desipramine 200 mg at bedtime for 3 months. They tell the nurse that some nights they forget to take the medication but do not feel bad the next day. The patient thinks they must not need the medication anymore. How should the nurse respond?

Case Study 2

An adolescent patient who has been irritable and refusing to go to school or eat meals for several months is admitted to an adolescent psychiatric unit. Cognitive behavioral therapy is started, and the psychiatrist prescribes fluoxetine.

8. What precautions teaching would the nurse provide because of the risk of serotonin syndrome?

The patient's insurance allows only 10 days of inpatient hospitalization, and the patient is to be discharged to the care of their parents. All antidepressants have a boxed warning for suicide risk, especially in children and adolescents.

9. The nurse would caution the patient's parents that suicide risk is greatest at what point in antidepressant therapy?

10. What actions should be taken because of this risk?

11. What rationale would support the use of antidepressants in this case?

36 Drugs for Bipolar Disorder

STUDY QUESTIONS

True or False

For each of the following statements, enter T for true or F for false.

1. ___ All patients with bipolar disorder (BPD) alternate between mania and depression, but the length of episodes varies.
2. ___ BPD is a chronic condition.
3. ___ BPD requires treatment for the rest of the patient's life.
4. ___ Manic episodes are always distressing to the patient with BPD.
5. ___ The cause of BPD is an unstable personality.
6. ___ The pathophysiology of BPD may involve disruption of neuronal growth.
7. ___ The drug divalproex sodium can promote neuronal growth in the subgenual prefrontal cortex.
8. ___ Antipsychotic drugs should not be used in BPD unless the patient has symptoms of psychosis.

CRITICAL THINKING, PRIORITIZATION, AND DELEGATION QUESTIONS

✳9. A patient is admitted with an acute mixed episode of BPD. The patient is started on divalproex sodium and bupropion. Which is the priority nursing concern?
   a. Electrolyte imbalances
   b. Hydration
   c. Safety
   d. Toxicity

▶10. When administering lithium carbonate, which would be the expected outcome?
   a. Does not exhibit flight of ideas
   b. Exhibits pressured speech
   c. Sits long enough to watch a television program
   d. Sleeps 8 hours per night

▶11. A nurse is reviewing laboratory tests of a patient receiving lithium carbonate for long-term management of BPD. Which result should the nurse report to the provider immediately?
   a. Albumin 4.5 g/dL
   b. Creatinine 2.7 mg/dL
   c. Sodium 132 mEq/L
   d. Potassium 4 mEq/L

▶12. The nurse is caring for an acutely ill patient who is prescribed lithium carbonate for BPD. Which could increase lithium levels and cause toxicity? (**Select all that apply**.)
   a. Diuretics
   b. Ibuprofen
   c. Cetirizine
   d. Nadolol
   e. Imipramine

✳13. It would be a priority to consult the provider of lithium carbonate about monitoring lithium levels if the BPD patient is diagnosed with hypertension and prescribed which drug?
   a. Amlodipine
   b. Atenolol
   c. Bumetanide
   d. Valsartan

▶14. When administering divalproex sodium, which observation would be a reason to withhold the drug and contact the provider? (**Select all that apply**.)
   a. Abdominal pain
   b. Dark-colored urine
   c. Pale conjunctiva
   d. Petechial rash
   e. Pale stool color

✳15. A patient with BPD is prescribed carbamazepine 200 mg twice a day. Trough levels drawn 30 minutes before the next prescribed dose are 6 mcg/mL. Which is the appropriate nursing action?
   a. Administer the drug.
   b. Assess for seizure activity.
   c. Consult the provider.
   d. Elevate the bed's side rails.

▶16. The complete blood count (CBC) on a patient who is scheduled to receive the first dose of carbamazepine includes hemoglobin 14.5 g/dL, platelets 170,000/mm^3, reticulocyte count 2%, and white blood cell (WBC) 6600/mm^3. Which action should the nurse take?
   a. Administer the drug.
   b. Hold the medication.
   c. Consult the provider.
   d. Assess the patient.

✳17. A patient with BPD is taking lamotrigine, and the nurse notes a rash along with vesicles in the patient's oral cavity. Which is the appropriate nursing action?
   a. Administer the drug.
   b. Hold the medication.
   c. Leave a message for the provider.
   d. Consult the provider immediately.

DOSE CALCULATION QUESTIONS

18. Lithium carbonate 0.6 g three times a day is prescribed. How many capsules should be administered if 300-mg capsules are available?

19. Divalproex sodium is available as a syrup containing 250 mg/5 mL. How many milliliters should be administered if the prescribed dose is 375 mg three times a day?

CASE STUDY

A patient with a history of BPD has stopped taking their prescribed divalproex sodium. They are brought to the hospital because they have become increasingly hyperexcitable over the past 5 days. They have talked on the phone almost continuously because they say they are trying to start a business. The patient has called friends and relatives all over the country at all hours of the night to tell them the news. They went on a spending spree to buy new clothes and equipment for the business venture and accumulated almost $10,000 worth of bills before they were caught writing bad checks. The patient's partner was called when they tried to purchase a car, and the bank reported that the patient had insufficient funds to cover the check. The patient was brought to the hospital in an acute manic state. On admission, they move about restlessly, waving their arms in a threatening manner while loudly berating their partner and the hospital staff. The patient demands to be released from "this jail" and curses the nurse who interviews them.

1. Why might this patient have stopped taking their medication?

2. Lithium carbonate 300 mg is prescribed four times a day. Why must lithium be taken in divided daily doses?

3. The patient complains that they cannot play cards or write a letter. What should the nurse do?

4. The nurse has explained to the patient and family the importance of monitoring plasma lithium levels every 2–3 days until therapeutic levels have been reached and maintained and every 1–3 months once the maintenance-level dose has been established. When should the patient contact the provider for additional monitoring?

5. What measures can the nurse teach the patient to prevent fluctuations in lithium levels?

6. What is the therapeutic range of plasma lithium for maintenance therapy, and at what point are lithium levels critical?

7. Adherence to drug therapy is often an obstacle to managing BPD. How can the nurse increase the likelihood of this patient taking their medication and participating in therapy as prescribed?

8. What teaching does the nurse need to provide to the patient and family relating to prescribed and over-the-counter drugs that relate to the patient's medical history?

9. What nonpharmacologic measures can the nurse teach the patient and family that may help modulate mood?

37 Sedative-Hypnotic Drugs

STUDY QUESTIONS

Matching

Match the effect of benzodiazepines with the affected area of the brain.

1. ___ Cerebral cortex and hippocampus
2. ___ Cortical areas
3. ___ Limbic system
4. ___ Supraspinal motor areas
   a. Anterograde amnesia and confusion
   b. Muscle relaxation
   c. Promote sleep
   d. Reduce anxiety

True or False

For each of the following statements, enter T for true or F for false.

Benzodiazepine-like drugs

5. ___ can intensify the effects of alcohol.
6. ___ are classified as Schedule IV substances.
7. ___ produce moderate muscle relaxation.
8. ___ are used to prevent seizures.
9. ___ prolong periods of uninterrupted sleep.
10. ___ promote falling asleep.
11. ___ have a rapid onset.
12. ___ reduce rapid eye movement (REM) sleep.
13. ___ may cause rebound insomnia.
14. ___ can cause significant rebound insomnia if suddenly discontinued.

CRITICAL THINKING, PRIORITIZATION, AND DELEGATION QUESTIONS

15. Which sites of action of benzodiazepines produce their effects? (**Select all that apply**.)
    a. Limbic system
    b. Cortical areas
    c. Pineal gland
    d. Mimic γ-aminobutyric acid (GABA)
    e. Cerebellum

16. The nurse knows which is true about most benzodiazepines?
    a. They are absorbed very slowly.
    b. They intensify the effects of GABA.
    c. Metabolites are not pharmacologically active.
    d. Benzodiazepines are short-acting.

*17. A patient asks for a sleeping pill at 2200. They state that they can fall asleep but awaken during the night and have difficulty getting back to sleep. The medication administration record (MAR) lists triazolam 0.125 mg at hour of sleep (hs) as needed. Which action should the nurse take?
    a. Administer the as-needed triazolam.
    b. Request a prescription for estazolam.
    c. Contact the provider to increase triazolam.
    d. Teach the patient about sleep hygiene.

*18. The nurse in the emergency department administers progressive doses of flumazenil to a patient who has overdosed on a benzodiazepine and alcohol. Which is a priority nursing action?
    a. Ensuring adequate fluids
    b. Monitoring breathing
    c. Reducing anxiety
    d. Assessing renal function

*19. Which is the nursing priority when administering a long-lasting benzodiazepine?
    a. Gastric distress
    b. Potential for abuse
    c. Respiratory depression
    d. Safety

20. When providing morning care for a patient who received zolpidem the night before, the nurse should monitor for symptoms of which common adverse effect?
    a. Dizziness
    b. Hypertension
    c. Sweating
    d. Tremors

21. A patient falls asleep without difficulty but frequently awakens during the night. The nurse would consult the prescriber if which drug was prescribed for sleep? (**Select all that apply**.)
    a. Eszopiclone
    b. Ramelteon
    c. Temazepam
    d. Zaleplon
    e. Suvorexant

22. Tolerance to barbiturates does **NOT** produce cross-tolerance to which substance?
    a. Alcohol
    b. Benzodiazepines
    c. Cannabis
    d. Opiates

23. The nurse should assess for which symptoms in a patient with a suspected barbiturate overdose?
    a. Hyperthermia
    b. Hypoventilation
    c. Hypertension
    d. Dilated pupils

*24. Following an overdose on a barbiturate, which is priority for the nurse to monitor?
    a. Bowel sounds
    b. Deep tendon reflexes
    c. Peripheral pulses
    d. Oxygen saturation

25. Which antidepressants are effective in treating depression-associated insomnia? (**Select all that apply**.)
    a. Bupropion
    b. Doxepin
    c. Fluoxetine
    d. Fluvoxamine
    e. Trazodone

26. A patient occasionally uses diphenhydramine for insomnia. Which should the nurse include in patient education to prevent a very common adverse effect?
    a. Increase fiber in the diet.
    b. Limit fluid intake.
    c. Eat a low-fat diet.
    d. Take the medication with food.

*27. The nurse is caring for a hospitalized patient who states that they have difficulty falling asleep when away from home. Which intervention should the nurse employ first?
    a. Assess for a possible reason for insomnia.
    b. Discuss the benefits of melatonin for insomnia.
    c. Medicate with prescribed as-needed zolpidem.
    d. Teach the patient about sleep hygiene.

28. Which statement is true regarding the use of melatonin for insomnia?
    a. Research suggests melatonin is highly effective.
    b. Melatonin is not regulated by the FDA.
    c. The drug is not effective in blinded studies.
    d. Studies have shown melatonin prevents jet lag.

DOSE CALCULATION QUESTIONS

29. Zolpidem 10 mg as needed at hs is prescribed. Available are 5-mg immediate-release tablets. How many tablets would be administered at one dose?

30. Flumazenil 0.2 mg is ordered for a patient with a benzodiazepine overdose, followed by a second dose of 0.3 mg 60 seconds later by intravenous push. The drug is available in 0.1 mg/mL. How much drug should the nurse administer for each dose?

CASE STUDIES

Case Study 1

A college student comes to the outpatient department of a local mental health center. They express worries about upcoming exams and state they cannot sleep, cannot concentrate on studies, have felt their heart pounding, are dizzy, and have trouble catching their breath. These symptoms are unusual for the student and began several weeks ago.

1. What additional data should the nurse collect about the patient's symptoms?

2. Why is it imperative that patients on benzodiazepines be cautioned against combining them with alcohol?

3. What information should be included in the nurse's health teaching plan for this patient?

Case Study 2

A patient who has been receiving benzodiazepine therapy for a long time has been notified that their insurance will no longer cover the medication.

4. What are possible effects of sudden discontinuation of the drug?

5. What can the nurse do to help this patient if they can no longer afford a drug to treat insomnia?

38 Management of Anxiety Disorders

STUDY QUESTIONS

True or False

For each of the following statements, enter T for true or F for false.

1. ___ Social anxiety, generalized anxiety, obsessive-compulsive, panic, and posttraumatic stress disorders are all primary anxiety disorders.
2. ___ Benzodiazepines are approved for use for three major anxiety disorders—generalized anxiety disorder (GAD), obsessive-compulsive disorder, and phobias.
3. ___ Cognitive behavioral therapy combined with drug therapy is effective for panic disorder.
4. ___ Depression often coexists with anxiety disorders.
5. ___ GAD is an acute condition.
6. ___ Onset of relief from anxiety with lorazepam and buspirone is rapid.
7. ___ Principal adverse effects of buspirone include sedation and psychomotor slowing.
8. ___ Serotoninergic reuptake inhibitors (SRIs) are effective against anxiety even when depression is not present.
9. ___ Supportive, cognitive behavioral, and/or relaxation therapy is usually all that is needed in mild to moderate anxiety disorders.
10. ___ Symptoms of situational anxiety may be intense, but they are temporary.

Completion

Fill in the blank with the disorder being described.

11. Anxiety when patient thinks they cannot leave a room or situation: ____________
12. Chronic uncontrollable worrying: ____________ ____________ ____________
13. Intense irrational fear of embarrassment: ____________ ____________ ____________
14. Persistent uncontrollable thinking and repetitive actions: ____________ ____________ ____________
15. Reexperiencing, avoidance, and/or emotional, numbing, and hyperarousal: ____________ ____________ ____________ ____________
16. Sudden anxiety attacks that may include fear of dying or going crazy: ____________ ____________

CRITICAL THINKING, PRIORITIZATION, AND DELEGATION QUESTIONS

✳17. A nurse is admitting a patient who is scheduled for outpatient surgery. The patient was instructed to take their levothyroxine with a sip of water in the morning before coming to the hospital. The patient revealed that they were extremely anxious, so they also took a lorazepam, but only with the same sip of water "about 1 hour ago." Which is the priority nursing action?
   a. Assessing for substance use disorder related to benzodiazepines
   b. Documenting the administration of lorazepam
   c. Ensuring that the patient understands the preoperative teaching
   d. Notifying anesthesia of the medications taken this morning

18. The nurse is preparing to administer buspirone to a patient who has been taking the drug for 2 months. Which teaching should be included when administering the drug?
   a. Importance of administering on an empty stomach
   b. Safety precautions because sedation is common
   c. Teaching to avoid drinking grapefruit juice
   d. Discussing not discontinuing this drug suddenly

►19. A patient has been taking paroxetine for anxiety for 3 months. The nurse expects that the drug has been most effective in reducing which of the following symptoms? (**Select all that apply.**)
   a. Nervous stomach
   b. Palpitations
   c. Poor concentration
   d. Tension headache
   e. Worrying

✳20. A patient with a history of GAD has been admitted with exacerbated chronic obstructive pulmonary disease (COPD). Which drug would need consultation with the provider prior to administering?
   a. Alprazolam
   b. Buspirone
   c. Duloxetine
   d. Paroxetine

21. The nurse is caring for a patient who has been diagnosed with panic disorder. Teaching should include which information?
    a. Avoid strenuous exercise in the morning.
    b. Drug therapy helps avoidance behavior.
    c. It is important to maintain regular sleep habits.
    d. Symptoms of panic usually only last 1–2 hours.

✳22. It is a priority for the nurse to report a history of suicide attempts in the past if the patient was currently prescribed which drug?
    a. Clomipramine
    b. Clonazepam
    c. Fluoxetine
    d. Imipramine

23. The nurse notes that a patient becomes very upset when any object in the room is rearranged. The nurse would expect to find which diagnosis in the patient's history?
    a. Obsessive-compulsive disorder
    b. Panic disorder symptoms
    c. Social anxiety disorder
    d. GAD

▶24. When the nurse administers sertraline to a patient for social anxiety disorder, which outcome would indicate that therapy has achieved the desired effect?
    a. Goes on errands without experiencing palpitations
    b. Presents teaching projects to other patients
    c. Rides in elevators without experiencing anxiety
    d. Touches people without fear of contamination

DOSE CALCULATION QUESTIONS

25. Buspirone 7.5 mg orally (PO) twice a day is ordered. Available are 5-mg tablets. How many tablets should the nurse administer per dose?

26. What is the safe dose range of lorazepam intravenous push for a 121-lb adult patient when the recommended dose is 0.02–0.06 mg/kg?

CASE STUDY

A patient with a 70-pack-year history of tobacco use is admitted with exacerbated COPD. During care, the patient states they are afraid they are going to be fired for missing work, will not make their household payments on time, and are sure they have cancer. The patient has not been sleeping and has difficulty completing daily tasks because of weakness and fatigue. Additionally, the patient reports palpitations. On exam, you note cold, clammy hands, and they wring their hands when talking.

1. What should the nurse do first?

2. The nurse tries nonpharmacologic interventions to relieve the patient's anxiety, without success. The provider orders alprazolam 0.5 mg three times a day. What should the nurse include in teaching about this benzodiazepine drug?

3. The patient's adult child comes to visit and expresses concern about their parent receiving a benzodiazepine drug. They state that their parent has a history of alcohol use disorder but has not had a drink for several years. How should the nurse respond to this information?

4. A consult is ordered, and the patient is diagnosed with GAD and a history of alcohol use disorder. Routine alprazolam is discontinued, and buspirone 7.5 mg twice a day is ordered. Why is this drug a good choice for this patient?

5. The patient reports that the drug is not working the same as alprazolam, and asks if they can take an extra dose of buspirone. How should the nurse respond?

6. The patient is referred for cognitive behavioral therapy to augment drug therapy. What are the principles of this therapy?

39 Central Nervous System Stimulants and Attention-Deficit/Hyperactivity Disorder

STUDY QUESTIONS

Matching

Match the drug with its description.

1. ___ Amphetamine
2. ___ Dexmethylphenidate
3. ___ Lisdexamfetamine
4. ___ Modafinil
5. ___ Methylphenidate
6. ___ Methylxanthine
7. ___ Theophylline
   a. Found in coffee, tea, soda, and energy drinks
   b. The drug is not effective if injected or inhaled
   c. A 50:50 mixture of dextroamphetamine and levoamphetamine
   d. Has stimulant effects but is used for bronchodilation
   e. Approved for promoting wakefulness in patients with excessive sleepiness
   f. The dosage is one-half the dosage of methylphenidate
   g. Structurally dissimilar from the amphetamines, but the pharmacologic actions are essentially the same

True or False

Indicate whether these statements relating to atomoxetine are true, T, or false, F.

8. ___ It is approved for use for attention-deficit/hyperactivity disorder (ADHD) in adults.
9. ___ It has a moderate potential for abuse.
10. ___ It has a small risk of liver injury.
11. ___ It takes at least a week before therapeutic effects develop.
12. ___ Patients doing well on stimulant drugs should be switched to Strattera because it is safer and more effective.
13. ___ Patients with an atypical form of the CYP2D6-metabolizing enzyme of cytochrome P450 need higher doses of the drug to be effective.
14. ___ Sexual dysfunction, suicidal thinking, and growth delay are possible adverse effects in children.

CRITICAL THINKING, PRIORITIZATION, AND DELEGATION QUESTIONS

15. Central nervous system (CNS) stimulants are appropriately used for which condition? (**Select all that apply**.)
    a. ADHD
    b. Obesity
    c. Depression
    d. Narcolepsy
    e. Diabetes

▶16. The elementary school nurse cares for a 5-year-old child who receives a CNS stimulant drug for ADHD. The child comes into the office complaining of not feeling well. Which assessment finding would be a concern?
    a. Blood pressure 120/84 mm Hg
    b. Heart rate 100 beats/min
    c. Oxygen saturation 96%
    d. Weight gain of 2 lb since last year

17. A patient asks the nurse why their physician will not prescribe amphetamines to help them lose weight. The patient states one of their parents took them and lost weight. Which is the appropriate nursing response?
    a. "These drugs are ineffective for weight loss."
    b. "They are not long prescribed due to bradycardia."
    c. "Amphetamines can cause physical dependence."
    d. "Stimulant drugs can unmask latent bipolar disorder."

▶18. A patient with a history of narcolepsy, treated with dextroamphetamine extended release (ER), is day 1 postoperative following a right knee replacement. The patient has become somnolent and difficult to arouse. Which action should the nurse take?
    a. Consult the provider.
    b. Administer doxapram.
    c. Continue nursing care.
    d. Restrain the patient.

19. A child who has been prescribed methylphenidate ER for ADHD is having difficulty swallowing the medication. Which is a logical nursing action?
    a. Crush the medication and mix it in a small amount of applesauce.
    b. Notify the provider because the medication must be taken whole.
    c. Open the capsule and sprinkle the beads in a small amount of soft food.
    d. Open the capsule and dissolve the contents in sweet-flavored liquid.

20. A fifth-grade student with ADHD has been prescribed a transdermal methylphenidate patch. They normally awaken at 6:30 a.m., attend school from 8:00 a.m. until 3:15 p.m., and do homework as soon as they get home from school. The student goes to bed at 9:00 p.m. The nurse will teach the parents which is the best time to apply the patch?
    a. 5:30 a.m.
    b. 7:00 a.m.
    c. 4:00 p.m.
    d. 9:00 p.m.

21. The nurse teaches a parent to apply a transdermal methylphenidate patch to unbroken skin on which part of the child's body?
    a. Arm
    b. Back
    c. Gluteus
    d. Hip

22. A nurse's aide is experiencing a headache aura. Caffeine often helps prevent a full-blown migraine. They ask the nurse which item has the most caffeine. Which is the best response?
    a. Cola, 12 oz
    b. Iced tea, 12 oz
    c. Chocolate bar, 1.5 oz
    d. Orange soda, 12 oz

23. Research suggests that caffeine consumption during human pregnancy is associated with
    a. Birth defects
    b. Low birth weight
    c. Spontaneous abortion
    d. Preterm birth

24. Modafinil has been prescribed for a 22-year-old female who works rotating shifts. When teaching about this drug, the nurse should include which instructions?
    a. Take on an empty stomach to enhance absorption.
    b. Maintain orthostatic blood pressure precautions.
    c. Take immediately after waking to avoid insomnia.
    d. Use a second form of birth control while taking drug.

*25. When a school-aged child is prescribed clonidine for ADHD, it is a priority to teach parents to report to the provider if the child experiences which symptom?
    a. Difficulty completing homework
    b. Dizziness with position changes
    c. Weight gain greater than 2 lb in 1 year
    d. Pulse less than 70 beats/min

DOSE CALCULATION QUESTIONS

26. The recommended initial dose of caffeine citrate for neonatal apnea is 20 mg/kg IV administered over 30 minutes. Caffeine citrate 60 mg has been prescribed for a neonate who weighs 6 lb 12 oz. Is the dose safe?

27. Caffeine citrate comes in a concentration of 20 mg/mL. What is the infusion rate in drops per minute if 60 mg is to be administered over 30 minutes and the drip factor is 60 drops/mL?

CASE STUDIES

Case Study 1

The school nurse cares for a seventh-grade child who recently was diagnosed with ADHD, combined type. The parents rejected the diagnosis previously because they do not like the idea of their child using medication. The child is prescribed methylphenidate 10 mg three times a day. The parents speak with the nurse when they deliver the medication and medication administration forms to the school. They verbalize concern that they will be "drugging" their child and ask why behavioral therapy would not be sufficient.

1. Based on current research, how will the nurse explain the rationale for drug therapy?

2. The nurse has been administering the second dose at 11:00 a.m. The nurse is planning for the individual education plan (IEP) meeting with teachers, a counselor, and parents. They note that the child has not been gaining weight. The child admits that they are not very hungry. In the meeting, the nurse learns that the parents give the child methylphenidate at 6:30 a.m. The child eats breakfast at school. The last dose is administered at 5:00 p.m. with dinner. What changes can be made to help improve the appetite of this child?

3. Most teachers at the IEP meeting share that the child's behavior has improved since starting medication. However, the student's organization and study skills are still very weak. Based on the expected therapeutic response to methylphenidate, what information can the nurse provide?

4. The fourth-period (10:15–11:00 a.m.) teacher states that the child is very sleepy in class. What could be happening to cause this sleepiness?

5. Several weeks later, the child's parents come to see the nurse, stating that the pediatrician has recommended that their child be switched to methylphenidate ER 20 mg once a day. The parents are concerned because this is a newer drug, and they don't know enough about it. How should the nurse respond?

6. The child does well at school on methylphenidate ER but has difficulty once home getting homework done and socially at after school activities. The provider puts the child on methylphenidate osmotic-release oral system. How does the nurse explain the difference between methylphenidate osmotic-release oral system and methylphenidate ER?

7. What teaching should be provided about administration of methylphenidate osmotic-release oral system?

Case Study 2

A young adult is seeking medical help for amphetamine dependence. They were prescribed amphetamines for weight loss several years ago and lost 100 lb. The patient is 5 feet 6 inches tall and weighs 130 lb. The patient continued taking amphetamines after reaching their goal weight and now wants to stop taking the drug but says they cannot do it alone. When they stop taking the amphetamines, they experience withdrawal symptoms and become frightened, so they continue to use the drug.

8. What signs and symptoms would you expect the patient to exhibit when using amphetamines?

9. It is important to decrease the amphetamine slowly, since the patient has previously experienced withdrawal symptoms. What withdrawal symptoms should the nurse be alert for when a patient is withdrawing from amphetamine use, and what nursing interventions can help the patient cope with these symptoms?

40 Substance Use Disorders I: Basic Considerations

STUDY QUESTIONS

Completion

1. ____________________ is when a particular dose elicits a smaller response than it did with initial use.
2. When a person is ______________ ______________ on a drug, abstinence syndrome will develop if the drug is stopped.
3. ______________ ______________ is the intense subjective need for a particular psychoactive drug.
4. When a person experiences ______________ ______________, symptoms are often opposite of the normal effects of the drug.
5. Higher doses of a drug are needed in ____________________ because the person has misused another drug, usually in the same class.
6. ____________________ is when one drug can prevent withdrawal from another drug.
7. ____________________ is the neurotransmitter involved in the reward circuit of the brain.
8. Substance use disorder (SUD) is a(n) ____________ ____________________, ________________ illness.

CRITICAL THINKING, PRIORITIZATION, AND DELEGATION QUESTIONS

9. Which statements are true regarding SUD? (**Select all that apply**.)
   a. SUD involves psychological harm.
   b. It involves reinforcement of pleasure.
   c. The brain's reward circuit is activated.
   d. Reduces intensity of unpleasant experiences.
   e. Physical dependence is present.
10. Which psychological factors are associated with tendencies toward drug abuse? (**Select all that apply**.)
   a. Impulsivity
   b. Anxiety disorders
   c. Rebelliousness
   d. Antisocial personality
   e. Developmental delay
11. Which are drugs the nurse can administer and that have the highest potential for abuse and dependence?
   a. Schedule I
   b. Schedule II
   c. Schedule III
   d. Schedule IV
   e. Schedule V
12. A patient has been prescribed hydrocodone 5 mg acetaminophen 325 mg, a schedule IV drug. Which is a federal regulation regarding refills of this drug?
   a. No refills are allowed
   b. Refilled every 6 months
   c. May be refilled five times
   d. Dispensed without prescription
13. When there are different laws on the state and federal levels regarding prescribing controlled substances, which of the following laws takes precedence?
   a. The most restrictive law
   b. The least restrictive law
   c. The federal law
   d. The state law

CASE STUDY

The nurse is working on a drug and alcohol detoxification unit. Describe how the nurse's expertise can be applied to address the following issues of SUD.

1. Diagnosis and treatment of toxicity

2. Diagnosis and treatment of secondary medical complications

3. Facilitating withdrawal

4. Educating and counseling drug abusers in hope of maintaining long-term abstinence

41 Substance Use Disorders II: Alcohol

STUDY QUESTIONS

True or False

For each of the following statements, enter T for true or F for false.

1. ___ The pattern of drinking alcohol is more important than type of alcohol when evaluating cardiovascular effects.
2. ___ Moderate alcohol consumption may decrease the risk of type 1 diabetes mellitus.
3. ___ Alcohol consumption speeds the development of osteoporosis.
4. ___ A person with chronic obstructive pulmonary disease (COPD) should never drink alcohol because even 1–2 drinks can slow respirations.
5. ___ Persons with alcohol use disorder may take antacids on a regular basis.
6. ___ Persons with chronic alcohol use disorder develop nonviral hepatitis more often than cirrhosis.
7. ___ Diuresis that occurs with alcohol consumption occurs because of increased release of antidiuretic hormone (ADH).
8. ___ Alcohol enhances sexual desire and performance.
9. ___ Moderate alcohol intake is a risk factor for several common cancers.
10. ___ Valid research suggests drinking a maximum of 1–2 drinks a week is safe during pregnancy.
11. ___ Alcohol is an effective treatment for insomnia.
12. ___ Low to moderate alcohol use may protect against dementia.

Matching

Match the substance with the effect when combined with alcohol.

13. ___ High alcohol intake counteracts effects.
14. ___ Increases risk of injury to gastrointestinal (GI) mucosa.
15. ___ Increases risk of liver damage.
16. ___ Intensifies central nervous system (CNS) depression.
17. ___ Produces nausea and vomiting; can produce death.
    a. Acetaminophen
    b. Antihypertensives
    c. Benzodiazepines
    d. Disulfiram
    e. Nonsteroidal antiinflammatory drug (NSAID)

CRITICAL THINKING, PRIORITIZATION, AND DELEGATION QUESTIONS

18. The nurse is caring for a patient with a history of chronic alcohol use disorder. The patient is prescribed thiamin to prevent Wernicke encephalopathy. The nurse should assess for which symptoms of this disorder? (**Select all that apply.**)
    a. Abnormal ocular movements
    b. Confabulation
    c. Confusion
    d. Polyneuropathy
    e. Nystagmus
19. Research on older adults suggests that consumption of one alcoholic drink per day has been associated with which effect?
    a. Atrophy of the cerebrum
    b. Development of dementia
    c. Improving the quality of sleep
    d. Preservation of cognitive functioning
20. Research suggests that moderate alcohol consumption has which positive effect?
    a. Prolongation of life
    b. Increased incidence of myocardial infarction (MI)
    c. Higher incidence of heart failure
    d. Heightened risk of mortality

►21. A patient who has been a heavy drinker for 30 years is admitted with constant, severe midepigastric pain radiating to the flank. Which is a priority for the nurse to report to the provider?
    a. Amylase 500 international units/L
    b. Brain natriuretic peptide (BNP) 33 pg/mL
    c. Bilirubin 1 mg/dL
    d. Protein 6.5 g/dL

22. For the average person with normal liver functioning, alcohol levels in the blood will begin to increase if a person consumes which drink in 1 hour? (**Select all that apply**.)
    a. One Margarita on the Rocks
    b. One 1.5-oz shot of whiskey
    c. One 8-oz glass of wine
    d. One 24-oz glass of craft beer
    e. One 8-oz wine cooler

23. Chronic alcohol consumption produces tolerance to which class of drugs or drug? (**Select all that apply**).
    a. Opioids
    b. Anesthetics
    c. Barbiturates
    d. Benzodiazepines
    e. Chloral hydrate

24. Which benzodiazepine regimen has been shown to protect against seizures and breakthrough symptoms of alcohol withdrawal while promoting speedier withdrawal?
    a. As needed in response to symptoms
    b. In combination with another drug
    c. Around the clock on a fixed schedule
    d. In declining doses on a fixed schedule

25. Which symptom suggests acetaldehyde syndrome in a patient taking disulfiram?
    a. Hypertension
    b. Bradycardia
    c. Chest pain
    d. Mydriasis

26. Disulfiram reactions can occur if a patient is exposed to alcohol and takes which antimicrobial medication?
    a. Azithromycin
    b. Gentamicin
    c. Metronidazole
    d. Cefazolin

27. Which explains the use of naltrexone to assist with abstinence in a patient with a history of alcohol use disorder?
    a. Results in vomiting when combined with alcohol.
    b. Lower doses of opioids are required to control pain.
    c. Anxiety is the most common side effect of the drug.
    d. Reduces the high experienced by persons drinking alcohol.

28. Which is the reason naltrexone for intramuscular (IM) injection needs to be administered only once a month?
    a. It has a long half-life.
    b. It is lipid soluble.
    c. It is slowly absorbed from the muscle.
    d. This prevents adverse effects.

*29. Which teaching is priority when a patient is prescribed acamprosate?
    a. Importance of seeking help if thoughts of self-harm occur
    b. The full effects do not occur for about a week
    c. Increase fiber in the diet if diarrhea occurs
    d. Value of including psychosocial support in therapy

DOSE CALCULATION QUESTIONS

30. Disulfiram 125 mg orally at bedtime is prescribed for a patient motivated to abstain from alcohol. Available are 250-mg tablets. The nurse will teach the patient to self-administer how many tablets per dose?

31. Diazepam 10 mg intravenous push is prescribed for a patient in alcohol withdrawal. Available is 5 mg/mL to be administered over 3 minutes. To make it easier to inject the drug over this period of time, the nurse decides to dilute the drug to a total of 3 mL. How much diluent should the nurse add to the drug solution in the syringe to achieve a total of 3 mL?

CASE STUDIES

Case Study 1

The nurse is caring for a patient with a history of alcohol use disorder and cirrhosis of the liver who is admitted with GI bleeding from ulcers.

1. What would be appropriate nursing diagnoses and related assessments for this patient?

2. The patient's blood alcohol level is 0.320%. Chlordiazepoxide was ordered at 100 mg IM STAT followed by high doses via the oral route with the dose decreasing every 3 days. What is the rationale for this treatment regimen?

3. What would be an appropriate nursing outcome for this patient relating to the reason for administering chlordiazepoxide?

4. The patient has been admitted once before for detoxification. They were discharged at that time on a maintenance dose of chlordiazepoxide. Based on the believed effects of alcohol on the CNS, why would this patient relapse?

5. After detoxification, the patient states they are motivated to quit. The patient asks for disulfiram to help them refrain from drinking. What teaching should the nurse provide to the patient and family about this drug?

Case Study 2

Senior-level student nurses have just finished clinical hours in a local hospital emergency department (ED) and are having a postconference. They are discussing a 21-year-old patient who was brought in during their shift and was resuscitated in the ED after acute overdose of alcohol. A fellow college student accompanying the patient reported that they drank four shots in 15 minutes while playing a drinking game. The students had not eaten anything for more than 3 hours before starting the game.

6. The nursing students identify which priority nursing problem for this patient?
   a. Airway clearance
   b. Anxiety
   c. Knowledge deficit
   d. Sensory perceptual alterations

7. The parents of the patient arrived at the ED. The patient's father asked how this could happen. He states that he has had more than five drinks in an evening and has been fine. What factors should the nurse identify as having contributed to the patient's extreme intoxication?

8. Why would discussion about alcohol's effects on the heart, liver, stomach, and kidneys not be likely to motivate this patient to abstain from alcohol?

9. Developmentally, discussion of what adverse effects of alcohol might motivate this young patient to drink responsibly?

42 Substance Use Disorders III: Nicotine

STUDY QUESTIONS

True or False

For each of the following statements, enter T for true or F for false.

1. ___ Tobacco is a drug that, when used exactly as directed, kills adults and children.
2. ___ Medical costs from smoking are greater than nonmedical costs (e.g., lost productivity).
3. ___ The prevalence of smoking in the United States in the 21st century is approximately 30%.
4. ___ Tobacco smoke contains nicotine, carbon monoxide, hydrogen cyanide, ammonia, nitrosamines, and tar.
5. ___ Nicotine in cigar smoke is absorbed primarily from the mouth.
6. ___ It takes approximately 5 minutes for the nicotine from inhaled smoke to reach the brain of a fetus.
7. ___ Nicotine elevates blood pressure (BP) and heart rate in new and chronic smokers.
8. ___ Nicotine slows gastric motility, which is why new smokers often vomit.
9. ___ The effects of nicotine on the pleasure system are mild compared to the effects of cocaine and amphetamines.
10. ___ Nicotine replacement is worth consideration during pregnancy.
11. ___ Research suggests that gradual reduction in tobacco use prolongs withdrawal symptoms.
12. ___ Nicotine is the active ingredient in some insecticides.
13. ___ The risk of chronic obstructive pulmonary disease (COPD) and death from myocardial infarction equals that of those who have never smoked for 20 years after quitting.
14. ___ Health care providers can predict which smoking cessation product will be best for a particular patient.
15. ___ Counseling increases the chance that smoking cessation drugs will be effective.
16. ___ E-cigarettes are effective devices to promote smoking cessation.
17. ___ Vaping can lead to lung injury and death.
18. ___ The most common side effects of bupropion ER are dry mouth, insomnia, and headache.

CRITICAL THINKING, PRIORITIZATION, AND DELEGATION QUESTIONS

19. A 9-month-old child is admitted to the emergency department after eating a cigarette. Which assessment finding would be of most concern?
    a. Apical pulse 145 beats/min
    b. Blood pressure 66/48 mm Hg
    c. Respirations 15/min
    d. Temperature 37°C
20. Which nicotine product produces the most similar effect on the pleasure system as tobacco use?
    a. Chewing gum
    b. Lozenges
    c. Nasal spray
    d. Transdermal patch
21. Which statement, if made by a patient who is planning to use nicotine gum for smoking cessation, suggests the need for more teaching?
    a. "Chewing releases the nicotine."
    b. "I might burp more often when using the gum."
    c. "I should chew after eating to avoid upset stomach."
    d. "I should chew the gum slowly."
22. When using a transdermal nicotine patch, which instructions should the person be given?
    a. Change the patch daily following brand instructions.
    b. Change the site of application once a month.
    c. Report mild redness and itching at the patch site.
    d. Apply the patch to a clean, dry area on the hip.
23. The nurse is teaching a patient how to use nicotine nasal spray. Which instructions should the nurse include in teaching? (**Select all that apply**.)
    a. Administer two sprays per dose.
    b. Use up to five doses per hour.
    c. Take up to 60 doses per day.
    d. Direct the spray away from the nasal septum.
    e. Hold the vial in your dominant hand.
24. The nurse will withhold which smoking cessation drug and contact the provider if the patient exhibits seizure activity?
    a. Bupropion
    b. Nicotine patch
    c. Nicotine lozenge
    d. Nortriptyline

25. Which should be included in the teaching for a patient prescribed bupropion ER?
    a. How to manage dry mouth symptoms
    b. Increase fiber to reduce constipation
    c. The drug may cause rapid weight gain
    d. Do not combine the drug with a nicotine patch

26. Why should e-cigarettes not be used for smoking cessation? (**Select all that apply**.)
    a. The doses of nicotine vary.
    b. Products with known efficacy are available.
    c. Vapor contains contaminants.
    d. The FDA does not regulate e-cigarettes.
    e. They have been shown to be ineffective.

DOSE CALCULATION QUESTIONS

27. Bupropion 300 mg extended release (ER) is prescribed. Bupropion 150 mg ER is available. How many tablets should the nurse administer?

28. Varenicline 500 mcg is prescribed for the first 3 days of smoking cessation therapy. Available are 0.5-mg tablets. How many tablets should the patient self-administer?

CASE STUDY

You are talking with your patient about smoking cessation. Your patient states they have been smoking since they were a teenager and have tried to quit before, "but it never works, so why bother now?"

1. What is your best response to your patient?

2. After further discussion, your patient agrees to try again; how do you determine what the best course of action is to facilitate smoking cessation?

3. Your patient states they have tried quitting "cold turkey," gum, patches, and, most recently, varenicline. What would be the best therapeutic option this time?

43 Substance Use Disorders IV: Major Drugs of Abuse Other Than Alcohol and Nicotine

STUDY QUESTIONS

True or False

For each of the following statements, enter T for true or F for false.

1. ___ In an effort to decrease opioid deaths, naloxone is available in the community setting as an autoinjector.
2. ___ Health care providers are at greater risk for opioid abuse than teachers, engineers, or architects.
3. ___ Heroin is the most commonly abused opioid among street users.
4. ___ Among regular users of barbiturates, very little tolerance develops to respiratory depression.
5. ___ Opioid drug abusers must be hospitalized during withdrawal because opioid withdrawal syndrome can be life-threatening.
6. ___ A patient who is stable after receiving a dose of naloxone for a life-threatening overdose of heroin is still at risk for death if naloxone dosing is not repeated.
7. ___ Buprenorphine is only available through certified opioid treatment programs.
8. ___ When administered as intended, sublingual Suboxone is unlikely to precipitate withdrawal.
9. ___ Naltrexone is a drug that blocks the desired effects of opioids that can be administered as a depot injection once a month.
10. ___ Methadone therapy should not be offered to a patient who admits that they are not interested in detoxification at this time.
11. ___ Sudden withdrawal of opioids is more likely to cause severe symptoms and possible death than sudden withdrawal of barbiturates.
12. ___ A person who requires increased doses of barbiturates will also need higher doses of morphine in order to achieve adequate pain relief after surgery.
13. ___ During surgery, a person who has developed tolerance to barbiturates might be awake and experiencing pain despite anesthesia but might be unable to speak or move due to muscle paralysis.
14. ___ Naloxone can reverse the physical effects of opioids, barbiturates, cocaine, and methamphetamines.
15. ___ Research suggests that psychological dependence on methamphetamines is greater than physical dependence.
16. ___ Marijuana has several approved medical uses.
17. ___ Chronic use of lysergic acid diethylamide (LSD) produces tolerance and physical dependence.
18. ___ LSD can cause permanent visual disturbances.
19. ___ Deaths associated with LSD are primarily related to the effect on the heart.
20. ___ Dissociative drugs were developed for use in surgery.
21. ___ Phencyclidine (PCP) can prevent muscle contraction and cause hypothermia.
22. ___ There is no known effective treatment for PCP overdose.

CRITICAL THINKING, PRIORITIZATION, AND DELEGATION QUESTIONS

✱23. Which is the priority concern when caring for a person with methamphetamine use disorder who is experiencing withdrawal syndrome?
   a. Central nervous system (CNS) depression
   b. Preventing respiratory arrest
   c. Relapsing back to methamphetamine use
   d. Timing of doses of bupropion

✱24. A patient who has a history of heroin use disorder is brought into the emergency department (ED) unresponsive with pinpoint pupils. The nurse assesses that the patient has stopped breathing. In addition to supporting respirations, the patient is prescribed intravenous (IV) naloxone HCl. The nurse notes an improvement in level of consciousness, respiratory rate, and effort within minutes of administration of naloxone. Which is the priority action by the nurse 30–40 minutes after administration of the drug?
   a. Assessing the patient for withdrawal symptoms
   b. Identifying the abused opioid
   c. Monitoring of pulse and blood pressure (BP)
   d. Reassessing for respiratory depression

►25. Which experience by the patient is the most accurate indicator to the nurse that the dose of methadone prescribed to minimize withdrawal syndrome is inadequate?
a. Difficulty arising in the morning
b. Experiences daily vomiting
c. Exhibits fatigue throughout the day
d. The patient states that the dose is inadequate

►26. A patient has been prescribed sublingual buprenorphine-naloxone for long-term management of heroin addiction. Which would occur if the patient crushed, dissolved, and injected the drug IV?
a. An overdose
b. Heroin-induced euphoria
c. Respiratory depression
d. Withdrawal symptoms

27. Which has been associated with maintenance therapy with methadone?
a. Early death
b. Social isolation
c. Lack of motivation
d. No need to buy opioids

✳28. A patient with a suspected barbiturate overdose is brought into the ED unresponsive with pinpoint pupils. Which nursing intervention is priority?
a. Administering phenobarbital
b. Maintaining respirations
c. Preventing withdrawal symptoms
d. Starting an IV line

►29. When responding to acute overdose of cocaine, which outcome would best indicate that therapy has been successful?
a. BP stable at 110/70 mmHg
b. No adventitious lung sounds
c. Sensory perceptions normal
d. Temperature 99.5°F

30. A patient has been admitted with adverse effects of taking methylenedioxymethamphetamine (MDMA; also known as ecstasy). Which assessment finding would warrant consulting the provider regarding possible administration of dantrolene?
a. Extreme anxiety
b. Hallucinations
c. Spasmodic jerking
d. Suicidal thoughts

31. Which are potential effects of high doses of dextromethorphan? (**Select all that apply**.)
a. Disorientation
b. Euphoria
c. Hallucinations
d. Paranoia
e. Sedation

►32. Which is an appropriate concern when a patient has taken excessive amounts of amyl nitrate?
a. Confusion
b. Constipation
c. Dehydration
d. Safety

33. Which finding suggests that a 14-year-old patient may have huffed nail polish remover?
a. BP 135/82 mm Hg
b. Apical pulse 48 beats/min
c. Respirations 16/min
d. Temperature 102.2°F (39°C)

DOSE CALCULATION QUESTIONS

34. A patient with known opioid addiction is prescribed buprenorphine/naloxone, 4 mg/1 mg sublingual. Available are buprenorphine/naloxone 2-mg/0.5-mg sublingual tablets. How many tablets should be administered?

35. Dantrolene 1 mg/kg is prescribed for an 80-kg patient experiencing malignant hyperthermia associated with MDMA use. The drug is available as 20 mg/mL. The drug is prescribed to be administered by IV push over 2 minutes. How many milliliters should the nurse administer?

CLINICAL JUDGMENT CASE STUDY

At an inpatient substance use disorder support group, a new member shares their story of drug abuse.

HEALTH HISTORY	NURSE'S NOTES	PHYSICIAN'S ORDERS	LABORATORY PROFILE

Time: 10:40 hrs
Patient began drinking in high school and, by tenth grade, was getting drunk several times a week. They married an alcoholic and drank with them for many years. The patient then began taking diazepam with alcohol. They stated they experienced hangovers in the mornings, so they would have a beer or two and some amphetamines to "get themself together." They would also take a few aspirin for the headache and go to work feeling sick. As a rule, they would leave work at 5:00 p.m., stop by the liquor store, go home to watch TV, drink, and take a few diazepam to calm down. After a few years of this, they began to buy crack cocaine and could not do their job because they were either high or needed a fix, so they were fired. The patient stayed home, drank, and found they were having difficulty buying drugs. They would get into violent arguments with their partner, who physically abused them. They finally left their partner and sought help at a shelter. They tried to stop using drugs many times over the years but could only stop for a few days before they began to feel ill. They started stealing to support their habit. After being arrested for stealing, they were required to enter a treatment program.

While talking, the patient was intermittently crying. They did not make eye contact with others in the support group. They rubbed their hands on their upper arms as if cold, then on their thighs, sighed and yawned frequently. The patient swung their crossed ankles back and forth while sitting in the chair. After sharing, they sneezed repeatedly and asked for Kleenex to wipe their nose.

Vital signs on return to room: BP 110/72, pulse 68, respirations 14, temperature 99.0°F, oxygen saturation on room air, 98%.

Which assessments should the nurse perform to assess for drug withdrawal? **(Select one, some, or all that apply**.)

a. Gooseflesh
b. Fever
c. Yawning
d. Rhinorrhea
e. Constipation
f. Violent sneezing
g. Headache
h. Muscle spasm

44 Diuretics

STUDY QUESTIONS

Matching

Match the terms and descriptors.

1. ___ Most significant regulator of urine composition
2. ___ Moves passively following osmotic gradient
3. ___ Filtered and then reabsorbed by active transport
4. ___ Nonselective process that does not regulate urine composition
5. ___ Uses pumps selective for organic acids and organic bases for active transport
   a. Filtration
   b. Reabsorption
   c. Active tubular secretion
   d. Solutes
   e. Water

True or False

For each of the following statements, enter T for true or F for false.

This food is a good source of potassium when a patient is receiving a potassium-wasting diuretic.

6. ___ Bananas
7. ___ Beans
8. ___ Cheese
9. ___ Red meat
10. ___ Oranges
11. ___ Pork
12. ___ Raisins
13. ___ Spinach
14. ___ Yogurt

Completion

15. The kidney produces approximately _______ mL of filtrate each day.
16. More than _______ % of the water, electrolytes, and nutrients that are filtered at the glomerulus undergo reabsorption.
17. Most diuretics work by blocking ______________ ______________ and ______________ reabsorption.
18. Diuretics that produce the most significant diuresis affect reabsorption in the ______________ ______________ of the ______________ ______________ ______________ of the ______________ ______________ ______________ ______________.
19. Diuretics can affect blood levels of ______________, ______________, ______________, ______________, ______________, ______________, ______________, ______________, ______________, ______________, and ______________.

CRITICAL THINKING, PRIORITIZATION, AND DELEGATION QUESTIONS

20. Antidiuretic hormone affects kidney reabsorption of which substance?
   a. Glucose
   b. Potassium
   c. Sodium
   d. Water

►21. A liter of water weighs approximately 1 kg. A patient with heart failure (HF) who weighs 176 lb has been prescribed a loop diuretic with the goal of loss of 1000 mL of additional urine output in the next 24 hours. If the goal is met, not taking any other factors affecting weight into consideration, which is the expected weight?
   a. 170 lb
   b. 172 lb
   c. 174 lb
   d. 175 lb

22. A patient with chronic kidney disease has been retaining fluid despite dialysis. Which diuretic would the nurse expect to administer?
    a. Bumetanide
    b. Hydrochlorothiazide
    c. Metolazone
    d. Spironolactone
23. Which food is a good source of potassium when a patient is prescribed a potassium-wasting diuretic? (**Select all that apply**.)
    a. Baked potato
    b. Dried fruit
    c. Lamb
    d. Nuts
    e. Spinach

✳24. A patient with left-sided HF has been prescribed a loop diuretic. Which assessment most accurately reflects a therapeutic effect of this drug?
    a. Blood pressure (BP) 132/84 mm Hg
    b. Normal heart sounds
    c. Clear lung sounds
    d. Pulse 80 and regular

✳25. A patient who has been diagnosed with HF and a known history of type 2 diabetes mellitus (T2DM) has been prescribed furosemide 20 mg by mouth once a day. It is important for the nurse to assess this patient for which symptom?
    a. Paresthesias
    b. Diaphoresis
    c. Weakness
    d. Vomiting

✳26. The nurse takes orthostatic BP readings before administering diuretics to a group of patients. It would be a priority to teach orthostatic BP precautions to a patient with which change in BP readings?
    a. Drop in systolic BP (SBP) of 20 mm Hg
    b. 10 mm Hg decrease in SBP
    c. SBP increase of 5 mm Hg
    d. Increase in SBP of 15 mm Hg

27. Which laboratory test results should the nurse monitor when a patient is prescribed a loop diuretic? (**Select all that apply**.)
    a. Electrolytes
    b. Glucose
    c. Lipid profile
    d. Uric acid
    e. Platelets

✳28. A patient has been prescribed furosemide. The nurse would report which symptom to the provider?
    a. Feeling tired
    b. Bradycardia
    c. Muscle cramping
    d. Palpitations

29. Which over-the-counter medication can alter the effects of diuretics?
    a. Acetaminophen
    b. Ibuprofen
    c. Famotidine
    d. Ferrous sulfate

30. Which is the recommended diuretic for initial therapy of essential hypertension?
    a. Loop
    b. Osmotic
    c. Potassium sparing
    d. Thiazide

31. Which symptom suggests ototoxicity when a patient has been prescribed a loop diuretic?
    a. Photophobia
    b. Telangiectasia
    c. Tinnitus
    d. Xeroderma

✳32. The nurse is reviewing the lab values for a patient who has been prescribed lithium carbonate for bipolar disorder and furosemide for HF. Which result would be a reason for concern?
    a. Chloride 100 mEq/L
    b. Magnesium 1.8 mEq/L
    c. Potassium 4.1 mEq/L
    d. Sodium 128 mEq/L

33. Which new symptom suggests hypokalemia when a patient is prescribed a thiazide or loop diuretic?
    a. Confusion
    b. Muscle weakness
    c. Hypotension
    d. Painful great toe

34. A patient who is prescribed valsartan does not mention that they are taking an oral contraceptive that contains the potassium-saving ingredient drospirenone. They are admitted to the emergency department (ED) with chest pain. Which finding suggests that the combination of drugs is causing hyperkalemia?
    a. Dyspepsia
    b. Abnormal heart rhythm
    c. Muscle spasticity
    d. Diaphoresis

✳35. Which laboratory result should be reported to the provider if a patient with diabetes is prescribed hydrochlorothiazide 50 mg once a day and metformin/glyburide 500 mg/2.5 mg twice a day?
    a. Blood glucose 90 mg/dL
    b. Hemoglobin A1c 8.2%
    c. Potassium 4 mEq/L
    d. Sodium 136 mg/dL

∗36. A 20-year-old patient has been prescribed spironolactone for primary polycystic ovary syndrome (POS). Developmentally, which would be a priority nursing diagnosis?
   a. Activity intolerance related to loss of sodium
   b. Altered body image related to hirsutism
   c. Decisional conflict related to treatment options
   d. Fluid volume excess related to excessive salt intake

37. Because of the risk of hyperkalemia, the nurse consults the provider and monitors potassium levels if a patient is prescribed spironolactone and a drug with which suffix? (**Select all that apply**.)
   a. -floxacin
   b. -olol
   c. -pril
   d. -sartan
   e. -statin

∗38. It is a priority for the nurse to question a patient about which home feature when a patient has been prescribed a diuretic?
   a. Central air
   b. Forced air furnace
   c. Water softener
   d. City water

DOSE CALCULATION QUESTIONS

39. Furosemide 40 mg orally once a day is prescribed. Available is furosemide 80-mg tablets. How many tablets will the nurse administer?

40. Your 330-lb patient is prescribed furosemide 0.1 mg/kg intravenous (IV) × 1 prior to starting an infusion. Your pharmacy stocks furosemide 40 mg/5 mL. How many milligrams will you administer? How fast will the furosemide be pushed?

CASE STUDY

An older adult has been taking spironolactone 100 mg/day for about 6 years to control moderate hypertension and mild HF. They come to the ED with bilateral crackles in the lower and middle lobes and a BP of 190/120 mm Hg. They are short of breath, very anxious, tachycardic, and diaphoretic. Their family assures you that the patient has been taking their medication. The family tells you the patient has been getting worse over the past 2 weeks since having friends bring her favorite lunch of hot dogs and potato chips every day. Pulmonary edema is diagnosed. Orders include STAT IV push furosemide 40 mg and morphine sulfate 2 mg, 3 L of oxygen via nasal cannula, electrolytes, and complete blood count, and an indwelling Foley catheter.

1. How will furosemide help relieve this patient's symptoms?

2. What information must the nurse know about furosemide administration before administering the drug via IV push?

3. Why was the Foley catheter ordered?

4. It has been 45 minutes since the patient received furosemide. The Foley catheter is in place. The patient says they are very thirsty. What assessments should be made at this point?

5. Lab results, drawn before they received any medication, have returned. The sodium is 140 mEq/L, chloride is 110 mEq/L, and potassium is 3.5 mEq/L. Knowing that they received their furosemide after these lab values were drawn, what should be included in the nurse's plan of action?

6. The patient improves significantly within the first 6 hours. BP is 138/90 mm Hg, pulse 102, and respirations 20, and rales are heard only in lung bases bilaterally. The patient asks you how this could have happened since they had been taking their medicine as prescribed. What should the nurse discuss with the patient as possible reasons for their condition?

7. What nursing assessments would be made on at least a daily basis while the patient is in the hospital?

8. The patient continues to improve and is being discharged home on furosemide 20 mg twice a day and spironolactone 50 mg daily. What teaching should be provided regarding dietary patterns, activity, and signs and symptoms of further problems?

9. What information should the nurse provide to prevent problems with drug interactions?

10. The patient will need to be started on digoxin. What must the nurse remember now that the patient is on digoxin and furosemide? What laboratory values need to be monitored?

45 Agents Affecting the Volume and Ion Content of Body Fluids

STUDY QUESTIONS

Completion

1. Cirrhosis of the liver can cause ________________ ______________.
2. Diuretics and chronic kidney disease can cause ______________ ______________.
3. Extensive burns can cause ______________________ ______________.
4. Vomiting and diarrhea can cause ______________ ______________.
5. Total osmolality of plasma is about two times the osmolality of ______________.
6. A normal saline with potassium infusion increases excretion of bicarbonate in ______________ ______________.
7. Treatment of severe ________________________ ____________________includes rebreathing CO_2.
8. Sodium bicarbonate is used to treat ______________ ________________.

Matching

Match the conditions with the appropriate descriptor.

9. ___ Metabolic acidosis
10. ___ Respiratory acidosis
11. ___ Metabolic alkalosis
12. ___ Respiratory alkalosis
    a. Can occur with salicylate poisoning.
    b. Lung changes from smoking are a risk for this condition.
    c. May be associated with prolonged gastric suctioning.
    d. May be caused by hysteria.

CRITICAL THINKING, PRIORITIZATION, AND DELEGATION QUESTIONS

*13. Which is priority when infusing an intravenous (IV) solution in cases of isotonic contraction?
   a. Assess for crackles in the lung fields.
   b. Monitor the heart rate apically.
   c. Augment the IV fluid with oral.
   d. Infuse 0.45% sodium chloride.

14. Which is why IV solutions of 5% dextrose in water are technically isotonic in the bag but hypotonic in the body?
   a. The body uses the dextrose for energy.
   b. Kidneys rapidly excrete the dextrose.
   c. Dextrose is a nonabsorbable sugar.
   d. It is metabolized in the blood to H_2O and CO_2.

►15. A teen with bulimia who abuses laxatives is admitted to the hospital after experiencing extreme leg weakness. Potassium chloride 40 mEq by mouth twice a day has been prescribed. The nurse reviews the most recent laboratory results before administering the drug. Results include Na 137 mEq/L, K 3.5 mEq/L, and Cl 100 mEq/L. Which is the appropriate nursing action?
   a. Page the provider STAT.
   b. Administer the medication.
   c. Hold the medication.
   d. Leave a message for the provider.

►16. The nurse is administering furosemide and sustained-release potassium chloride to a patient with heart failure (HF). The nurse notes that the patient is chewing the potassium chloride. The patient states they cannot swallow the large pill. Which action should the nurse take?
   a. Crush the pill and mix it with applesauce or pudding.
   b. Allow the patient to continue chewing the pill.
   c. Contact the provider for a change in formulation.
   d. Request a GI consult for upper GI studies.

*17. Which assessment finding would be a priority to report to the provider when a patient is taking potassium tablets?
   a. Black stool
   b. Constipation
   c. Muscle weakness
   d. Nausea

*18. Which laboratory result would be a priority to report to the provider when a patient is receiving IV fluids containing potassium?
   a. Blood urea nitrogen 28 mg/dL
   b. Creatinine 4.2 mg/dL
   c. Potassium 3.5 mEq/L
   d. Serum glucose 220 mg/dL

▶19. A patient with diabetes is admitted with hyperosmolar hyperglycemic syndrome (HHS). Their serum glucose level is 750 mg/dL, and blood pH is 7.41. An infusion of regular insulin in normal saline (0.9% NaCl) is prescribed to lower the patient's blood sugar. When administering the IV insulin, the nurse needs to assess the patient for which symptoms?
   a. Skeletal muscle weakness
   b. Seizures
   c. Hypotension
   d. Peaked T waves on ECG

20. Which medication can increase the risk of hyperkalemia if prescribed with potassium? (**Select all that apply**.)
   a. Amlodipine
   b. Atenolol
   c. Furosemide
   d. Ramipril
   e. Spironolactone

✳21. Which is the priority action when a patient is diagnosed with hyperkalemia?
   a. Administer sodium polystyrene sulfonate.
   b. Initiate continuous cardiac monitoring.
   c. Question the patient about medical history.
   d. Dietary teaching about high-potassium foods.

✳22. The night shift nurse receives a call from the laboratory about a patient's magnesium level of 1 mEq/L. When calling the results to the on-call provider, it is imperative to include the patient's history of which disorder?
   a. Chronic obstructive pulmonary disease
   b. Atrioventricular heart block
   c. Gastroesophageal reflux disease
   d. Rheumatoid arthritis

23. Because of the risk of neuromuscular blockade when administering magnesium, the nurse must have immediate access to which injectable medication?
   a. Calcium gluconate
   b. Potassium chloride
   c. Sodium chloride
   d. Sodium polystyrene sulfonate

DOSE CALCULATION QUESTION

Sodium bicarbonate three vials (50-mEq/50-mL vials) is ordered for your 110-pound patient who has been admitted with salicylate poisoning and a salicylate level of 90 mg/dL and urinary pH at 6. The sodium bicarbonate is to be added to 850 mL of dextrose 5% in water (D5W) and infused at 2 mEq/kg/h for 4 hours.

24. What rate in milliliters per hour should be programmed into the IV pump?

CASE STUDIES

Case Study 1

A patient is admitted with prolonged diarrhea. An IV solution of 0.45% sodium chloride with 40 mEq of potassium chloride is prescribed at 150 mL/h.

1. What laboratory tests does the nurse need to monitor when administering potassium supplements?

2. What assessments does the nurse need to perform to ensure the safe infusion of the potassium solution?

3. What measures should the nurse take to ensure accurate infusion of the prescribed dose of fluid and electrolytes?

4. What assessments should the nurse perform to assess for possible fluid overload?

Case Study 2

A postoperative patient has been nothing by mouth (NPO) for 4 days with a nasogastric tube set to low intermittent suction. The patient develops muscle cramping and disorientation. Serum Mg is 1.0 mEq/L. The provider orders an IV solution of 10% magnesium sulfate to infuse at 100 mL/h.

5. What should the nurse do before initiating this IV therapy?

6. The provider changes the infusion rate to 90 mL/h. What critical assessment should the nurse perform while administering magnesium?

7. What assessment findings would warrant the nurse stopping the infusion and consulting the provider?

46 Review of Hemodynamics

STUDY QUESTIONS

True or False

For each of the following statements, enter T for true or F for false.

1. ___ Arteries readily stretch in response to pressure changes.
2. ___ Arterioles regulate blood flow to tissue.
3. ___ Cardiac output is determined by heart rate times the amount of blood ejected from the heart with each beat.
4. ___ Conditions that decrease chest expansion with breathing decrease blood return to the heart.
5. ___ Conditions that cause an inability of skeletal muscle to contract can cause peripheral edema.
6. ___ Normal adult blood volume is 8 L.
7. ___ Stimulation of the vagal nerve, such as bearing down to defecate, speeds the heart rate.
8. ___ As diameter of the ventricles increases, there is a corresponding increase in contractile force.
9. ___ The heart of a normal adult pumps the entire blood volume in approximately 1 minute.
10. ___ Most of the blood in the body is in the arteries and the heart.
11. ___ Vasodilation increases resistance to blood flow.

Matching

Match the terms and descriptors.

12. ___ Afterload
13. ___ Aldosterone (renin-angiotensin-aldosterone system)
14. ___ Baroreceptors
15. ___ β_1-Adrenergic receptors
16. ___ Cardiac output
17. ___ C-natriuretic peptide
18. ___ Preload
19. ___ Muscarinic receptors
20. ___ Natriuretic peptides: atrial natriuretic peptide (ANP) and brain natriuretic peptide (BNP)
21. ___ Sinoatrial node
22. ___ Stroke volume
23. ___ Systemic filling pressure

a. Amount of blood pumped out of the heart in 1 minute
b. Constricts vessels and increases water retention
c. Force that returns blood to the heart
d. Force with which the ventricles of the heart contract
e. The amount of stretch in the ventricle before it contracts
f. Pressure in the aorta that the heart must overcome to eject blood out of the heart
g. Pressure sensors in the aortic arch and carotid sinus
h. Primarily promotes vasodilation
i. Shift fluid from vascular to extravascular compartment, increase diuresis, dilate arterioles and veins
j. Where stimulation of heartbeat originates
k. Stimulation of these receptors decreases heart rate
l. Stimulation of these receptors increases heart rate

CRITICAL THINKING, PRIORITIZATION, AND DELEGATION QUESTIONS

24. Individuals who have plaque lining their arteries experience an increase in vessel resistance. The nurse should assess for which reaction that is the body's attempt to compensate?
    a. Bradycardia
    b. Hypertension
    c. Peripheral edema
    d. Tachypnea

25. Drugs that can be used to lower blood pressure decrease venous resistance by which action? (**Select all that apply**.)
    a. Venous dilation
    b. Reduced right atrial pressure
    c. A reduction in blood volume
    d. Decreased cardiac contractility
    e. Increased blood viscosity

►26. A patient with early heart failure (HF) has an average heart rate of 90 beats/min and a stroke volume of 55 mL. Which statement is true about this patient's cardiac output?
    a. Extremely low.
    b. Low.
    c. High.
    d. Normal.

✳27. The nurse is researching a drug. The handbook states that it decreases afterload. Before the nurse administers this medication to a patient, which assessment is priority?
    a. Blood pressure
    b. Apical pulse
    c. Respirations
    d. Temperature

✳28. Which is the mechanism by which natriuretic peptides reduce cardiac preload? (**Select all that apply.**)
    a. Increased heart rate
    b. Increased vascular permeability
    c. Constriction of arterioles
    d. Sodium loss
    e. Loss of water

►29. The nurse is reassessing a patient 1 hour after administering a vasodilator to treat hypertension. Assessment findings include BP 116/70 mm Hg (down from 145/88 mm Hg), pulse 88 (up from 80 beats/min), and respirations 22 (up from 20). Which action should the nurse take? (**Select all that apply**.)
    a. Collect additional data.
    b. Document the findings.
    c. Explain orthostatic BP precautions.
    d. Page the prescriber STAT.
    e. Raise all four bed side-rails for safety.
    f. Reassess the vital signs within 1 hour.

✳30. A patient who has a high incidence of orthostatic hypotension is receiving a vasodilator. Before administering the medication and after the patient has rested supine for 5 minutes, the nurse assesses the BP and pulse. Results are BP 145/80 mm Hg and pulse 68 beats/min. The nurse assists the patient to stand, ensuring safety and, after 1 minute, reassesses the BP and pulse. Which reading is of most concern to the nurse?
    a. BP 110/70 mm Hg, pulse 92 beats/min
    b. BP 126/70 mm Hg, pulse 78 beats/min
    c. BP 134/70 mm Hg, pulse 72 beats/min
    d. BP 140/82 mm Hg, pulse 70 beats/min

CASE STUDIES

Case Study 1

A patient newly diagnosed with coronary artery disease (CAD) has been prescribed a nitroglycerin patch 12 hours on and 12 hours off. The nurse is explaining the medication to the patient. Nitroglycerin is a drug that causes extensive venous vasodilation. The drug handbook states that the therapeutic effect is to decrease the workload of the heart. The patient wants to know how this helps their heart.

1. How should the nurse explain this effect?

2. The patient verbalizes understanding of nitroglycerin but states that they are afraid to take off the patch because they might have a heart attack. Which is the rationale for removing nitroglycerin patches after 10–12 hours?
    a. Absorption becomes decreased.
    b. Skin irritation occurs.
    c. Decreases side-effects.
    d. Minimizes tolerance to the drug.

Case Study 2

The student nurse is caring for a patient with HF. The heart is enlarged and weak, and its muscle fibers are stretched beyond the point of effective recoil. The student nurse must do a teaching project.

3. Describe how the student nurse could use a balloon to demonstrate the pathophysiology of HF to the patient.

47 Drugs Acting on the Renin-Angiotensin-Aldosterone System

STUDY QUESTIONS

Matching

1. ___ Catalyzes the conversion of angiotensin I into angiotensin II.
2. ___ Reduces levels of angiotensin II, leading to arterial dilation and reduced blood volume.
3. ___ Inhibits the conversion of angiotensinogen into angiotensin I.
4. ___ Blocks access of angiotensin II to its receptors in blood vessels.
5. ___ Produces selective blockade of aldosterone receptors, leading to excretion of sodium and water.
6. ___ Causes retention of sodium and excretion of potassium and hydrogen.
7. ___ Facilitates formation of angiotensin I from angiotensinogen.
8. ___ Regulates blood pressure (BP), blood volume, and fluid and electrolyte balance.
9. ___ Acts directly on vascular smooth muscle to cause contraction.
   a. Aldosterone
   b. Aldosterone receptor antagonist
   c. Angiotensin II
   d. Angiotensin-converting enzyme (ACE; kinase II)
   e. ACE inhibitor
   f. Angiotensin II receptor blocker (ARB)
   g. Direct renin inhibitor (DRI)
   h. Renin-angiotensin-aldosterone system (RAAS)
   i. Renin

CRITICAL THINKING, PRIORITIZATION, AND DELEGATION QUESTIONS

10. The nurse recognizes that the generic names of ARB drugs end in which suffix?
    a. -mycin
    b. -olol
    c. -pril
    d. -sartan
11. The nurse recognizes that the generic names of ACE inhibitor drugs end in which suffix?
    a. -mycin
    b. -olol
    c. -pril
    d. -sartan
12. The nurse teaches a patient how drugs that block the effects of angiotensin II are beneficial for heart failure patients. Which statement indicates a need for further teaching?
    a. "The drug improves cardiac function by decreasing electrical conduction through heart tissue."
    b. "The drug can help heart function by increasing excretion of sodium and water by the kidneys."
    c. "The drug can decrease the formation of pathologic changes in cardiac structure."
    d. "The drug can help heart function by preventing pathologic changes to blood vessels."
13. Which stimulates renin release by the kidneys? (**Select all that apply**.)
    a. Dehydration
    b. Hemorrhage
    c. Hypernatremia
    d. Renal artery stenosis
    e. Hypotension
14. Which adverse effect can a patient experience from taking an ACE inhibitor? (**Select all that apply**.)
    a. Dehydration
    b. Dry cough
    c. Hyperkalemia
    d. Hyponatremia
    e. Neutropenia

▶15. Which laboratory results should the nurse review before administering lisinopril? (**Select all that apply**.)
    a. Creatinine
    b. Blood glucose
    c. Sodium
    d. Potassium
    e. Uric acid

✳16. It would be a priority to teach orthostatic BP precautions to a patient before the first dose of an ACE inhibitor if laboratory tests include which result?
    a. Blood glucose 95 mg/dL
    b. Creatinine 1.2 mEq/L
    c. Potassium 4.1 mEq/L
    d. Sodium 132 mg/dL

17. The nurse receives laboratory test results, including aspartate aminotransferase (AST) 22 IU/L, alanine aminotransferase (ALT) 33 international units/L, blood urea nitrogen (BUN) 32 mg/dL, and creatinine 2.2 mg/dL, for a patient who is scheduled to receive an ACE inhibitor drug. Which ACE inhibitor could be administered without concern of toxicity?
    a. Captopril
    b. Enalapril
    c. Fosinopril
    d. Lisinopril

*18. A patient who is prescribed an ACE inhibitor complains of tongue swelling and is experiencing obvious dyspnea. Which is the priority nursing action?
    a. Administer epinephrine.
    b. Assess BP.
    c. Assess lung sounds.
    d. Consult the prescriber.

▶19. Which side effect of ACE inhibitors is related to an accumulation of bradykinin?
    a. Hyperkalemia
    b. First-dose hypotension
    c. Renal insufficiency
    d. Hacking cough

20. A patient who has been taking an ACE inhibitor for hypertension is concerned because she has just discovered that she is 7 weeks pregnant. The nurse knows research suggests that if the patient stops taking the ACE inhibitor, which is the risk for adverse effect on the fetus?
    a. Unknown
    b. Low
    c. Medium
    d. High

*21. When a patient is prescribed an ACE inhibitor, it is a priority to teach the patient to contact their prescriber before taking which OTC drug?
    a. Omeprazole
    b. Mucinex
    c. Senokot
    d. Ibuprofen

22. ARB drugs are similar to ACE inhibitors, but they do not have which adverse effect?
    a. Cancer
    b. Cough
    c. Fetal harm
    d. Kidney disease

23. Which are side effects of spironolactone? (**Select all that apply.**)
    a. Gynecomastia
    b. Hypokalemia
    c. Hypotension
    d. Hirsutism
    e. Impotence

24. Which is an adverse effect of eplerenone?
    a. Flushed skin
    b. Diarrhea
    c. Irritability
    d. Spasticity

*25. When taking a history from a patient who is prescribed an ACE inhibitor, ARB, or eplerenone, which question would be most important for the nurse to ask?
    a. "Are you bothered by a frequent cough?"
    b. "Do you eat fruits on a daily basis?"
    c. "Do you have iron-deficiency anemia?"
    d. "What do you use to season your food?"

DOSE CALCULATION QUESTION

26. Aliskiren is available as 150-mg tablets. How many tablets are administered for a 300-mg dose?

CASE STUDY

An older adult is admitted to the medical unit with complaints of a 10-lb weight gain over the past week, swollen ankles, and increasing shortness of breath. Although furosemide was partially effective in reducing fluid overload, the provider chooses to add an ACE inhibitor. The patient is prescribed captopril 2.5 mg by mouth three times a day. Their BP is currently 140/74 mm Hg. The patient has a history that includes an anterior myocardial infarction 12 months ago and renal artery stenosis involving the right kidney.

1. What question should the nurse ask when consulting the provider about this new medication order?

2. What teaching should the nurse provide about the timing of the doses of captopril?

3. What assessments and actions should the nurse perform when administering the first dose of captopril?

4. What teaching should the nurse provide to the patient and family about reasons to contact the prescriber?

5. The patient's spouse has a friend who used to take captopril, but the friend's provider discontinued the ACE inhibitor and prescribed the newer drug valsartan. The patient's partner would like the patient to be prescribed valsartan because it is "newer and better." How should the nurse respond?

48 Calcium Channel Blockers

STUDY QUESTIONS

Completion

1. Verapamil blocks calcium channels in ___________ ___________ and in the ___________.
2. Calcium channel blockers (CCBs) act selectively on ___________ ___________ and ___________, and ___________ of the heart.
3. Dihydropyridine CCBs primarily affect _________ ______________.
4. The three net effects of the CCBs verapamil and diltiazem on the heart are _________________, _________________ _________________ _________________, and _________________ _________________ _________________.
5. The suffix of the generic name of dihydropyridine CCBs is _______________________.

CRITICAL THINKING, PRIORITIZATION, AND DELEGATION QUESTIONS

✳ 6. In addition to assessing BP, which is the priority assessment before administering diltiazem?
   a. Ankle edema
   b. Apical pulse
   c. Peripheral pulses
   d. Respiratory rate

7. Which is a direct effect of verapamil blocking calcium channels in the heart and blood vessels?
   a. Increased arterial pressure
   b. Coronary perfusion is increased
   c. Atrioventricular (AV) nodal conduction is increased
   d. Constriction of peripheral arterioles

8. The nurse is caring for a patient scheduled to receive verapamil and atenolol at 0900. It is important for the nurse to assess for which potential adverse effect when administering both drugs? (**Select all that apply**.)
   a. Pulmonary edema
   b. Muscle pain
   c. Shortness of breath
   d. Urinary output of at least 45 mL/h
   e. Weight gain of 3 lb in 24 hours

9. The drop in BP produced by the CCB activates baroreceptors and stimulates the sympathetic nervous system. Which of these CCBs is most likely to have the adverse effect of reflex tachycardia?
   a. Diltiazem
   b. Nifedipine
   c. Verapamil
   d. Isradipine

▶10. The nurse is caring for a patient who is scheduled to receive verapamil extended release (ER) 180 mg and atenolol 50 mg at 0900. The patient has had a gastric tube (G-tube) inserted, and drugs are to be administered via the tube. Which action should the nurse take before administering these two drugs?
   a. Administer at least 2 hours apart.
   b. Consult the provider.
   c. Crush both tablets separately.
   d. Flush the G-tube between drugs.

✳11. A patient is prescribed diltiazem. It would be a priority to withhold the drug and contact the provider if which assessment finding is present?
   a. BP 150/85 mm Hg
   b. Constipation
   c. Orthostasis
   d. Pulse 50 beats/min

▶12. Which dermatologic finding in an older adult would warrant consultation with the provider regarding the administration of diltiazem?
   a. Burrows between the fingers
   b. Generalized eczematous eruptions
   c. Scaling plaques on the elbows
   d. Cheesy plaque on the tongue

13. The nurse is teaching their patient about the most common side-effects of verapamil. Which effects should be included in the teaching? (**Select all that apply**.)
   a. Constipation
   b. Dizziness
   c. Headache
   d. Edema
   e. Reflex tachycardia

14. A patient on a surgical unit has been prescribed intravenous (IV) diltiazem for atrial fibrillation. Which is the appropriate nursing action?
    a. Move the resuscitation cart into the patient's room.
    b. Arrange for continuous cardiac monitoring.
    c. Continuously monitor oxygen saturation.
    d. Hanging the IV medication by gravity feed.

15. Which assessment finding is an indication of verapamil toxicity?
    a. Bradycardia
    b. Edema
    c. Cough
    d. Dyspnea

►16. The medication administration record states that a patient should receive diltiazem ER 120 mg once a day. The hospital formulary includes diltiazem sustained release (SR). Which is the appropriate nursing action?
    a. Administer the medication as ordered.
    b. Withhold the medication.
    c. Use the patient's home medication.
    d. Contact the provider about the issue.

17. Which drug might be prescribed to counteract the reflex tachycardia associated with administration of a dihydropyridine CCB?
    a. Digoxin
    b. Enalapril
    c. Furosemide
    d. Metoprolol

18. A patient who has experienced reflex tachycardia while taking nifedipine 20 mg three times a day has had their prescription changed to nifedipine ER 60 mg once a day. The patient asks the nurse how taking the same medication once a day instead of three times a day will help prevent palpitations. Which is the appropriate nursing response?
    a. "The ER formulation is less potent than the other."
    b. "Blood levels of ER formulas become therapeutic slower."
    c. "SR formulas cause a more gradual drop in BP."
    d. "Nifedipine ER suppresses the automaticity of the heart."

19. A patient has been prescribed ER nifedipine. Teaching regarding administration should include which instruction?
    a. Take with a snack before bed.
    b. Do not crush or chew tablet.
    c. It is best to take with grapefruit juice.
    d. Administer on an empty stomach.

*20. Which indicates nifedipine toxicity and should be reported to the provider? (**Select all that apply**.)?
    a. Palpitations
    b. Constipation
    c. Syncope
    d. Dyspnea
    e. Nausea

DOSE CALCULATION QUESTIONS

21. Diltiazem is prescribed for IV infusion for a patient in atrial fibrillation. A dose of 5 mg/h has been prescribed. The pharmacy has supplied the drug at a concentration of 0.45 mg/mL. How many milliliters per hour will the nurse program into the IV infusion pump?

22. The recommended initial dose of diltiazem IV push is 0.25 mg/kg for adult patients. What is the recommended safe dose for a patient who weighs 178 lb?

CASE STUDY

An older adult patient who is a nonsmoker with a history of hypertension, esophageal cancer, and type 2 diabetes mellitus comes to the emergency department with fatigue and extreme shortness of breath. They are diagnosed with atrial fibrillation. The provider orders verapamil 5 mg IV push.

1. The nurse is administering the verapamil IV push. While administering the medication, the nurse notes a sudden reduction in heart rate and prolongation of the PR interval on the cardiac monitor. What should the nurse do?

2. Thirty minutes after injecting the IV verapamil, the patient requests assistance with getting up and using the toilet to void. What should the nurse do?

3. The patient is stabilized, and the provider has prescribed verapamil 120 mg three times a day. The nurse is reviewing the patient's laboratory tests. Which laboratory value would require consultation with the provider regarding administration of verapamil? (**Select all that apply and explain why**.)
   a. ALT 250 units/L
   b. BUN 28 mg/dL
   c. Creatinine 3.2 mg/dL
   d. Fasting blood glucose (FBG) 250 mg/dL
   e. Hemoglobin (Hgb) 10 mg/dL
   f. International normalized ratio (INR) 1.8
   g. Potassium (K^+) 3.3 mEq/L
   h. Sodium (Na^+) 146 mg/dL

4. The nurse is reviewing the patient's prescribed medications. In addition to verapamil 80 mg three times a day, the patient is taking nateglinide 120 mg, a medication that increases production of insulin by the pancreas and lowers the blood sugar to treat the patient's diabetes mellitus. Both verapamil and nateglinide are metabolized by the CYP3A4 hepatic enzyme. Verapamil inhibits the action of this enzyme. Because of this interaction, the nurse knows the patient is at increased risk for hypoglycemia. What symptoms suggest that the patient's blood glucose has dropped below normal?

5. What teaching should the nurse provide that can prevent problems with common adverse effects of verapamil?

49 Vasodilators

STUDY QUESTIONS

True or False

For each of the following statements, enter T for true or F for false.

1. ___ Hydralazine reduces the work of the heart by reducing afterload.
2. ___ Hydralazine lowers blood pressure by causing vasodilation and diuresis.
3. ___ An adverse effect of minoxidil is impairment in tissue perfusion.
4. ___ The effects of an intravenous (IV) infusion of nitroprusside end within minutes of stopping the infusion.
5. ___ Nitroglycerin is used to treat angina because it dilates arterioles in the heart, allowing more oxygen to get to heart muscle cells.
6. ___ Orthostatic hypotension is more likely to occur when a patient is receiving a drug that dilates veins than one that dilates arterioles.
7. ___ Reflex tachycardia only occurs with drugs that dilate both arterioles and veins.
8. ___ Drugs with the suffix "-lol" are used to slow the heart when reflex tachycardia occurs.
9. ___ When a patient is receiving nitroprusside, the nurse would report a thiocyanate level greater than 0.1 mg/mL.

CRITICAL THINKING, PRIORITIZATION, AND DELEGATION QUESTIONS

✳10. The nurse is caring for a patient prescribed hydralazine. Which assessment finding would be a priority to report to the provider?
   a. Temperature 99.0ºF (37.22ºC)
   b. Blood pressure 132/80 mm Hg
   c. Apical pulse 118 beats/min
   d. Respirations 18 breaths/min

11. A frequent adverse effect of hydralazine is increased blood volume. Which drug is often prescribed to prevent this adverse effect?
   a. Atenolol
   b. Furosemide
   c. Isosorbide dinitrate
   d. Minoxidil

✳12. Which adverse effect may be observed when caring for a patient who is prescribed minoxidil?
   a. Abnormal hair growth
   b. Bradycardia
   c. Fluid volume deficit
   d. Dark colored urine

►13. A patient with severe hypertension is prescribed minoxidil. The nurse would notify the provider if which symptom was found on assessment?
   a. Headache
   b. 3+ peripheral edema
   c. Fatigue
   d. Sweating

14. The nurse caring for an older adult prescribed a vasodilator should monitor the older adult for which problem?
   a. Kidney dysfunction
   b. Delirium
   c. Falls
   d. Seizures

✳15. Laboratory test results on a patient receiving hydralazine include elevated antinuclear antibodies (ANA). When notifying the provider of these lab results, it is a priority to include which assessment finding?
   a. Fatigue
   b. Headache
   c. Respirations 22/min
   d. Temperature 101°F (38.3°C)

►16. The nurse is administering nitroprusside in a cardiac care unit. The provider also orders administration of oral antihypertensives. The patient's blood pressure is still elevated but dropping slowly. Which is the appropriate nursing action?
   a. Administer both medications.
   b. Hold both medications.
   c. Hold the oral antihypertensive only.
   d. Consult the provider about the orders.

►17. Which action must be taken when nitroprusside is used to lower blood pressure (BP) in hypertensive emergencies?
   a. Administer the drug rapidly to lower BP.
   b. Provide thiosulfate supplementation.
   c. Simultaneously begin an oral antihypertensive.
   d. Monitor plasma cyanide levels.

▶18. A patient who weighs 165 lb is receiving IV nitroprusside sodium at 300 mcg/min. The nurse should monitor the patient for which adverse effect?
  a. Adequate urinary output
  b. Joint and muscle pain
  c. Facial flushing
  d. Disorientation

DOSE CALCULATION QUESTIONS

19. What rate of infusion of nitroprusside would the nurse program into the IV pump if administering 3 mcg/kg per minute to a patient who weighs 176 lb if the drug dilution is 50 mg in 250 mL of 5% dextrose in water?

CLINICAL JUDGMENT CASE STUDY

HEALTH HISTORY	NURSE'S NOTES	PHYSICIAN'S ORDERS	LABORATORY PROFILE

Time: 1040 hrs

Patient is admitted via the emergency department (ED) with a frontal headache, dyspnea, chest pain, and generalized complaints of "not feeling well." They have a history of type 2 diabetes mellitus.

Blood pressure is 210/120 mm Hg, pulse 115 bpm, and respirations are 24 and labored. Lungs are clear anteriorly and posteriorly on auscultation. Heart rate is tachycardic with regular rhythm, normal S1 and S2. Skin is warm and clammy. Speech is rapid, and the patient keeps asking if they are having a heart attack.

The patient is 5′11″ tall and weighs 93 kg. The patient's partner is at the bedside and repeatedly telling the patient to relax and let the nurse do their job.

Orders received for IV nitroprusside, to begin at 0.5 mcg/kg/min, increasing by 0.5 mcg/kg/min every 5 minutes.

While administering nitroprusside, the nurse knows to monitor the patient for ___(1)_______, ___(2)_______, and ___(3)_______, which are significant adverse effects of the drug.

(1)	(2)	(3)
Gynecomastia	Cyanide poisoning	Cardiac tamponade
Reflex tachycardia	Heart failure	Systemic lupus erythematosus (SLE)-like syndrome
Hypertrichosis	Sodium retention	Thiocyanate toxicity
Hypotension	Water retention	Pericardial effusion

50 Drugs for Hypertension

STUDY QUESTIONS

Matching

Match the statement with the class of antihypertensive drug.

1. ___ Because of their ability to conserve potassium, these drugs can play an important role in an antihypertensive regimen.
2. ___ Have direct suppressant effects on the heart, reducing reflex tachycardia.
3. ___ Because venous dilation is minimal, the risk of orthostatic hypotension is low.
4. ___ Blood pressure (BP) reduction results from dilation of arterioles and veins, reduction of heart rate and contractility, and suppression of renin release.
5. ___ Promotes renal excretion of sodium and water and renal retention of potassium.
6. ___ Act directly on renin to inhibit conversion of angiotensinogen into angiotensin I.
7. ___ Produce much greater diuresis than the thiazides.
8. ___ First-line drugs for hypertension.
9. ___ Are less effective in African Americans than in Whites.
10. ___ Act within the brainstem to suppress sympathetic outflow to the heart and blood vessels.
11. ___ Depletes norepinephrine from postganglionic sympathetic nerve terminals.
12. ___ Fall into two groups: dihydropyridines and nondihydropyridines.
13. ___ Prevent sympathetically mediated vasoconstriction.
14. ___ Have low incidence of inducing cough.
15. ___ Prevent formation of angiotensin II, thereby preventing angiotensin II-mediated vasoconstriction and aldosterone-mediated volume expansion.

a. Adrenergic neuron blockers
b. Aldosterone antagonists
c. α_1-Blockers
d. α/β-Blockers
e. Angiotensin-converting enzyme inhibitors (ACEIs)
f. Angiotensin receptor blockers (ARBs)
g. β-Adrenergic blockers
h. Centrally acting α_2 agonists
i. Calcium channel blockers (CCBs)
j. Direct-acting vasodilators
k. Direct renin inhibitors
l. Loop diuretics
m. Nondihydropyridine CCBs
n. Potassium-sparing diuretics
o. Thiazide diuretics

CRITICAL THINKING, PRIORITIZATION, AND DELEGATION QUESTIONS

16. Hypertension in which patient would be classified as primary hypertension?
    a. Patient with diabetes who is in end-stage renal failure
    b. Adult with hyperthyroidism
    c. African American female who is postmenopausal
    d. Young adult male with an adrenal tumor
17. When possible, the nurse should assess the patient's BP with the patient in which position?
    a. Lying flat in bed
    b. Head elevated at least 45 degrees
    c. Sitting with arm hanging straight
    d. Arm at same level as heart
18. ▶ Which is true concerning the adverse effects of antihypertensive drugs?
    a. They affect adherence.
    b. They are life-threatening.
    c. They are necessary if the drug is effective.
    d. They cause loss of weight.
19. The teaching plan for a patient taking antihypertensive drugs should include which information? (**Select all that apply**.)
    a. Smoking can reduce the effectiveness of antihypertensive drugs.
    b. Eating fresh produce can help lower BP.
    c. Soda has substantial amounts of sodium without a salty taste.
    d. Calcium intake of 2500 mg/day helps lower BP.
    e. It is important to keep taking the drug even if you feel good.

20. When administering an antihypertensive drug to a patient who has a history of hypertension and type 2 diabetes mellitus, which is an appropriate outcome for therapy?
    a. BP 95/60 to 110/70 mm Hg
    b. BP 110/70 to 130/80 mm Hg
    c. BP 135/80 to 145/90 mm Hg
    d. BP 128/80 to 138/90 mm Hg

►21. Which laboratory results should be reported to the provider if a patient is receiving a thiazide diuretic?
    a. Blood urea nitrogen (BUN) 20 mg/dL
    b. Hemoglobin A1c 5.5%
    c. Potassium (K^+) 3.2 mEq/L
    d. Uric acid 20 mg/dL

22. A patient who is on which diuretic should be taught to avoid use of potassium-containing salt substitutes and excessive consumption of bananas and orange juice?
    a. Ethacrynic acid
    b. Furosemide
    c. Hydrochlorothiazide
    d. Spironolactone

23. β-Adrenergic blockers with intrinsic sympathomimetic activity decrease the incidence of which adverse effect?
    a. Bradycardia at rest
    b. Bronchoconstriction
    c. Heart block
    d. Hypoglycemia

✳24. Which is priority when a patient starts therapy with an α_1-blocker?
    a. Adequate exercise
    b. Hydration
    c. Safety
    d. Urinary output

25. A patient would most likely experience reflex tachycardia if receiving which antihypertensive drug?
    a. ACE inhibitors
    b. β-Blockers
    c. Direct-acting vasodilators
    d. Nondihydropyridine calcium channel blockers

✳26. Which is the priority action when caring for a patient who has just been prescribed a drug for hypertension?
    a. Identifying obstacles to adherence
    b. Teaching how the drug works
    c. Demonstrating how to assess BP
    d. Telling the patient their target BP

27. Which teaching is necessary to prevent one of the most serious adverse effects when taking clonidine for hypertension?
    a. Change positions slowly.
    b. Do not stop the drug suddenly.
    c. Exercise regularly.
    d. Use sugar-free candy.

28. Which drug class is recommended as first-line treatment for an African-American patient with hypertension?
    a. ACE inhibitor
    b. Calcium channel blocker
    c. Diuretic
    d. Vasodilator

29. Excessively elevated BP, in a patient with acute congestive heart failure, must be lowered in which period of time?
    a. 30 minutes
    b. 60 minutes
    c. 90 minutes
    d. 120 minutes

30. A positive human chorionic gonadotropin (hCG) would be of most concern if the patient is prescribed which drug?
    a. Captopril
    b. Hydrochlorothiazide
    c. Methyldopa
    d. Propranolol

31. Which is the best treatment for severe preeclampsia?
    a. Delivery of the fetus
    b. Labetalol
    c. Lisinopril
    d. Fluids

32. Which magnesium level is within the target range for a patient treated for eclampsia?
    a. 1 mEq/L
    b. 2 mEq/L
    c. 5 mEq/L
    d. 8 mEq/L

✳33. It would be priority to monitor capillary blood sugar rather than rely on symptoms that suggest hypoglycemia, if a patient is prescribed which class of antihypertensive drugs?
    a. ACE inhibitor
    b. β-Blocker
    c. Loop diuretic
    d. Thiazide diuretic

CASE STUDY

A 28-year-old African American female is admitted with a diagnosis of preeclampsia at 28 weeks gestation. This is the patient's second pregnancy; she experienced preeclampsia at 30 weeks with her previous pregnancy. Medical history includes type 1 diabetes and hypertension. On exam, the nurse obtains a BP of 160/94 mm Hg, heart rate of 94 bpm, respirations of 18 bpm, and a temperature of 98.2°F. Other findings include 2+ pitting edema in bilateral lower extremities. The 28-week-old fetus weighs 2 pounds and has a heart rate of 140 bpm.

1. What risk factors for preeclampsia does the patient have?
2. What is the drug of choice for lowering BP, including its dose and frequency?
3. If the patient develops seizures, then what drug would be administered? What monitoring parameters should be followed?

51 Drugs for Heart Failure

STUDY QUESTIONS

Matching

Match the patient symptoms of heart failure (HF) with the most appropriate patient problem.

1. ___ Faint peripheral pulses, decreased urine output
2. ___ Lack of exercise, high-fat diet
3. ___ Orthopnea, jugular venous distention (JVD)
4. ___ Palpitations, pallor
5. ___ Shortness of breath when walking to bathroom
   a. Motor function reduced
   b. Heart failure
   c. Fluid overload
   d. Need for health teaching
   e. Decreased tissue perfusion

Match the drug with its description.

6. ___ Improve left ventricle (LV) ejection fraction, reduce HF symptoms, increase exercise tolerance, decrease hospitalization, enhance quality of life, and reduce mortality.
7. ___ Produce profound diuresis; can promote fluid loss even when glomerular filtration rate (GFR) is low.
8. ___ Has profound effects on the mechanical and electrical properties of the heart; it has important neurohormonal effects.
9. ___ Block production of angiotensin II, decrease release of aldosterone, and suppress degradation of kinins, thereby improving hemodynamics and favorably altering cardiac remodeling.
10. ___ Indreases natriuretic peptides while suppressing the negative effects of the renin-angiotensin-aldosterone system (RAAS).
11. ___ Block aldosterone receptors in the heart and blood vessels.
12. ___ Produce moderate diuresis and is used when edema is not too great. Are ineffective when GFR is low; cannot be used if cardiac output is greatly reduced.
13. ___ Can improve LV ejection fraction, increase exercise tolerance, slow progression of HF, reduce the need for hospitalization, and prolong survival.
14. ___ Catecholamines that cause the activation of β_1-adrenergic receptors, increasing myocardial contractility, thereby improving cardiac performance.
15. ___ Increases myocardial contractility and promotes vasodilation through the inhibition of enzymes that degrade cyclic adenosine monophosphate (cAMP).
16. ___ Cardiovascular risk reduction in pateints with type 2 diabetes and atherosclerotic cardiovascular disease (ASCVD)
   a. Mineralocorticoid receptor antagonist
   b. Angiotensin-converting enzyme (ACE) inhibitors
   c. Angiotensin receptor blockers (ARBs)
   d. Beta-adrenergic receptor blockers (β-blockers)
   e. Cardiac glycosides
   f. Loop diuretics
   g. Sympathomimetic drugs
   h. Angiotensin receptor-neprilysin inhibitor
   i. Thiazide diuretics
   j. Phosphodiesterase inhibitors
   k. Sodium-glucose cotransporter 2 (SGLT-2) inhibitors

CRITICAL THINKING, PRIORITIZATION, AND DELEGATION QUESTIONS

17. Which statement, if made by a patient with HF, would indicate a need for further teaching?
   a. "If blood cannot get through my heart, the backup of fluid will make it hard for me to breathe."
   b. "My heart is stretching so much, it is losing the ability to squeeze out the blood."
   c. "The changes in my heart started when I began to feel tired and short of breath."
   d. "When my heart beats too fast, it cannot fill properly."
18. Which is the cause of the release of B-natriuretic peptide (BNP)?
   a. Tachycardia
   b. Atrial stretch
   c. Hypoxia
   d. Hypertrophy

19. The nurse would be most concerned if a patient with HF exhibits which sign? **(Select all that apply.)**
    a. Peripheral edema
    b. Urine output 35 mL/hr
    c. Jugular venous distension
    d. Weight gain of 3 pounds in 24 hrs
    e. Blood pressure 128/74 mm Hg

20. The nurse is caring for a patient with a history of heart failure. They are seen in the clinic for management. Upon questioning, the patient states that they are able to do some of the household chores, but now need assistance. They become short of breath going up stairs, after vacuuming the first floor of the house, they become short of breath and it feels like their heart is skipping beats, and they need to take a nap before they can vacuum the second floor. This patient is in which New York Heart Association Class?
    a. Class I
    b. Class II
    c. Class III
    d. Class IV

*21. A patient with HF is prescribed spironolactone and enalapril. It would be a priority to consult the provider regarding evaluation of the patient's potassium levels if the patient exhibited which symptom?
    a. Confusion
    b. Constipation
    c. Weakness
    d. Shallow respirations

*22. Which is a priority assessment when administering dopamine?
    a. Bowel sounds
    b. Capillary refill
    c. Temperature
    d. Urine output

23. The nurse is caring for a patient with heart failure and is on a maintenance infusion of milrinone. Their BNP is 675 pg/mL. Vital signs: blood pressure 156/86 mm Hg, temperature 97.8°F (36.5°C), pulse 122 beats per minute (bpm), and respirations 18 breaths per minute. Oxygen saturation is 94%. Lungs with bilateral rales. Bilateral lower extremities (LE) with 3+ pitting edema. Which would indicate a positive therapeutic response to the milrinone?
    a. Cough with frothy, white sputum
    b. Heart rate 132 bpm and irregular
    c. 1+ pitting edema bilateral LE
    d. Blood pressure 160/90 mm Hg

24. Isosorbide reduces the congestive symptoms of heart failure through which means?
    a. Relaxation of vascular smooth muscle
    b. Decreasing the conduction of impulses through the heart
    c. Decreasing the volume of blood in the vascular system
    d. Increasing myocardial remodeling

25. The nurse is preparing to administer hydralazine for HF. Because this drug has been associated with drug-induced lupus-like syndrome, it is a priority to report which symptom to the provider? **(Select all that apply.)**
    a. Facial rash
    b. Heartburn
    c. Joint pain
    d. Fever
    e. Diarrhea

26. A patient with heart failure and atrial fibrillation is taking digoxin 250 mcg PO daily. Which benefits can the patient expect by taking digoxin? **(Select all that apply.)**
    a. Prolonged life expectancy
    b. Increased exercise tolerance
    c. Reduced hospitalizations
    d. Symptom management
    e. Decreased urine output

►27. When a patient with HF is prescribed digoxin and furosemide, the nurse should carefully assess the patient for which symptom of digoxin toxicity?
    a. Anorexia
    b. Abdominal cramps
    c. Bone pain
    d. Muscle spasms

►28. Which findings in a patient with HF would warrant the nurse holding digoxin and notifying the provider?
    a. Blood pressure 100/76 mm Hg
    b. Digoxin level 2.4 ng/mL
    c. Heart rate 100 beats/min
    d. Potassium 5.3 mEq/L

29. The nurse would consult the provider if a patient in HF experiences pain and is prescribed which drug?
    a. Acetaminophen
    b. Imipramine
    c. Ibuprofen
    d. Morphine

30. A fixed dose of hydralazine and isosorbide has been approved to treat HF in people of which self-reported race?
    a. American Indian
    b. Asian
    c. Caucasian
    d. African American

*31. It is a priority to assess for digoxin toxicity if a patient's digoxin level is 1.3 ng/mL and the patient has which other laboratory result?
    a. BNP 1813 pg/mL
    b. International normalized ratio (INR) 1.5
    c. Potassium 3.0 mEq/L
    d. Sodium 150 mEq/L

32. Angiotensin receptor neprilysin inhibitors (ARNIs) may be used in place of which class of drugs, for patients with stage II–IV heart failure? **(Select all that apply.)**
    a. Aldosterone antagonists
    b. Angiotensin-converting enzyme inhibitors
    c. Angiotensin receptor blockers
    d. Direct renin inhibitors
    e. Potassium-sparing diuretics

DOSE CALCULATION QUESTIONS

33. Dobutamine HCl is prescribed at a rate of 2.5 mcg/kg per minute. The patient weighs 165 lb. The drug is available as 2 mg/mL of 5% dextrose. The IV pump is calibrated in milliliters per hour. What rate should the nurse program into the IV pump?

34. An IV bolus of 5 mg milrinone is prescribed for a patient who weighs 154 lb. Is the dose safe if the recommended dose is 25–75 mcg/kg?

CASE STUDIES

Case Study 1

An older adult patient with chronic HF who resides in a long-term care facility has been treated with digoxin 0.125 mg, furosemide 80 mg, and potassium chloride 20 mEq once a day for a long time. Recently, the provider added eplerenone 50 mg once a day to the medication regimen.

1. When consulting the provider about this patient, what questions might the nurse ask?

2. Why is it important for the nurse to monitor electrolyte and digoxin levels in this patient?

3. The long-term care night shift nurse noted that the patient has become increasingly restless, "coughs all night," and seems very fatigued when the staff is providing care. The patient's appetite has been poor, even for things they normally enjoy. Assessment findings include BP 90/70 mm Hg, alternating weak and strong pulse at a rate of 118 beats/min, S_3 ventricular gallop, rales throughout lung fields, and a 5-lb weight gain in the last week. What action should the nurse take?

4. The patient is admitted to an acute care facility. Based on the knowledge of digoxin and its relationship to potassium, how could these blood levels have contributed to the patient's decompensation?

Case Study 2

An older adult patient is a direct admission to the nursing unit with abdominal pain, nausea, and extreme weakness. The patient has a history of diabetes, chronic kidney disease, and sleep apnea. Admission nursing assessment findings include oxygen saturation 92% on room air, temperature 99.3°F, BP 174/110 mm Hg, pulse 96 and irregular, point of maximal impulse (PMI) shifted to the left, JVD 4.5 cm above the angle of Louis, 3 + pitting edema in the lower extremities, and tenderness in the right upper quadrant (RUQ) with abdominal palpation.

5. What patient problem is most appropriate for this patient?

6. The nurse obtains laboratory results from tests drawn on admission, including BNP 1275 pg/mL, K^+ 5.4 mEq/L, creatinine 2.7 mg/dL, and blood urea nitrogen (BUN) 42 mg/dL. The nurse contacts the provider, who orders a STAT electrocardiogram, which shows S-T changes. What action should the nurse take at this point?

7. The patient is transferred to the coronary care unit. Oxygen is administered along with furosemide, nitroglycerin, and enalapril. What is the rationale for administration of these drugs?

8. The patient is stabilized and is transferred to the nursing unit. Prescribed drugs include carvedilol, enalapril, and furosemide. What laboratory values does the nurse need to monitor when a patient is receiving these drugs?

9. What teaching should the nurse provide to prepare this patient for discharge?

10. The patient lives in an apartment building with 12 stairs to climb to his apartment. After climbing the stairs, they need to rest because due to short of breath. The patient can, however, perform most activities of daily living. According to the New York Heart Association (NYHA), what is this patient's HF classification?

52 Antidysrhythmic Drugs

STUDY QUESTIONS

Completion

1. *Arrhythmia* is not as accurate a term as *dysrhythmia* because arrhythmia literally means ____________________ of a heart rhythm.
2. *Dysrhythmia* means ____________________ heart rhythm.
3. *Bradydysrhythmia* is the term for a dysrhythmia that is ____________________ than normal.
4. *Tachydysrhythmia* is the term for a dysrhythmia that is ____________________ than normal.
5. More rapid depolarization of Purkinje fibers results in synchronized ____________________ contraction.

Matching

Match the electrolyte with the effect of blocking rapid potentials.

6. ___ Blocking this ion slows impulse conduction.
7. ___ Blocking this ion reduces myocardial contractility.
8. ___ Blocking this ion delays repolarization.
   a. Calcium
   b. Potassium
   c. Sodium

Match the antidysrhythmic drug class with its action.

9. ___ Delay repolarization of fast potentials by blocking potassium (K^+) channels
10. ___ Reduce calcium (Ca^+) entry during fast and slow depolarization and depress phase 4 repolarization of slow potentials
11. ___ Slow impulse conduction in atria and ventricles by blocking sodium (Na^+) channels
    a. Class I
    b. Classes II and IV
    c. Class III

CRITICAL THINKING, PRIORITIZATION, AND DELEGATION QUESTIONS

*12. Which is the priority patient problem for a patient with a dysrhythmia?
   a. Reduced perfusion
   b. Fluid balance
   c. Ischemia
   d. Dyspnea

13. Multiple P waves before the QRS complex on an electrocardiogram (ECG) indicate which condition?
   a. Atria are depolarizing faster than the ventricles.
   b. Atrial impulses to the ventricles are being slowed.
   c. Ventricles are depolarizing faster than the atria.
   d. Ventricular impulses to the atria are being slowed.

14. Ectopic foci can dominate the pace of the heart if the discharges of the ectopic stimuli have which characteristic?
   a. Atrial in origin
   b. Faster than the sinoatrial (SA) node
   c. From the ventricles
   d. Slower than the SA node

►15. A patient has been prescribed an antidysrhythmic drug that prolongs the QT interval on an ECG. The nurse should teach the patient the importance of reporting which symptom that suggests that torsades de pointes may be occurring?
   a. Ankle edema
   b. Feeling faint
   c. Headache
   d. Shortness of breath

16. Instructing a patient on the Valsalva maneuver is asking the patient to perform which activity?
   a. Bear down as if having a bowel movement.
   b. Breathe through pursed lips.
   c. Pant like a dog.
   d. Tighten the pelvic floor muscles.

►17. A focused nursing assessment of a patient with atrial fibrillation should always include assessment of which changes?
   a. Appetite
   b. Bowel pattern
   c. Deep tendon reflexes
   d. Mental status

18. Which laboratory result for international normalized ratio (INR) would indicate that warfarin therapy has achieved the desired effect in a patient with atrial fibrillation?
    a. INR between 0.9 and 1.1
    b. INR between 2 and 3
    c. INR between 5 and 9
    d. INR greater than 10

19. The nurse responds quickly when a ventricular tachydysrhythmia is identified because this type of dysrhythmia impairs which ability of the heart?
    a. Contract rapidly enough to meet body needs
    b. Eject an adequate amount of blood
    c. Close valves properly
    d. Open valves properly

20. A patient with a dysrhythmia, type 2 diabetes mellitus (T2DM), and heart failure (HF) is prescribed quinidine, metformin, furosemide, and digoxin. The nurse should be vigilant in monitoring for which early adverse effect of digoxin toxicity that may occur with this combination of drugs?
    a. Nausea
    b. Clammy skin
    c. Excessive thirst
    d. Double vision

*21. Which of these assessment findings, if identified in a patient receiving quinidine, is of greatest priority to report to the prescriber?
    a. Blood pressure 150/88 mm Hg
    b. Tinnitus
    c. Sudden dyspnea
    d. Three soft stools in 8 hours

22. A patient asks the nurse why they were instructed to take quinidine with food. Which is an appropriate response by the nurse?
    a. Decreases GI symptoms
    b. Increases absorption
    c. Prevents cinchonism
    d. Prevents tachycardia

►23. The nurse monitors the telemetry of a patient receiving a continuous IV infusion of quinidine at 0.02 mg/kg/min. The nurse notes that the QRS complex was widened 25% from pre–drug therapy findings. Which is the priority nursing action?
    a. Administer a β-blocker.
    b. Continue nursing care.
    c. Discontinue monitoring the ECG.
    d. Notify the prescriber immediately.

24. The nurse should assess patients receiving long-term therapy with procainamide for which adverse effect? **(Select all that apply.)**
    a. Dyspnea
    b. Chest pain
    c. Palpitations
    d. Thrombocytopenia
    e. Edema

*25. Which anticholinergic effect of disopyramide would be priority to report to the prescriber?
    a. Blurred vision
    b. Dry mouth
    c. No bowel movement × 2 days
    d. Postvoid residual of 350 mL

26. Because of extensive first-pass effect, the nurse expects to administer lidocaine in which manner?
    a. Via nasogastric tube
    b. Intravenously
    c. Orally with water
    d. Sustained-release formula

*27. Which adverse effect of propafenone, if occurring for 3–4 days, would be of most concern to the nurse?
    a. Abdominal pain
    b. Anorexia
    c. Dizziness
    d. Vomiting

28. The nurse is preparing to administer acebutolol. Which assessment would indicate the need for immediate consultation with the prescriber?
    a. Apical pulse 105 beats/min
    b. Bronchial wheezes
    c. Blood glucose 220 mg/dL
    d. 1+ pitting edema

29. The patient must be informed of possible damage to the lungs when prescribed oral therapy with which drug?
    a. Amiodarone
    b. Dofetilide
    c. Propafenone
    d. Propranolol

30. In addition to monitoring the heart rate and rhythm, which must the nurse continuously monitor when administering IV amiodarone?
    a. Blood pressure
    b. Level of consciousness
    c. Intravenous site
    d. Respiratory effort

31. Propranolol is contraindicated in patients with which conditions? **(Select all that apply.)**
    a. Sinus bradicardia
    b. Asthma
    c. Heart failure
    d. High degree heart block
    e. QT prolongation

32. Which laboratory results would increase the risk of cardiotoxicity when a patient is prescribed digoxin?
    a. Potassium 3.2 mg/dL
    b. Potassium 5.3 mg/dL
    c. Sodium 132 mg/dL
    d. Sodium 148 mg/dL

✳33. Which is a priority for the nurse to teach a patient prescribed verapamil?
    a. Drink 2500 mL of fluid each day.
    b. Increase fiber in the diet.
    c. Take orthostatic BP precautions.
    d. Report bruising.

34. Which nursing action is most appropriate when administering adenosine IV?
    a. Administer oxygen.
    b. Check apical heart rate.
    c. Evaluate for edema
    d. Monitor cardiac rhythm.

35. In which case does the need for antidysrhythmic drugs exceed the risks of adverse effects?
    a. Dysrhythmia is prolonged.
    b. QT interval is excessively long.
    c. Ventricular pumping is ineffective.
    d. SA node discharges at a rate 160 beats/min.

DOSE CALCULATION QUESTIONS

36. A patient who weighs 165 lb is prescribed IV diltiazem. The recommended initial bolus dose is 0.25 mg/kg. What is the recommended dose for this patient?

37. One gram of lidocaine in 250 mL of 5% dextrose in water at a rate of 2 mg/min is prescribed. The IV pump is calibrated in milliliters per hour. What rate should be programmed into the pump?

CASE STUDY

An older adult underwent open-heart surgery 5 days ago and postoperatively developed a cerebrovascular accident (CVA). The patient has a history of hypertension, kidney dysfunction, alcohol use disorder, and a two-pack-per-day smoking habit. They are progressing well postoperatively without any further complications. A physical therapist and nurse assisted the patient to transfer to a recliner. Following transfer, the patient stated that their heart felt "like it was racing."

1. What assessment should the nurse perform?

The nurse checks on the patient because the monitor showed a heart rate of 185 beats/min. The nurse asks the patient to bear down to stimulate the vagus nerve and slow the heart rate. After obtaining a full set of vital signs, the nurse calls the provider. The provider orders a STAT 12-lead ECG. The provider arrives on the unit, examines the 12-lead ECG, and diagnoses ventricular tachycardia. A bolus dose of lidocaine 100 mg is ordered.

2. What precautions must the nurse take before and during administration of the IV bolus dose?

3. The bolus dose is followed by an infusion of a solution of lidocaine. What patient data can the nurse provide to assist the prescriber with determining the amount of fluid with which to dilute the lidocaine?

4. What should be included when the nurse reports to the prescriber the patient's response to lidocaine?

53 Drugs That Help Normalize Cholesterol and Triglyceride Levels

STUDY QUESTIONS

Completion

1. Cholesterol is required for synthesis of certain __________ and ___________ ________.
2. The ________________ is the primary source of endogenous cholesterol in the body.
3. When trying to lower blood cholesterol, it is important to reduce intake of _______________ fats.
4. ________________ serve as carriers for transporting lipids in blood.
5. *Hydrophilic* means ______________________ __________________, and *hydrophobic* means __________________ __________________.
6. Lovaza is approved as an adjunct to dietary measures to reduce levels of triglycerides greater than _____________ mg/dL.
7. Vascepa is recommended for patients taking a statin with a triglyceride level greater than _____________ mg/dL.
8. The recommendation for regular physical activity is _____________ to _____________ minutes on most days.

CRITICAL THINKING, PRIORITIZATION, AND DELEGATION QUESTIONS

9. A patient who is a one-pack-per-day smoker for 15 years with a family history of coronary heart disease (CHD) has been prescribed a lipid-lowering medication. Which outcome would be most important for this patient?
   a. Cholesterol total less than 200 mg/dL
   b. HDL greater than 40 mg/dL
   c. LDL less than 100 mg/dL
   d. Triglycerides less than 150 mg/dL
10. A patient has received instructions regarding cholesterol and the body. Which statement made by the patient would indicate they need further teaching?
    a. "Drugs that decrease the liver's ability to produce cholesterol should be taken at night."
    b. "Drugs to prevent the absorption of cholesterol are the most effective drugs."
    c. "It is very important to limit the amount of saturated fat in my diet."
    d. "My cholesterol can be high even if I eat a low-fat diet and exercise regularly."
11. Recent laboratory results for a patient include HDL 85 mg/dL, LDL 145 mg/dL, and triglycerides 630 mg/dL. Which assessment should the nurse perform?
    a. Abdominal
    b. Respiratory
    c. Integument
    d. Cardiac
12. The nurse has reviewed the laboratory results for a patient who is scheduled to receive lovastatin 40 mg. Results include aspartate aminotransferase (AST) 122 units/L, alanine aminotransferase (ALT) 155 units/L, creatine kinase (CK) 250 units/L, HDL 45 mg/dL, and LDL 245 mg/dL. Which action should the nurse take?
    a. Administer the drug.
    b. Hold the drug.
    c. Assess for abdominal pain.
    d. Notify the provider.
13. A patient has been diagnosed with hypercholesterolemia. The provider has ordered simvastatin 20 mg, once a day at hour of sleep, to be started after laboratory results are obtained. Which laboratory result should be reported to the provider?
    a. ALT 57 international units (IU)/L
    b. Creatinine 1.4 mg/IU/dL
    c. C-reactive protein (CRP) 3 mg/dL
    d. Human chorionic gonadotropin 287 IU/L
14. A patient who is receiving lovastatin experiences chest pain. CK level is 580 units/mL (CK-MM 99%) and troponin T 0.02 g/mL. It is priority for the nurse to monitor the functioning of which organ?
    a. Brain
    b. Heart
    c. Kidneys
    d. Lungs
15. The nurse is teaching a patient starting treatment with evolocumab. Which would indicate the patient understands their instructions?
    a. "Redness and pain at the injection site are normal."
    b. "The drug will be given by intramuscular injection."
    c. "The home health nurse will fill my syringes."
    d. "I should call my health care provider if I develop a rash."
16. The nurse has been caring for a patient with dehydration. The patient has been taking colesevelam and reports nausea. Which is the most common adverse effect of this drug?
    a. Bloating
    b. Flatulence
    c. Constipation
    d. Indigestion

17. A patient has been prescribed cholestyramine in addition to hydrochlorothiazide. The hydrochlorothiazide should be administered at which time in relation to the cholestyramine?
    a. 1 hour after
    b. 1 hour before
    c. 2 hours after
    d. 2 hours before

18. The nurse would be most concerned about which patient?
    a. One experiencing a rash while on lovastatin.
    b. A patient on cholestyramine reporting constipation
    c. While on colesevelam a patient experiencing dyspepsia
    d. Right upper quadrant pain in a patient receiving gemfibrozil

19. Which laboratory test result would be of concern if noted in a patient prescribed ezetimibe?
    a. ALT 35 IU/L
    b. Blood urea nitrogen 20 mg/dL
    c. Platelets 75,000/mm^3
    d. White blood cell 10,000/mm^3

20. A patient with a history of atrial fibrillation is prescribed gemfibrozil and warfarin. Which international normalized ratio (INR) result suggests that the warfarin dose is therapeutic?
    a. INR 1
    b. INR 3
    c. INR 6
    d. INR 10

21. The nurse would teach the patient strategies to prevent constipation if the patient was prescribed which drug for dyslipidemia?
    a. Atorvastatin
    b. Colestipol
    c. Gemfibrozil
    d. Niacin

22. Which statement suggests that the patient prescribed colesevelam needs additional teaching?
    a. "The powder can be mixed in applesauce."
    b. "I can take it at the same time as my other drugs."
    c. "Colesevelam can be taken as a dry powder."
    d. "It is a good idea to drink water with the drug."

23. Proprotein convertase subtilisin/kexin type 9 (PCSK9) inhibitors are indicated for which patients:
    a. One who cannot tolerate taking statin drugs
    b. Patients with type 2 diabetes with peripheral neuropathy
    c. A history of familial hypercholesterolemia
    d. Primary treatment in those with known CAD

24. Adenosine triphosphate-citrate lyase (ACL) inhibitors can contribute to the development of which adverse effect? **(Select all that apply.)**
    a. Hypercalcemia
    b. Hyperuricemia
    c. Hyperkalemia
    d. Pancreatitis
    e. Tendon rupture

25. Icosapent ethyl is indicated to reduce ASCVD events in patients with diabetes by targeting:
    a. Total cholesterol
    b. LDL cholesterol
    c. Triglycerides
    d. HDL cholesterol

DOSE CALCULATION QUESTIONS

26. Colesevelam is supplied as 625-mg tablets. How many tablets should the nurse administer if the prescribed dose is 1.9 g?

27. Gemfibrozil 600 mg has been prescribed twice daily. Available are 600 mg tablets. How many tablets should be administered each dose?

CASE STUDY

A patient with type 2 diabetes has been prescribed simvastatin because, despite good nutrition and exercise resulting in A1c within acceptable levels, their LDL cholesterol has not dropped below 150 mg/dL. The patient asks why they need additional bloodwork (liver function test [LFT], CK, and human chorionic gonadotropin [hCG]) before the provider will prescribe the drug.

1. How should the nurse respond?

2. What teaching should the nurse provide about birth control?

3. The patient asks how they would know if liver or muscle cell damage was occurring. What should be included in the explanation?

4. Why is it important to teach the patient to report chest pain and to describe the characteristics and whether it is worsened by coughing or laughing?

5. The patient calls after getting the prescription filled. They state that the nurse told them to take the drug in the evening, but the pharmacy information states that it can be taken at any time. How should the telephone triage nurse respond?

54 Drugs for Angina Pectoris

STUDY QUESTIONS

Completion

1. Angina pectoris occurs when the ____________ supply to the ________________ is inadequate.
2. Cardiac oxygen demand is determined by heart rate, contractility, ____________________, and ____________________.
3. Arterial blood flow to myocardial cells occurs during the ____________________ phase of a heartbeat.
4. The most common drug used to decrease platelet activity is ____________________.

CRITICAL THINKING, PRIORITIZATION, AND DELEGATION QUESTIONS

✳5. Which is the priority patient problem for a patient with angina pectoris?
   a. Heart failure
   b. Decreased gas exchange
   c. Decreased tissue perfusion: cardiopulmonary
   d. Dyspnea

6. Which is the goal of drug therapy for chronic stable angina?
   a. Constrict coronary arteries to increase blood pressure
   b. Decrease myocardial need for oxygen during stress
   c. Increase myocardial blood flow during systole
   d. Prevent coronary artery spasms with activity

7. A patient asks the nurse why nitroglycerin can be administered in so many ways. Which is the basis of the nurse's response?
   a. Does not undergo first-pass effect in the liver.
   b. Has very few adverse effects when given by different routes.
   c. Is an inactive compound, so route does not matter.
   d. Delay hepatic metabolism and prolong therapeutic effects.

8. A patient who has been using a nitroglycerin patch for angina has recently been prescribed verapamil. Which statement, if made by this patient, would suggest that the patient understood teaching about the new drug?
   a. "I need to take this drug because nitroglycerin causes my blood pressure to go up."
   b. "If I experience erectile dysfunction from verapamil, I can take sildenafil."
   c. "This drug prevents my heart from racing, which happens with nitroglycerin."
   d. "Adding verapamil will make the nitroglycerin work better."

▶9. A patient is prescribed a nitroglycerin patch that is to be applied at 0900 hrs and removed at 2100 hrs. When preparing to administer the 0900 hrs patch, the nurse notes that a nitroglycerin patch is still in place. Which is the appropriate nursing action?
   a. Leave the old patch on until the nursing supervisor is contacted.
   b. Consult with the prescriber regarding application of a new patch.
   c. Remove the old patch and apply the new patch to a different site.
   d. Change the timing of the medication to remove the patch at 0900 hrs.

10. When collecting data from a patient who is not obtaining relief from sublingual nitroglycerin tablets, the nurse should ask whether the patient allows the tablet to completely dissolve in their mouth. Which is the basis for letting the tablet completely dissolve in the mouth?
   a. If swallowed, the liver inactivates the drug before it works.
   b. Dissolving the tablet in the mouth decreases drug tolerance.
   c. Prevents the small intestine from absorbing the drug.
   d. Speeds excretion of the drug via the kidneys and urine.

11. Which is important for the nurse to teach a patient who has been prescribed sublingual nitroglycerin tablet on an as-needed basis?
   a. Discard unused tablets after 12 months.
   b. Store the tablets in a cabinet in the bathroom.
   c. Keep a few tablets in their pocket for emergency use.
   d. Store in the original container with lid tightly closed.

▶12. When assessing a patient who is scheduled to receive the second dose of newly prescribed sustained-release nitroglycerin, the patient reports a headache. Which action should the nurse take?
   a. Administer as-needed analgesic.
   b. Crush the medication to speed absorption.
   c. Notify the prescriber of the headache.
   d. Withhold the medication.

13. The nurse is aware that which nitroglycerin preparation has a rapid onset?
   a. Sublingual tablets
   b. Sustained-release capsule
   c. Topical ointment
   d. Transdermal patch

▶14. The nurse is talking to a patient about smoking cessation. Which statement indicates the patient understands the benefits of quitting?
  a. "Smoking only increases my risk for heart attack by 25%, so why quit?"
  b. "Smoking cessation does little to reduce the risk for heart attack."
  c. "Smoking cessation will significantly reduce my risk for heart attack."
  d. "I will still have angina, even if I quit smoking; why stop now?"

15. The nurse recognizes that a drug is a β-blocker if the generic name of the drug ends in which suffix?
  a. -cillin
  b. -olol
  c. -pril
  d. -sartan

16. Which is the reason β-blockers are useful to improve myocardial oxygen supply in angina?
  a. Dilate the coronary arteries.
  b. Increase cardiac contractility.
  c. Decrease cardiac oxygen demand.
  d. Reduce blood return to the heart.

17. The nurse would withhold a β_1-blocker and immediately contact the prescriber if it was discovered that the patient has a history of which condition?
  a. Asthma
  b. Heart block
  c. Hyperglycemia
  d. Sick sinus syndrome

18. Which drugs are used to suppress nitroglycerin-induced tachycardia? **(Select all that apply.)**
  a. Diltiazem
  b. Isosorbide
  c. Metoprolol
  d. Nifedipine
  e. Verapamil

✳19. Which would warrant notification of the provider when the nurse is caring for a patient who is receiving ranolazine?
  a. Estimated glomerular filtration rate (eGFR) 95 mL/min
  b. Penicillin allergy
  c. Normoglycemia
  d. Unexplained fainting

DOSE CALCULATION QUESTIONS

20. Nitroglycerin topical ointment (2%) is dispensed from a tube, and the length of the ribbon squeezed from the tube determines dosage. (One inch contains about 15 mg of nitroglycerin.) How many inches would equal 30 mg?

21. Intravenous (IV) nitroglycerin is prescribed at a rate of 5 mcg/min. The drug is available in a premixed glass bottle with 100 mg/L of 5% dextrose in water (D_5W). The IV pump is calibrated in milliliter/hour. At what rate should the nurse program the pump?

CASE STUDIES

Case Study 1

An older adult with a history of stable angina, asthma, and hypertension is admitted to the hospital with substernal chest pain that was not relieved by three sublingual nitroglycerin tablets. In the emergency department, the patient is prescribed diltiazem and an IV nitroglycerin drip.

1. What actions must the nurse take when administering IV nitroglycerin?

2. The patient's pain is relieved after receiving a dosage of 330 mcg/min. They are admitted to the coronary care unit. Vital signs are stable, and they are currently without pain. Cardiac enzyme levels do not suggest myocardial cell death. The electrocardiogram (ECG) shows normal sinus rhythm. The provider believes that the patient is having classic angina and not a myocardial infarction. Orders are received for the patient to be weaned from the nitroglycerin drip and nitroglycerin transdermal patches 10 mg/24 per hour started. The patient is also prescribed aspirin 81 mg, diltiazem-CD 30 mg, and ramipril 2.5 mg once a day. If the provider wants continuous administration of nitroglycerin when changing the patient from the nitroglycerin drip to the patch, should the nurse apply the nitroglycerin patch?

3. What teaching should the nurse provide about administration of the nitroglycerin patch?

4. The patient has the nitroglycerin drip turned off, the nitroglycerin patch is applied, and the diltiazem-CD is administered. They ask the nurse what may have been the reason that the nitroglycerin sublingual tablets did not work. Based on knowledge of nitroglycerin sublingual tablets, what factors may have contributed to why the nitroglycerin tablets did not relieve the anginal pain?

5. The nurse asks the patient's partner to bring the patient's supply of sublingual nitroglycerin tablets to the hospital. The partner shows the nurse a small plastic pill container. "Heart pills" is handwritten on a masking tape label. What teaching does the nurse need to provide?

6. The patient states that they will not need to get any more nitroglycerin sublingual tablets now that they are using the nitroglycerin patches. How should the nurse respond?

7. The nurse is reconciling medications during discharge instructions. The patient admits to adherence issues with taking his antihypertensive drug therapy because of experiencing erectile dysfunction. They ask what the nurse thinks about sildenafil. What information should the nurse provide?

Case Study 2

A farmer who lives in a remote area was admitted with chest pain. They have been diagnosed with angina and are being discharged with a prescription for sublingual nitroglycerin tablets.

8. What teaching should the nurse provide about administration and storage of this drug?

9. The provider has written instructions that this patient should take the nitroglycerin before participating in stressful activity. What teaching should the nurse provide, considering that farm work includes operation of potentially dangerous equipment?

10. The provider has instructed this patient to continue to take nitroglycerin up to three tablets 5 minutes apart, take an aspirin, and seek emergency medical care if relief is not obtained after administration of the first sublingual nitroglycerin tablet. The patient's partner states that an older family member took nitroglycerin and had been instructed to seek medical care if relief was not experienced after taking three tablets. Why are the provider's instructions logical for this patient?

11. The patient has been instructed to take one baby aspirin tablet per day. The patient verbalizes that this seems silly because one baby aspirin tablet will not do much to relieve chest pain. How should the nurse respond?

55 Anticoagulant, Antiplatelet, and Thrombolytic Drugs

STUDY QUESTIONS

True or False

For each of the following statements, enter T for true or F for false.

1. ___ Patients who take anticoagulant, antiplatelet, and thrombolytic drugs are at risk for bleeding.
2. ___ Pregnant or nursing patients should never be prescribed heparin.
3. ___ Anticoagulant and antiplatelet drugs only affect the formation of clots, not removal.
4. ___ When given at prescribed doses, anticoagulant and antiplatelet drugs can cause unintended bleeding.
5. ___ *Hemostasis* is a synonym for clot.
6. ___ *Aggregation* means clustering.

CRITICAL THINKING, PRIORITIZATION, AND DELEGATION QUESTIONS

7. A patient asks why heparin cannot be administered orally. Which is the basis of the nurse's response?
   a. It has a prolonged half-life when administered orally.
   b. It can only be prepared as an oral solution and is bitter tasting.
   c. It is destroyed by proteases in the gastrointestinal tract.
   d. Heparin is large and negatively charged, limiting absorption.

✳8. Which of these laboratory test results would be a priority to report to the provider if a patient is prescribed heparin?
   a. Activated partial thromboplastin time (aPTT) 75 seconds
   b. Blood urea nitrogen (BUN) 22 mg/dL
   c. Platelet count 40,000/mm^3
   d. White blood cell (WBC) 11,000/mm^3

9. Which action should the nurse take when a patient who has been receiving heparin tells the nurse that she thinks she could be pregnant?
   a. Administer the heparin.
   b. Withhold the heparin.
   c. Confirm pregnancy status.
   d. Consult the provider.

▶10. Which teaching older adults, teaching should be provided for the patient to prevent a common adverse effect of long-term anticoagulant therapy?
   a. Use disposable razors.
   b. Reduce risk of falls.
   c. Avoid vigorous exercise.
   d. Use TUMS for heart burn.

▶11. A patient is scheduled for a below-knee amputation at 1000. Heparin 5000 units is scheduled to be administered subcutaneously (subQ) at 2100 the evening prior to surgery and 0900 the morning of surgery. Which is the appropriate nursing action?
   a. Administer both doses of the drug as ordered.
   b. Contact the provider regarding the 2100 dose.
   c. Withhold the medication.
   d. Contact the provider regarding the 0900 dose.

12. A 110-lb patient who has just received a subcutaneous dose of 4000 units of heparin has developed hemoccult-positive stool. A STAT aPTT is 155 seconds. The provider orders protamine sulfate. Which is the recommended dose of protamine?
   a. 10 mg
   b. 20 mg
   c. 40 mg
   d. 60 mg

13. Which aPTT result suggests that heparin therapy is in the therapeutic range?
   a. 30–40 seconds
   b. 40–50 seconds
   c. 60–80 seconds
   d. 90–120 seconds

14. Intravenous heparin 5000 units every 6 hours is prescribed. Doses are scheduled at 1200, 1800, 2400, and 0600. If following monitoring recommendations, the nurse will enter a laboratory request for the aPTT specimen to be obtained at which times?
   a. Once daily
   b. Twice daily
   c. One hour after dosing
   d. An hour before each dose

►15. A victim of trauma is prescribed heparin after open reduction and internal fixation (ORIF) of multiple fractures. Which symptom would be of greatest concern to the nurse after beginning subcutaneous heparin therapy?
   a. Bruising at injection site
   b. Severe headache
   c. Temperature 100°F (37.8°C)
   d. Bleeding gums

16. The nurse would consult the provider if which drug was prescribed with no order for monitoring of aPTT?
   a. Fragmin
   b. Heparin
   c. Warfarin
   d. Lovenox

17. Which statement applies to enoxaparin? **(Select all that apply.)**
   a. It costs less than unfractionated heparin.
   b. Dosing may be based on the patient's weight.
   c. Used to prevent PE following STEMI
   d. Protamine sulfate is an effective antidote.
   e. Twice-daily dosing is every 12 hours.

✳18. An older adult, weighing 143 lb, was admitted with a hip fracture and is scheduled for an ORIF of the hip the next day. Which is a priority to report to the provider if the patient is prescribed enoxaparin?
   a. Warfarin is ordered to start in 2 days
   b. Estimated glomerular filtration rate 85 mL/min
   c. International normalized ratio (INR) 1.2
   d. Spinal anesthesia will be administered for surgery.

19. Observations and research suggest that which OTC product might increase the effects of warfarin and increase the risk of bleeding? **(Select all that apply.)**
   a. Acetaminophen
   b. Disulfiram
   c. Cimetidine
   d. Rifampin
   e. Amiodarone

20. The nurse should teach patients who are prescribed warfarin to eat consistent amounts of which food? **(Select all that apply.)**
   a. Citrus fruits
   b. Liver
   c. Canola oil
   d. Mayonnaise
   e. Red meat

►21. Which should the nurse teach a patient concerning precautions before dental surgery when the patient is prescribed long-term warfarin therapy?
   a. No action is needed.
   b. Inform the dentist of INR results.
   c. Stop warfarin 3 days before dental surgery.
   d. Reduce warfarin dose for 3 days before surgery.

22. For how long after warfarin therapy has been discontinued should the nurse maintain precautions to prevent bleeding?
   a. 6 hours
   b. 8–12 hours
   c. 2.5 days
   d. 5 days

✳23. It would be of greatest priority to consult the provider if the nurse notes which laboratory test result for a patient who is prescribed dabigatran?
   a. Alanine aminotransferase (ALT) 65 IU/L
   b. Estimated glomerular filtration rate 14 mL/min
   c. Human chorionic gonadotropin (hCG) 2 mIU/mL
   d. Aspartate transferase (AST) 10 IU/L

✳24. Which assessment is priority when a patient is prescribed bivalirudin?
   a. Orthostatic vital signs
   b. Intake and output
   c. Pain with movement
   d. Percent meals eaten

25. The nurse is teaching a patient about rivaroxaban prescribed after right knee replacement surgery. Which statement made by the patient suggests understanding of the teaching?
   a. "I should use a soft toothbrush and electric razor."
   b. "I should not touch the needle when injecting this drug."
   c. "I only need to have a blood test once a month."
   d. "If I have sudden shortness of breath, I should just sit down."

26. Which statement, if made by a patient who has been prescribed low-dose aspirin therapy, would indicate a need for further teaching?
   a. "I need to tell my pharmacist I am taking aspirin."
   b. "I should develop a plan to quit smoking."
   c. "I should not use a drug that reduces stomach acid."
   d. "Enteric-coated aspirin eliminates the risk of GI bleeding."

27. A patient with acute coronary syndrome (ACS) who is taking clopidogrel vomits greenish-brown liquid with dark brown particles. Which action should the nurse take?
   a. Complete a head-to-toe assessment.
   b. Request an order for an emesis Hematest.
   c. Call the provider for an antiemetic.
   d. Stop administration of the clopidogrel.

28. The nurse is caring for a patient with a history of PUD who routinely takes omeprazole. The provider orders clopidogrel daily. Which is the appropriate nursing action?
   a. Only administer omeprazole.
   b. Hold the omeprazole.
   c. Administer both drugs.
   d. Withhold both drugs.

29. The nurse receives the laboratory report on the genetic testing of a patient prescribed warfarin. The results indicate the patient has the varient gene that codes for CYP2C9. Which does the nurse anticipate concerning the administration of warfarin?
    a. Reduction in dose
    b. Increase in dose
    c. Discontinuation of drug
    d. No change in dose

▶30. The nurse is reviewing the laboratory test result of a patient who has been prescribed heparin for the past week. The platelet count is 75,000/mm^3. Which is the nursing priority?
    a. Assessing adequate cardiac output
    b. Evaluating effective airway clearance
    c. Maintaining skin integrity
    d. Preventing thrombus formation

31. A patient who received abciximab as an adjunct to percutaneous coronary intervention (PCI) develops a hard lump at the access site and pain in the leg. Which nursing action would be appropriate? **(Select all that apply.)**
    a. Administer oxygen.
    b. Apply pressure over site.
    c. Maintain bed rest.
    d. Outline any bleeding dressing.
    e. Prepare for a CT scan.

32. Which is the advantage of rivaroxab over warfarin? **(Select all that apply.)**
    a. Few drug-food interactions.
    b. Has once daily dosing.
    c. Has an antidote for overdose.
    d. No blood tests are needed.
    e. Has a rapid onset.

33. The nurse teaches a patient who has been prescribed cilostazol that the risk of bleeding is increased if the patient includes which food in the diet?
    a. Cabbage
    b. Dairy products
    c. Grapefruit juice
    d. Green vegetables

*34. Which instruction is priority when teaching the family of a patient who is at risk for myocardial infarction?
    a. Drugs can open clogged circulation.
    b. It is important that they donate blood.
    c. Seek immediate medical care when symptoms start.
    d. Thrombolytic drugs carry a significant risk of bleeding.

35. Which is true concerning anti–factor Xa heparin assay? **(Select all that apply.)**
    a. It indirectly measures heparin and its activity.
    b. The test is not affected by other physiologic variables.
    c. Therapeutic levels range from 03 to 0.7 IU/mL.
    d. One drawback of the assay is increased cost over aPTT.
    e. Cannot be used to guide titration of IV heparin.

36. Protease-activated receptor-1 (PAR-1) antagonists are used in conjunction with aspirin or clopidogrel to decrease thrombotic events in patients with a history of which condition? **(Select all that apply.)**
    a. Venous occlusive disease
    b. Myocardial infarction
    c. Carotid stenosis
    d. Peripheral arterial disease
    e. Pulmonary embolus

DOSE CALCULATION QUESTIONS

37. A patient who received 5000 units of heparin subQ at 0900 develops hematemesis at 1030. The provider orders 50 mg of protamine sulfate via slow IV push injection. Protamine sulfate is available as 10 mg/mL. How many milliliters will the nurse administer?

38. The nurse calculates the safe dose of tirofiban for a 220-lb patient undergoing balloon angioplasty. The drug comes in a solution of 12.5 mg/250 mL. The IV pump is calibrated in milliliters per hour. What rate will the nurse enter into the IV pump per hour?

CASE STUDY

A young adult who weighs 132 lb is admitted for treatment of a deep vein thrombosis (DVT) in the right thigh. The patient has a job that requires frequent long airplane trips. The patient's partner asks why the patient's primary care provider did not prescribe low-dose aspirin to prevent DVTs.

1. How should the nurse respond?

2. The patient is initially ordered a heparin drip by the emergency department provider. What is the most common adverse effect of heparin, and what symptoms of this adverse effect should be monitored by the nurse?

3. The patient's primary care provider discontinues the IV heparin and orders enoxaparin 60 mg subQ every 12 hours. How much time should elapse between the nurse discontinuing the heparin drip and starting the subQ enoxaparin? Why?

56 Management of ST-Elevation Myocardial Infarction

STUDY QUESTIONS

Completion

1. The medical term for a heart attack is ___________________ ___________________.
2. The abbreviation for a myocardial infarction (MI) with complete blockage of the coronary artery is ___________________.
3. In myocardial infarction, the heart muscle is ___________________ secondary to local ischemia.
4. Myocardial infarctions where there is partial blockage of the coronary artery are called non-___________________ MI.
5. In addition to age, genetics, and sedentary lifestyle, risk factors for ST-elevation myocardial infarction (STEMI) include ___________________, ___________________, ___________________, ___________________, and ___________________.
6. Almost all coronary occlusions occur at the site of a ruptured ___________________ ___________________.
7. In acute MI, if blood flow is not restored in ___________________ minutes, cell death begins.
8. Remodeling of the myocardium that occurs with MI is driven in part by local production of ___________________.
9. Intracellular proteins released when cardiac muscle cells are damaged are called ___________________ and ___________________.
10. There is some evidence that ___________________ may be harmful.

CRITICAL THINKING, PRIORITIZATION, AND DELEGATION QUESTIONS

11. Research suggests which treatment improves outcomes in STEMI? **(Select all that apply.)**
    a. Aspirin
    b. β-Blocker
    c. Ibuprofen
    d. Morphine
    e. Sublingual (SL) nitroglycerin
    f. Oxygen

12. Which is an expected response within minutes of administering intravenous (IV) morphine during a STEMI? **(Select all that apply.)**
    a. Decrease in chest pain
    b. Improved hemodynamics
    c. Increase in depth of respirations
    d. Inversion of the T wave on ECG
    e. Central nervous system excitation

13. A protocol in the emergency department (ED) is to administer four chewable 81-mg aspirin tablets (total, 324 mg) to patients with suspected MI. A student nurse asks the nurse why four chewable aspirin tablets are administered instead of two regular aspirin tablets (650 mg). Which is the appropriate response from the nurse?
    a. "The aspirin will start to absorb before it reaches the stomach."
    b. "Chewable forms of aspirin are rapidly absorbed through the buccal mucosa."
    c. "Chewing breaks the tablet into smaller particles, which absorb quickly in the gut."
    d. "Exceeding 325-mg doses can offset the antiplatelet effects of lower doses."

*14. A patient who is experiencing an acute STEMI is prescribed metoprolol 50 mg by mouth every 6 hours. The nurse would contact the provider about which finding?
    a. Altered taste
    b. Insomnia
    c. Rhinorrhea
    d. Wheezing

15. The ED triage nurse answers the call of a patient who has a history of angina pectoris and chronic obstructive pulmonary disease (COPD). The patient reports chest pain that has not been relieved by three doses of nitroglycerin. The patient had been told by their physician that they should take chewable aspirin should this occur, but they do not have any aspirin. Which instructions should the nurse provide?
    a. Call 911.
    b. Call your PCP.
    c. Take ibuprofen.
    d. Use home oxygen.

▶16. Which drug prescribed for acute STEMI should be withheld and the provider consulted immediately if the patient's pulse is 118 beats/min?
   a. Aspirin
   b. Atenolol
   c. Morphine
   d. Nitroglycerin

17. By which mechanism does nitroglycerin decrease the workload of the heart?
   a. Dissolving existing clots
   b. Preventing clot formation
   c. Slowing the heart rate
   d. Reducing venous return

18. When caring for a patient during a STEMI who is prescribed alteplase, the nurse would question the provider if which drug was also prescribed?
   a. Abciximab
   b. Clopidogrel
   c. Lisinopril
   d. Heparin

19. Which laboratory result in the history of a patient who is experiencing STEMI would be most important to report to the provider who has just ordered captopril?
   a. Potassium 4.2 mg/dL
   b. Glucose 150 mg/dL
   c. Creatinine 2.3 mg/dL
   d. Troponin T (TnT) 0.8 ng/mL

DOSE CALCULATION QUESTION

20. IV morphine 4 mg is prescribed for a STEMI patient. Available is 5 mg/mL. How many milliliters of morphine should be administered?

CASE STUDY

A middle-aged adult on vacation is admitted to the ED with severe, crushing chest pain. The pain radiates to the left arm, and they are experiencing diaphoresis, weakness, and nausea. The ECG shows elevated ST segments in the inferior leads. TnT is elevated three times above lower limits, and the total creatine kinase (CK) and the CK-MB isoenzyme are slightly elevated. The provider diagnoses STEMI and decides to start thrombolytic therapy with alteplase (tPA).

1. What assessments should the nurse monitor related to the risk of intracranial bleeding?

2. The nurse is directed to interview the patient's partner. What information does the nurse need to obtain to assist the provider with deciding if thrombolytic therapy is appropriate?

3. The following medications are ordered. What is the purpose of these drugs, and what assessment should the nurse perform relating to administration of these drugs?
   a. Aspirin (ASA) 81-mg chewable tablets, four tablets STAT
   b. IV morphine 4 mg followed by 2 mg every 10 minutes as needed to control pain
   c. Metoprolol 5 mg IV every 2 minutes for three doses, then 50 mg orally every 6 hours × 48 hours
   d. Nitroglycerin IV drip 10 mcg per minute
   e. Lisinopril 5 mg for the first 2 days followed by 10 mg daily

4. Why is it important for the nurse to assess if this patient has taken sildenafil in the past 24 hours?

5. The patient is being discharged with prescriptions for metoprolol succenate extended release 100 mg once a day, lisinopril 10 mg daily, aspirin 81 mg once a day, and warfarin 5 mg once a day. The patient's partner asks why the patient must have bloodwork (international normalized ratio [INR]) done every week. How should the nurse respond?

6. When explaining warfarin therapy, the nurse shares the patient's INR results, which most recently were 1.8. The normal INR is 0.9–1.1 for the hospital's laboratory. How can the nurse explain that the target INR is 3, which appears to be abnormal?

57 Drugs for Hemophilia

STUDY QUESTIONS

True or False

For each of the following statements, enter T for true or F for false.

1. ___ Hemophilia always produces a severe bleeding disorder.
2. ___ Hemophilia can result from a spontaneous gene mutation.
3. ___ Hemophilia interferes with the formation of a platelet plug.
4. ___ Hemophilia is inherited on the Y chromosome.
5. ___ Every boy born to a mother who is a carrier of the defective gene has a one-in-two chance of inheriting the disease.
6. ___ Hemophilia never occurs in females.
7. ___ One hundred percent of daughters of people with hemophilia are carriers of the disease.
8. ___ Treatment with clotting factor replacement is costly.

CRITICAL THINKING, PRIORITIZATION, AND DELEGATION QUESTIONS

*9. The nurse is caring for a 3-year-old patient who was admitted after a car accident. Laboratory tests indicate that the patient has 0.4% of the normal amount of clotting factor VIII. Which symptom would be of most concern to the nurse?
   a. Blood pressure 72/58 mm Hg
   b. Difficult to arouse
   c. Pulse 100 beats/min
   d. Swollen ankle

10. The nurse needs to give an intramuscular immunization to a patient with a history of mild hemophilia B. Which action should the nurse take?
   a. Administer the immunization as usual.
   b. Use the subcutaneous route to administer.
   c. Apply pressure for 5 minutes after the injection.
   d. Only give immunizations that come in the nasal route.

11. The parent of a child with hemophilia calls the pediatrician's office. The parent has forgotten which medication can be given to the child for mild pain and fever. The telephone triage nurse follows protocol and explains that the safest choice for patients with hemophilia is which drug?
   a. Acetaminophen
   b. Acetylsalicylic acid
   c. Celecoxib
   d. Ibuprofen

►12. Which patient problem would apply to all patients with hemophilia?
   a. Anxiety
   b. Coping
   c. Fatigue
   d. Injury

13. For each unit per kilogram of recombinant factor IX administered, the patient's normal factor IX should increase by which percentage?
   a. 0.1%
   b. 0.2%
   c. 1%
   d. 2%

14. For each unit per kilogram of recombinant factor VIII administered, the patient's normal factor VIII should increase by which percentage?
   a. 0.1%
   b. 0.2%
   c. 1%
   d. 2%

15. When the provider is determining the proper dose of factor concentrate, which is the most important patient factor to consider?
   a. Age
   b. Clinical response
   c. Factor levels
   d. Weight

*16. The nurse is administering factor concentrate to a child who begins to experience swelling around the face. Which is the priority intervention?
   a. Give diphenhydramine.
   b. Administer epinephrine.
   c. Slow the infusion.
   d. Call the provider.

17. The nurse knows that inhibitors to factor concentrate are most likely to occur in people with hemophilia of which descent? **(Select all that apply.)**
    a. African American
    b. Asian
    c. Hispanic
    d. Middle Eastern
    e. Native American

18. When a patient is receiving factor VIIa, the patient should be carefully assessed for what?
    a. Nausea
    b. Anorexia
    c. Chest pain
    d. Fatigue

DOSE CALCULATION QUESTIONS

19. A nurse in the perioperative area is caring for a 12-year-old child with hemophilia A who weighs 99 lb. What is the recommended number of units of recombinant factor VIII concentrate to raise the child's level to 50%?

20. Desmopressin 0.3 μg/kg is prescribed for a 66-lb child. The drug is available in a solution of 4 mcg/mL to be further diluted in 0.9% normal saline and infused over 30 minutes. How many milliliters will be drawn up to further dilute? What rate will be programmed into the IV pump if the solution of desmopressin was further diluted in 50 mL of 0.9% normal saline?

CASE STUDY

A 17-month-old child has been newly diagnosed with hemophilia A. Review of the chart indicates that the patient has not been immunized for hepatitis A.

1. What teaching needs to be provided relating to hepatitis immunization, and what information relating to immunizations does the nurse need to obtain regarding caregivers?

2. The patient's parents ask why aspirin should not be given to their child. What should the nurse explain?

3. The nurse provides a comprehensive list of over-the-counter drugs that contain salicylate. Which of these drugs would the nurse include on the list? Alka Seltzer, BC Powder, Doan Extra Strength, Anacin, Ecotrin, Kaopectate, Pepto-Bismol, Bufferin, Trilisate.

4. The home health nurse goes to the patient's home to teach the parents how to administer recombinant factor VIII concentrate via a central venous catheter. What are the nursing diagnoses that the nurse should consider when developing the plan of care for this family?

5. Administering factor concentrate carries a risk of complications. What should the nurse teach the caregiver to prepare for possible complications?

58 Drugs for Deficiency Anemias

STUDY QUESTIONS

Completion

1. Red blood cells (RBCs) which lack hemoglobin are called _____________.
2. In the bone marrow, RBCs are called _____________ after gaining hemoglobin.
3. _________________ are immature erythrocytes.
4. _________________ stimulates maturation of RBCs.
5. _____________ is required for hemoglobin synthesis.
6. _____________ is required to support DNA synthesis.
7. The oxygen storing molecule of muscle is called _____________.
8. The useful life of RBCs is _________________ _________________.
9. The major route of iron excretion is the _____________.
10. Aggregated ferritin is called _________________.
11. Iron deficiency anemia results in an increase in _________ ___________ ___________.
12. _________ _________ is the preferred drug for preventing iron deficiency anemia.
13. _____________ reduce the absorption of iron.

Match the term with its definition.

14. ___ Platelet
15. ___ Over sized erythroblast
16. ___ Over sized erythrocyte
17. ___ Pale
18. ___ Small-sized cell
    a. Thrombocyte
    b. Hypochromic
    c. Macrocyte
    d. Megaloblast
    e. Microcytic

CRITICAL THINKING, PRIORITIZATION, AND DELEGATION QUESTIONS

►19. The nurse is caring for a patient with cancer and anemia who is receiving chemotherapy that prevents the reproduction of rapidly dividing cells. Which laboratory result suggests that the anemia is becoming worse?
   a. Hemoglobin 10 mg/dL
   b. Hematocrit 26%
   c. RBC 3.8×10^{12}/L
   d. Reticulocyte count 0.002%

✳20. It is a priority for the nurse to assess for symptoms of anemia in a patient who has a history of which condition?
   a. Multiple sclerosis
   b. Chronic kidney disease
   c. Osteoarthritis
   d. Hypertension

21. Which mechanism normally prevents excessive buildup of iron in the body?
   a. Decreased intestinal absorption of iron
   b. Increased excretion of RBCs
   c. Incorporation of hemoglobin into RBCs
   d. Excretion of RBCs in urine and bile

22. Which food should the nurse include in dietary teaching for pregnant females concerning prevention of iron-deficiency anemia? **(Select all that apply.)**
   a. Squash
   b. Milk
   c. Fish
   d. Legumes
   e. Apples

23. In iron-deficiency anemia, the nurse would expect which laboratory test to be elevated?
   a. Hematocrit
   b. Hemoglobin
   c. Total IBC
   d. MCV

24. Which is a common patient problem for patients with iron-deficiency anemia?
   a. Decreased self-esteem
   b. Decreased gas exchange
   c. Heart failure
   d. Fatigue

▶25. The school nurse has been consulted by a fifth-grade teacher regarding a student who is pale, tires excessively as the day progresses, and whose academic performance has been declining. Which nursing action is appropriate?
   a. Send a letter home informing the parents that their child is anemic.
   b. Tell the child's parents their child needs to be seen by their pediatrician.
   c. Make an appointment to speak with the parents about noted concerns.
   d. Ask the child to tell their parents that you think they are anemic.

26. Which is the most common adverse effect of ferrous sulfate?
   a. Yellowing of teeth
   b. Dyspepsia
   c. Hypotension
   d. Thready pulse

27. A patient reports intolerable nausea and heartburn from taking an oral iron preparation. Which instructions should the nurse provide?
   a. Consult with the provider.
   b. Take an antacid with the iron.
   c. Swallow the iron with milk.
   d. Drink orange juice with the iron.

28. The nurse is providing care to a patient receiving an oral iron preparation. The patient's stool is greenish-black. Which is the appropriate nursing action?
   a. Administer the iron preparation.
   b. Consult the provider.
   c. Ask if this is a change in stool color.
   d. Hold the iron preparation.

✳29. A patient with peptic ulcer disease has developed severe anemia. Iron dextran has just been prescribed. The nurse has administered a test dose. It is a priority for the nurse to observe the patient for which adverse effect?
   a. Edema of the throat
   b. Development of hives
   c. Phlebitis at site of injection
   d. Tissue damage from extravasation

30. When iron must be administered by injection, which method of administration should be used?
   a. Intradermal
   b. Intrathecal
   c. Subcutaneous
   d. Z-track

✳31. The dialysis nurse has administered iron dextran and erythropoietin. Which is a priority nursing concern?
   a. Gastrointestinal cramping
   b. Infusion site discomfort
   c. Decreased tissue perfusion
   d. Taste alterations

✳32. A patient with chronic kidney disease (not on hemodialysis) has been taking ferrous sulfate as prescribed. They present to their provider reporting fatigue and shortness of breath. On exam, pallor and a heart rate of 118 beats per minute is noted. The nurse anticipates which drug will be ordered?
   a. Ferric pyrophosphate
   b. Ferumoxytol
   c. Pteroylglutamic acid
   d. Sodium-ferric gluconate complex

✳33. Which are potential causes of impaired absorption of vitamin B_{12}? **(Select all that apply.)**
   a. Alcohol use disorder
   b. Regional enteritis
   c. Tropical sprue
   d. Celiac disease
   e. B_{12}-intrinsic factor complex antibodies

✳34. It is a priority to teach the patient with pernicious anemia to report which issue?
   a. Fatigue
   b. Joint pain
   c. Paresthesias
   d. Fever

▶35. A patient with pernicious anemia complains of numbness and tingling of the hands and feet. Which data should the nurse collect before notifying the provider of the patient's concern?
   a. Blood pressure
   b. Deep tendon reflex
   c. Capillary glucose
   d. Skin color

36. Vitamin B_{12} deficiency and folic acid deficiency in adults, both forms of megaloblastic anemia, differ from each other in that B_{12} deficiency can result in which condition? **(Select all that apply.)**
   a. Damage to brain
   b. Impaired myoglobin production
   c. Pulmonary edema
   d. Spinal cord damage
   e. Cognitive impairment

▶37. When a patient is prescribed drugs that increase the production of RBCs, it is a priority to monitor the effect of changes in serum potassium on which system?
   a. Cardiovascular
   b. Endocrine
   c. Gastrointestinal
   d. Pulmonary

DOSE CALCULATION QUESTIONS

38. The pediatrician prescribes ferrous sulfate drops 25 mg twice a day. The child weighs 22 lb, and the recommended dose is 5 mg/kg per day. Is the dose safe and effective?

39. The ferrous sulfate drops are available as 75 mg in 0.6 mL. How much should the parents administer with each dose?

CASE STUDIES

Case Study 1

An 11-month-old child, who drinks 8-ounce bottles of whole milk five to six times a day, is diagnosed with iron-deficiency anemia.

1. What can the nurse teach the parents about factors contributing to the anemia and measures to change the factors that can be altered?

2. What should the nurse teach the parents about ferrous sulfate therapy?

Case Study 2

A young adult has had gastric bypass surgery and has lost 25 lb in the past 2 months. They go to their primary care provider with reports of fatigue and glossitis.

3. Because of a history of this surgery, the patient is at risk for what type of anemia? Why?

4. The patient is prescribed parenteral injections of vitamin B_{12} 30 mcg and folic acid 200 mcg daily for 1 week. They will then receive oral cyanocobalamin 10,000 mcg/day and folic acid 400 mcg/day. The patient tells the nurse that they had learned that oral administration of cyanocobalamin is ineffective. How should the nurse respond?

5. The patient discusses concerns about taking "all of these pills" every day. The provider discontinues the oral cyanocobalamin and prescribes intranasal cyanocobalamin 1 spray in one nostril once a week. What teaching will the nurse provide about intranasal administration of the drug?

6. The nurse teaches the patient to report which symptoms that suggest the adverse effect of hypokalemia that is possible when taking cyanocobalamin?

59 Hematopoietic Agents

STUDY QUESTIONS

Completion

1. _______________ is the hormone produced in the proximal tubules of the kidney in response to anemia or hypoxia.
2. Erythropoiesis-stimulating agents (ESAs) may reduce overall survival in _______________ patients.
3. Epoetin has been associated with an increase in _______________ _______________ when hemoglobin levels rise higher than 11 g/dL.
4. The dosage of epoetin alfa should be reduced when hemoglobin increases by more than ______ g/dL in 2 weeks.
5. When administering filgrastim, the nurse should review the complete blood count (CBC) ______ weekly.
6. Allergy to _______________ would be a contraindication to administration of sargramostim.
7. Romiplostim's action is to _______________ platelet production.
8. The nurse needs to assess for shortness of breath, chest pain, and change in level of consciousness when a patient is prescribed the thrombopoietin receptor agonists (TRAs) because these drugs increase the risk of _______________ _______________.

CRITICAL THINKING, PRIORITIZATION, AND DELEGATION QUESTIONS

9. Which new assessment finding would be priority to report to the provider when a patient is receiving epoetin alfa?
   a. Chest pain
   b. Fatigue
   c. Pallor
   d. Weak pulses
10. A patient with a history of type 2 diabetes mellitus (T2DM) and chronic kidney disease (CKD) is receiving epoetin alfa. Which is a realistic goal for therapy?
   a. Hgb 8 g/dL
   b. Hgb 10 g/dL
   c. Hgb 12 g/dL
   d. Hgb14 g/dL
11. When epoetin alfa is administered preoperatively to reduce the need for blood transfusion postoperatively, the nurse would question the provider if which additional drug was not prescribed?
   a. Ferrous sulfate
   b. Folate
   c. Furosemide
   d. Heparin

✳12. It would be a priority to report to the provider which assessment finding in a patient taking darbepoetin alfa?
   a. Blood pressure 170/98 mm Hg
   b. Pulse 100 beats/min
   c. Respirations 20
   d. Temperature 100.0°F (38°C)

►13. A chemotherapy patient who has received two injections in the past week of epoetin alfa is due for the next dose. The patient's hemoglobin has not increased. What should the nurse do?
   a. Hold the next dose.
   b. Administer the medication.
   c. Assess patient for renal failure.
   d. Assessing for neutralizing antibodies.

►14. Epoetin alfa 4000 units subcutaneous (subQ) is ordered at 0900 pending endogenous erythropoietin levels for an anemic HIV-infected patient receiving zidovudine. Lab results arrived at 0830, including endogenous erythropoietin level of 578 milliunits/mL. Which action should the nurse take?
   a. Administer the drug.
   b. Verify dosing with pharmacist.
   c. Hold the medication.
   d. Notify the provider.

✳15. Elevation of uric acid is an adverse effect of pegfilgrastim therapy. Which is the priority nursing assessment related to this adverse effect?
   a. Edema
   b. Fever
   c. Joint redness
   d. Tachycardia

▶16. The nurse is teaching the administration of filgrastim to the parent of a child with congenital neutropenia who weighs 88 lb. The prescribed dose is 240 mcg (6 mcg/kg). The medication is available in a concentration of 300 mcg/mL in 1.6-mL vials. Which administration method should the nurse teach the parent?
   a. 0.6 mL, discarding the vial after the first dose
   b. 0.6 mL, obtaining two doses from each vial
   c. 0.8 mL, discarding the vial after the first dose
   d. 0.8 mL, obtaining two doses from each vial

17. The nurse is teaching a patient about the pharmacologic therapy they are receiving before hematopoietic stem cells (HSCs) are harvested. The patient asks why they will receive plerixafor, when they have already been receiving filgrastim. Which is the appropriate nursing response?
   a. "It will help reduce the risk of infection after your bone marrow ablation."
   b. "The filgrastim hasn't increased your HSCs enough; this will help boost yield."
   c. "Plerixafor will ensure your HSCs repopulate your bone marrow quicker."
   d. "This drug will help keep your myeloid cancer from coming back."

18. Which are the advantages of using pegfilgrastim instead of filgrastim?
   a. It can be administered after chemotherapy.
   b. The course of therapy is one injection.
   c. Pegfilrastim does not cause bone pain.
   d. There is less elevation of uric acid.

▶19. Which would be a symptom of a significant adverse reaction to massive doses of sargramostim?
   a. Crackles
   b. Rhonchi
   c. Pleuritic pain
   d. Wheezes

20. Sargramostim must be administered no later than which amount of time after reconstitution?
   a. 2 hours
   b. 4 hours
   c. 6 hours
   d. 8 hours

✳21. What is a priority nursing concern for a patient with idiopathic thrombocytopenic purpura (ITP) who is prescribed eltrombopag?
   a. Fluid volume
   b. Impaired mobility
   c. Nutritional needs
   d. Safety

22. It is important to ask a patient who has just been prescribed eltrombopag about the use of which over-the-counter product?
   a. Analgesics
   b. Antacids
   c. Cough medicines
   d. Decongestants

DOSE CALCULATION QUESTIONS

23. A patient is prescribed sargramostim 250 mcg/m^2 after a bone marrow transplant. The patient weighs 50 kg and is 163 cm tall. The pharmacy delivers sargramostim 500 mcg/mL, which the nurse dilutes to a concentration of 10 mcg/mL. How much sargramostim should be administered?

24. A patient is receiving tbo-filgrastim. They weigh 128 lb. The drug is prescribed at 5 mcg/kg subQ daily to begin 24 hours after chemotherapy. Tbo-filgrastim comes in two prefilled syringes: 300 mcg/0.5 mL and 480 mcg/0.8 mcg/mL. Which prefilled syringe should be selected? How much be administered?

CASE STUDIES

Case Study 1

An older adult with T2DM for 40 years and CKD managed with hemodialysis for 5 years is anemic and has been prescribed epoetin alfa three times a week to help maintain erythrocyte count. The provider has ordered periodic laboratory tests, including blood urea nitrogen (BUN), creatinine, phosphorus, potassium, RBC indices, hemoglobin, transferrin saturation, ferritin, and uric acid. The patient is tired of "being jabbed" and asks the nurse why these tests must be done.

1. Describe the rationale for each test in a way the patient can understand.
   a. BUN/creatinine

b. Phosphorus

c. Potassium

d. Hemoglobin

e. RBC indices

f. Ferritin

g. Transferrin saturation

h. Uric acid

2. What adverse effects should the nurse assess in this patient?

3. The nurse is reviewing laboratory results for this patient. Hemoglobin is 13.5 g/dL. What should the nurse do?

Case Study 2

A patient is prescribed sargramostim 250 mcg/m^2 after a bone marrow transplant.

4. What is the rationale for this therapy?

5. What should the nurse do or not do if the patient experiences these adverse effects?
   a. Diarrhea

   b. Weakness

   c. Rash

   d. Bone pain

60 Drugs for Diabetes Mellitus

STUDY QUESTIONS

True or False

For each of the following statements, enter T for true or F for false.

1. ___ Most long-term complications of diabetes occur secondary to disruption of blood flow.
2. ___ The primary goal of treating diabetes is to prevent long-term complications and manage symptoms of hyperglycemia.
3. ___ Blood sugar control will best be achieved if the patient follows a plan created by the health care providers.
4. ___ Exercise improves cellular response to insulin.
5. ___ Clear solutions are always short acting.
6. ___ Insulin therapy with one long-acting agent that mimics the body's basal insulin secretion and another short-acting agent to cover eating most closely mimics normal functioning.
7. ___ Once a patient's blood sugar is stabilized, the patient will be able to maintain control with oral drugs.
8. ___ Administering insulin or sulfonylurea drugs and not eating can cause serious effects from the blood sugar going too low.
9. ___ Tight glucose control decreases the incidence of chronic kidney disease.
10. ___ Treatment can be monitored by blood or urine.
11. ___ Weight loss is always needed to decrease the patient's insulin requirements.

CRITICAL THINKING, PRIORITIZATION, AND DELEGATION QUESTIONS

12. Which complication of diabetes causes the most deaths?
    a. Cardiovascular effects
    b. Hypoglycemia
    c. Ketoacidosis
    d. Kidney damage

▶13. The nurse is caring for a patient with long-standing diabetes. The patient reports nausea, and states they have vomited twice in the past couple of hours. On exam, the patient has abdominal distention. The nurse suspects the patient has which diabetic complication?
    a. Gangrene
    b. Sensory neuropathy
    c. Nephropathy
    d. Gastroparesis

14. Which would be appropriate nursing interventions for a young adult patient who, for the first time, has a fasting plasma glucose level of 145 mg/dL? **(Select all that apply.)**
    a. Recommend 30 minutes of exercise, 5 days a week.
    b. Discuss healthy diet options with the patient.
    c. Explain the need for oral antidiabetic medication.
    d. Teach the patient how to do a urine dip for glucose.
    e. Schedule the patient for a second fasting glucose test.

15. Which type of diabetes often exists for years before diagnosis, but fasting blood glucose is not elevated because of hyperinsulinemia?
    a. Gestational diabetes
    b. Juvenile diabetes
    c. Type 1 diabetes
    d. Type 2 diabetes

✳16. It would be a priority for the nurse to respond to which symptom if exhibited by a patient who is receiving insulin therapy for diabetes?
    a. Fatigue
    b. Perineal itching
    c. Difficult to arouse
    d. Constant hunger

17. A patient who has type 2 DM has been unable to follow the recommended diet and exercise regimen. They tried to alter their laboratory test results by eating less than usual before having blood testing performed. Which test would be most accurate for this patient because it evaluates glucose control over the past 3 months?
   a. Fasting glucose
   b. Hemoglobin A1c
   c. Postprandial glucose
   d. Two-hour glucose tolerance

18. A patient with type 1 diabetes who has been using traditional insulin therapy has been prescribed intensive insulin therapy to achieve tighter glucose control. Which information should be included in the teaching?
   a. An insulin pump is used to provide the best glucose control.
   b. Requires four injections of a rapid-acting insulin each day and basal insulin.
   c. Is indicated for new patients with type 1 diabetes who have not experienced ketoacidosis.
   d. Effective in preventing macrovascular complications characteristic of type 2 DM.

19. A nurse administered 30 units of neutral protamine Hagedorn (NPH) insulin in the same syringe as 8 units of insulin aspart coverage so that the patient would need only one injection. The nurse monitors the patient for which symptom that may result from the administration?
   a. Diaphoresis
   b. Itching
   c. Thirst
   d. Vomiting

►20. When obtaining a new vial of NPH insulin from the refrigerator, the nurse notes that the suspension is partially frozen. Which action should the nurse take?
   a. Obtain a new vial from the pharmacy.
   b. Shake the vial vigorously to produce heat.
   c. Warm the suspension in warm water.
   d. Withdraw unfrozen portion and discard the rest.

►21. A patient is admitted in a state of diabetic ketoacidosis. The provider orders insulin detemir 0.1 mg/kg per hour to be administered by intravenous (IV) drip. Which action should the nurse take?
   a. Mix it with 100 mL of normal saline.
   b. Inject into 100 mL bag of dextrose 5% in water (D_5W).
   c. Infuse the solution prepared by pharmacy.
   d. Consult the provider STAT.

►22. The nurse has completed an initial assessment of their assigned patients and is preparing to administer insulin. All patients are alert and oriented. It is 8:07 a.m., and breakfast trays are scheduled to arrive at 8:45 a.m. The nurse should administer insulin as ordered to which patient first?
   a. Insulin aspart 5 units
   b. Insulin glulisine 7 units
   c. NPH insulin 34 units
   d. Regular insulin 5 units

23. A patient has been prescribed 5 units of insulin aspart and 25 units of insulin detemir to be administered at 8:00 a.m. Which action should the nurse take?
   a. Draw up the two insulins in different syringes.
   b. Draw up insulin aspart first and then detemir insulin in the same syringe.
   c. Draw up clear insulin, then cloudy insulin, in the same syringe.
   d. Draw up detemir insulin first and then insulin aspart in the same syringe.

24. Which special administration techniques must the nurse use when administering NPH insulin?
   a. Never mix with another insulin.
   b. Administer this insulin only at bedtime.
   c. Roll the vial gently to mix particles in solution.
   d. When mixing insulins, draw NPH into the syringe first.

25. The nurse is caring for a patient who is nothing by mouth (NPO) for a diagnostic test. Which dose of insulin should be administered?
   a. Fingerstick blood glucose (FSBG) 100 mg/dL; insulin aspart 5 units, NPH 34 units
   b. FSBG 190 mg/dL; regular insulin 4 units sliding scale
   c. FSBG 110 mg/dL; insulin detemir 26 units
   d. FSBG 80 mg/dL; NPH insulin 34 units

26. Research suggests that tight glucose control decreases the risk of which condition? **(Select all that apply.)**
   a. Cerebrovascular accidents
   b. Peripheral neuropathy
   c. Lower extremity amputation
   d. Diabetic nephropathy
   e. Ophthalmic complications

*27. When performing the initial morning assessment on a patient with diabetes, the nurse notes that the patient is diaphoretic and confused. The nurse checks the FSBG, which is 37 mg/dL. What is the priority assessment before administering orange juice?
   a. Blood pressure
   b. Deep tendon reflexes
   c. Swallowing reflex
   d. Temperature

28. A patient with type 2 DM that is controlled with diet and metformin also has severe rheumatoid arthritis (RA) and has been prescribed prednisone to control inflammation. Which is most likely to occur?
    a. Hypoglycemia
    b. Morbiliform rash
    c. Gastroparesis
    d. Hyperglycemia

►29. The college health nurse is caring for a college student with type 2 DM, who was brought to the health clinic after becoming intoxicated at a party. The student is prescribed metformin 850 mg once a day. The nurse assesses the student. Which assessment would be of most concern to the nurse?
    a. Faint peripheral pulses
    b. Respirations 32 breaths/minute
    c. Pulse 100 beats/min
    d. Severe frontal headache

30. After receiving teaching about the drug glipizide, which statement would suggest that the patient understood the teaching?
    a. "I need to notify my doctor if I have episodes of shakiness."
    b. "I should not have low blood sugar with this drug."
    c. "I can eat anything I want while on this drug."
    d. "This drug is less potent than the newer drugs."

31. Which laboratory test result increases the risk that a patient who is prescribed metformin might experience hypoglycemia?
    a. Alkaline phosphatase 142 IU/L
    b. Blood urea nitrogen (BUN) 24 mg/dL
    c. Estimated glomerular filtration rate (eGFR) 42 mL/min
    d. Glucose-6-phosphate dehydrogenase (G6PD) 2.4 U/g hemoglobin

32. Which assessment change from yesterday morning, in a patient prescribed pioglitazone, would be of most concern to the nurse?
    a. Abdominal pain
    b. Crackles throughout lung fields
    c. Drop in BP from 130/82 to 118/78 mm Hg
    d. Temperature 102.4°F

►33. Which situation would warrant the nurse not administering repaglinide and consulting the provider?
    a. Fasting blood glucose is 95 mg/dL.
    b. Glycosylated hemoglobin (A1c) is 5.5%.
    c. Patient is NPO for a colonoscopy.
    d. Patient is scheduled for hemodialysis at 10:00 a.m.

34. Which nursing outcome would be expected for a patient who is prescribed nateglinide?
    a. Bedtime FSBG 160 mg/dL
    b. Fasting blood glucose less than 90 mg/dL
    c. Glycosylated hemoglobin (A1c) 7%
    d. Postprandial blood sugar less than 150 mg/dL

35. Which nursing action is appropriate when a patient is prescribed bromocriptine for type 2 DM?
    a. Change positions slowly.
    b. Elevate the head after eating.
    c. Monitor fluid intake and output.
    d. Weigh daily.

36. Which are the only drugs currently used to treat type 2 DM during pregnancy and lactation? **(Select all that apply.)**
    a. Acarbose
    b. Glipizide
    c. Insulin
    d. Metformin
    e. Pioglitazone

37. The nurse is preparing to perform the last assessment of the 7:00 p.m. to 7:00 a.m. shift at 6:00 a.m. Several assigned patients have diabetes. The patient receiving which drug should be assessed for hypoglycemia first?
    a. Acarbose 50 mg three times a day with meals
    b. Glargine insulin 37 units at bedtime
    c. Metformin 500 mg twice daily
    d. NPH 35 units every morning

DOSE CALCULATION QUESTIONS

38. A 132-pound patient is prescribed an IV infusion of regular insulin at 0.1 units/kg per hour, which calculates to 6 units per hour. The insulin comes mixed as a solution of 25 units in 100 mL of normal saline. The IV pump calibration is in milliliters per hour. What rate should the nurse program for the continuous IV insulin drip?

CASE STUDY

The nurse educator is presenting a seminar on insulin to nursing students. What would be the best response to these questions?

1. Why are regular and rapid-acting insulins the only insulins administered IV?

2. If regular insulin is most like human insulin, why do doctors prescribe rapid-acting insulins such as insulin aspart and insulin glulisine?

3. How is using detemir or glargine insulin better than using NPH insulin?

4. What is the disadvantage of using basal glargine insulin?

5. Some prescribers order basal glargine insulin in the morning rather than in the evening, as the literature recommends. Why would they do this?

6. Patients sometimes need both basal and bolus doses of insulin at the same time. What could happen if the basal detemir or glargine insulin is mixed with a bolus of insulin aspart or other rapid- or fast-acting insulins?

7. What should the patient or nurse do if a vial of insulin aspart is cloudy?

8. What is inhaled human insulin used for?

61 Drugs for Thyroid Disorders

STUDY QUESTIONS

True or False

For each of the following statements, enter T for true or F for false.

1. ___ The 3 and 4 in T_3 and T_4 indicate the number of atoms of iodine in the molecule.
2. ___ Propylthiouracil is the first-line drug for hyperthyroidism.
3. ___ Free T_4 is the count of T_4 hormone not bound by protein.
4. ___ Maternal hypothyroidism has the most significant effects on the fetus in the third trimester when most fetal weight is gained.
5. ___ Assessment for congenital hypothyroidism should be done at the infant's 2-month checkup.
6. ___ Exophthalmos is not seen in all cases of hyperthyroidism.
7. ___ Synthetic thyroid preparations are better standardized than animal gland extracts.
8. ___ It is more important to take thyroid hormone replacement at the same time each day than with or without food.
9. ___ Levothyroxine and other thyroid hormones should not be taken to treat obesity.

CRITICAL THINKING, PRIORITIZATION, AND DELEGATION QUESTIONS

►10. The nurse is preparing to administer levothyroxine. Which laboratory value, if significantly low, would be a reason for the nurse to withhold the medication and consult the provider?
   a. Free T_3
   b. Free T_4
   c. TSH
   d. T_3

✻11. It is a priority for the nurse to teach a female who is pregnant and diagnosed with hypothyroidism that adequate thyroid hormone replacement therapy is critical during which stage of the pregnancy?
   a. First trimester
   b. Second trimester
   c. Third trimester
   d. Delivery

✻12. Which would be priority when a patient is admitted in a thyrotoxic crisis?
   a. Lowering the heart rate
   b. Providing adequate nutrition
   c. Raising the secretion of TSH
   d. Suppressing thyroid hormone secretion

13. Which statement, if made by a patient receiving the antithyroid drug propylthiouracil, would indicate a need for further teaching?
   a. "Taking this drug should make my heart stop feeling like it is racing."
   b. "I should gain weight while eating less when I am on this drug."
   c. "This drug should help decrease the bulging appearance of my eyes."
   d. "This drug should stop the feeling that I am always too hot."

✻14. Which assessment finding would be critical for the nurse to report to the provider immediately if noted in a patient admitted with urosepsis who has a history of Graves disease treated by an antithyroid drug?
   a. Blood in urine on urinalysis
   b. Burning when urinating
   c. Flank pain
   d. Temperature 104°F (40°C)

15. The nurse is caring for a patient who receives levothyroxine. Which over-the-counter (OTC) drugs should not be administered within 4 hours of the administration of levothyroxine? **(Select all that apply.)**
   a. Aluminum hydroxide
   b. Calcium carbonate
   c. Acetaminophen
   d. Ferrous sulfate
   e. Milk of magnesia

▶16. The nurse should monitor a patient taking warfarin and levothyroxine for which condition?
   a. Bleeding
   b. Dysrhythmias
   c. Insomnia
   d. Tachycardia

17. A patient who has hypothyroidism tells the nurse that their insurance company now requires that they use a generic drug if one is available. Up to now, they have been taking brand-name Synthroid. Which is the appropriate nursing response?
   a. Ask the pharmacist what is best.
   b. Discuss this change with their provider.
   c. Pay for the brand-name drug.
   d. Go ahead and use the generic brand.

18. A patient has received instructions regarding administration of levothyroxine. Which of these statements made by the patient would indicate that they understood the directions?
   a. "I should take the drug in the morning with breakfast."
   b. "Stomach upset occurs if the drug is taken with an antacid."
   c. "The drug should be taken on an empty stomach 60 minutes before breakfast."
   d. "Taking the drug with orange juice increases drug absorption."

✳19. It would be a priority to report which laboratory test result, in a patient taking methimazole, to the provider?
   a. Alanine aminotransferase (ALT) 50 IU/L
   b. Blood urea nitrogen (BUN) 24 mg/dL
   c. Fasting blood glucose (FBG) 138 mg/dL
   d. Human chorionic gonadotropin (hCG) 425 mIU/mL

▶20. Because of the risk of agranulocytosis, the nurse should teach the patient who has been prescribed methimazole to report which symptom?
   a. Anorexia
   b. Bleeding gums
   c. Pale conjunctiva
   d. Sore throat

21. A 34-year-old female patient is prescribed iodine^{131} for toxic nodular goiter. Which statement, if made by this patient, would indicate a need for further teaching?
   a. "Inadequate thyroid hormone secretion is a concern with this therapy."
   b. "I must stay at home during therapy to avoid exposing others to radiation."
   c. "It is important to use two reliable methods of birth control while on this drug."
   d. "This drug takes months before it is fully effective."

22. Which of these factors, if identified in a patient receiving Lugol solution, would be concerning to the nurse?
   a. Decrease in free T_3
   b. Weight gain of 2 lb in 2 weeks
   c. Beverages having a brassy taste
   d. Drug taken with grapefruit juice

▶23. Propranolol has been prescribed for a patient in a thyrotoxic crisis. Which is the expected outcome for this therapy?
   a. BP 110/80–90/60 mm Hg
   b. Free T_4 0.8–2.3 ng/dL
   c. Pulse 60–80 beats/min
   d. TSH 0.4–4 mU/L

DOSE CALCULATION QUESTIONS

24. Levothyroxine 50 mcg is prescribed for a 4-month-old child with congenital hypothyroidism who weighs 9 lb. Is this a safe dosage?

25. Levothyroxine 0.2-mg tablets are available. The patient has been prescribed 100 mcg. How many tablets should the nurse administer?

CASE STUDIES

Case Study 1

A young adult visits their provider with reports of unusual fatigue, lethargy, intolerance to cold, and weight gain. At the visit, vital signs are BP 100/58 mm Hg, P 62 beats/min, respiration 16, and temperature 97.8°F.

1. What thyroid disorder do these symptoms suggest?

2. What laboratory test results would the nurse expect to see for this patient if they are hypothyroid?

3. After appropriate history, physical examination, and laboratory studies, the patient is diagnosed with primary hypothyroidism and started on levothyroxine 112 mcg once a day. What teaching should the nurse provide about the expected timing for relief of symptoms?

4. What teaching should the nurse provide to this patient about administration of levothyroxine?

5. The nurse should teach about possible adverse effects of levothyroxine. What adverse effects warrant notifying the provider?

6. The patient tells the nurse that their sibling has asked for some of their thyroid pills to help lose weight. The patient wants to know if this would be a problem. How should the nurse respond?

7. The patient returns for their 1-year checkup and wonders if they still need the medication because they sometimes forget to take the drug and do not feel any different on those days. How should the nurse respond?

Case Study 2

Propranolol 10 mg and propylthiouracil 100 mg three times a day are prescribed for a young adult who was recently diagnosed with Graves disease.

8. What laboratory results would the nurse expect to see when reviewing this patient's chart?

9. The patient asks the nurse why two drugs have been prescribed. What information should the nurse provide regarding the need for both drugs?

10. The drug methimazole is less toxic than propylthiouracil. What would be a possible reason why the provider chose propylthiouracil for this patient?

11. What assessments should the nurse teach the patient to monitor, and what findings should be reported to the provider?

12. Six months later, the patient's heart rate, blood pressure, TSH, and free T_3 levels are within normal limits. The provider provides a plan for gradual decrease and then discontinuation of propranolol. Why was this drug dose tapered rather than discontinued if vital signs are normal?

62 Drugs Related to Hypothalamic and Pituitary Function

STUDY QUESTIONS

Matching

Match the hormones (abbreviations) with their functions.

1. ___ Helps regulate growth hormone (GH) release.
2. ___ Acts on the adrenal cortex to promote synthesis and release of adrenocortical hormones.
3. ___ Acts on the ovaries to promote ovulation and development of the corpus luteum and acts on the testes to promote androgen production.
4. ___ Acts on the ovaries to promote follicular growth and development and acts on the testes to promote spermatogenesis.
5. ___ Stimulates milk production after childbirth.
6. ___ Stimulates growth in practically all tissues and organs.
7. ___ Acts on the thyroid gland to promote synthesis and release of thyroid hormones.
8. ___ Promotes uterine contractions during labor and stimulates milk ejection during breastfeeding.
9. ___ Acts on the kidney to cause reabsorption of water.
   a. ACTH
   b. ADH
   c. FSH
   d. GH
   e. LH
   f. Oxytocin
   g. Prolactin
   h. Somatostatin
   i. TSH

CRITICAL THINKING, PRIORITIZATION, AND DELEGATION QUESTIONS

10. Which finding would the nurse expect in a child who has a deficiency in the secretion of GH?
    a. Cognitive deficiency
    b. Long trunk and short extremities
    c. Profuse sweating
    d. Short stature but normal proportions

▶11. Which assessment of a 7-year-old child indicates an increased risk for severe adverse effects of somatropin?
    a. Anterior cervical lymphadenopathy
    b. Body mass index (BMI) 35
    c. Dry, flaky skin on elbows
    d. Pulse 100 beats/min

✻12. It would be a priority to teach a child with Type 1 diabetes who has been prescribed growth hormone, and the child's parents, to seek medical care if which symptom occurs?
    a. Diaphoresis
    b. Tachycardia
    c. Irritability
    d. Blurred vision

▶13. Which of these assessment findings, if identified in a patient who is receiving pegvisomant, most likely suggests possible liver injury and should be reported to the provider?
    a. Headache
    b. Nasal congestion
    c. Malaise
    d. Tea-colored urine

▶14. Which assessment finding would be a reason to consult the provider regarding the administration of vasopressin? (**Select all that apply.**)
    a. Blood pressure 82/60 mm Hg
    b. Chest pain
    c. Estimated glomerular filtration rate (eGFR) 45 mL/min
    d. Headache
    e. Drowsiness

15. A patient who was recently diagnosed with hypothalamic diabetes insipidus and prescribed vasopressin reports weight gain of 1–2 lb per day for the past week. The nurse should recognize that this may indicate
    a. Failure to comply with directions for administration of the drug.
    b. Failure to limit water intake.
    c. Improper diagnosis.
    d. Inadequate drug dosage.

✻16. Which laboratory result would be a priority to report to the provider when a patient is prescribed pegvisomant for acromegaly?
    a. Amylase 150 IU/L
    b. Alanine aminotransferase (ALT) 275 IU/L
    c. A1c 6.8%
    d. Hemoglobin 13 g/dL

DOSE CALCULATION QUESTIONS

17. A child is prescribed somatropin 0.2 mg/kg per week subcutaneously (subQ) to be divided into three doses to be administered every other day. The nurse teaches the parents of the child, who weighs 30 kg, to administer how much somatropin at each dose?

18. Mecasermin 800 mcg is prescribed for a 44-lb child. The drug is available as 10 mg/mL. How much drug will the nurse administer?

CASE STUDIES

Single-Episode Case Study

HEALTH HISTORY	NURSE'S NOTES	PHYSICIAN'S ORDERS	LABORATORY PROFILE

1030:

Received patient in recovery status post–open reduction and internal fixation of right humerus. Patient sustained compound fracture falling from mountain bike.

Patient with history of diabetes insipidus secondary to long-term lithium treatment for bipolar disorder.

Friend who was present at the accident is waiting in the family room.

Patient is groggy but arouses to name and responds to questions appropriately. Lungs with diminished sounds in bilateral bases. Heart regular rate and rhythm with normal S_1 and S_2. Hypoactive bowel sounds throughout with mild abdominal distension. Pedal pulses are difficult to palpate, capillary refill is >5 seconds, and all extremities are cold. Warm blankets provided.

Intravenous of dextrose 5% in water (D_5W) infusing at 125 mL/hr via 18-gauge catheter in left forearm. IV site clean, dry, and intact.

Vital signs: BP 152/90, heart rate (HR) 98, respiration 18, temperature 99.0°F, oxygen saturation on 2 L per nasal canula 95%.

Orders received for vasopressin, 5 units now and 5 units every 4 hours as needed.

1. Highlight the assessment findings. Which would be a reason to withhold the drug and contact the provider?

63 Drugs for Disorders of the Adrenal Cortex

STUDY QUESTIONS

Matching

Match the term with its description.

1. ___ Androgens
2. ___ Glucocorticoids
3. ___ Mineralocorticoids

a. Influence carbohydrate metabolism and other processes
b. Modulate salt and water balance
c. Contribute to expression of sexual characteristics

True or False

For each of the following statements, enter T *for true or* F *for false.*

4. ___ Fludrocortisone is a potent mineralocorticoid that also possesses significant androgenic properties.
5. ___ When present chronically in high concentrations, glucocorticoids produce symptoms much like those of diabetes.
6. ___ Thin extremities from muscle wasting is a symptom of glucocorticoid excess.
7. ___ Glucocorticoid excess prevents the breakdown of fat for energy.
8. ___ Glucocorticoids raise blood pressure (BP) by allowing blood vessels to constrict and limiting capillary permeability and loss of fluid into tissues.
9. ___ Excess glucocorticoid secretion is associated with depression.
10. ___ Adverse effects of water retention and muscle wasting are expected when a patient takes glucocorticoid therapy because of insufficient secretion by the adrenals.
11. ___ Patients who take glucocorticoid therapy because of insufficient secretion by the adrenals are at risk for hypotension and hypoglycemia anytime they experience elevated levels of physical or emotional stress.
12. ___ Hydrocortisone is a preferred drug for all forms of adrenocortical insufficiency.
13. ___ Addison disease involves insufficient secretion of adrenocorticoids, and Cushing syndrome is excessive production of adrenocorticoids.
14. ___ Cushing syndrome is usually treated by the administration of drugs that suppress adrenal secretion of hormones.

CRITICAL THINKING, PRIORITIZATION, AND DELEGATION QUESTIONS

15. The adrenals of the full-term fetus release a burst of glucocorticoids during labor and delivery to accomplish which action?
   a. Accelerate maturation of lungs.
   b. Lower maternal BP.
   c. Prevent uterine contractions.
   d. Stimulate fetal weight gain.

16. Ideally, to follow the normal circadian pattern of glucocorticoid release, glucocorticoid replacement therapy would be administered at which time?
   a. Midmorning
   b. Just after waking
   c. Midafternoon
   d. Just before sleep

✳17. It would be a priority to report which finding when caring for a patient with Cushing syndrome?
   a. Blood glucose 235 mg/dL
   b. Creatinine 1.2 mEq/dL
   c. Potassium 4.0 mEq/dL
   d. Albumin 4 g/dL

►18. Untreated primary hyperaldosteronism would be most dangerous if a patient had a history of which condition?
   a. Aspiration pneumonia
   b. Bowel obstruction
   c. Rheumatoid arthritis
   d. Heart failure

19. Eplerenone and spironolactone are prescribed for patients with adrenal hyperplasia because these drugs accomplish which action?
   a. Cause greater excretion of water
   b. Increase renal reabsorption of hydrogen
   c. Influence the normalization of potassium levels
   d. Reduction in left ventricular fibrosis

*20. Which is the priority teaching for a patient who has been prescribed hydrocortisone for adrenal insufficiency?
   a. Ensure adequate sodium in the diet.
   b. Take extra doses of corticoids when ill.
   c. Include fresh vegetables in the diet.
   d. Maintain fall precautions.

*21. Which findings would be a priority to report to the provider if a patient was prescribed fludrocortisone?
   a. BP 135/88 mm Hg
   b. Flushed, dry skin
   c. Nausea and vomiting
   d. Weight gain of 2 lb in 24 hours

22. The nurse is caring for a patient who is scheduled for an adrenalectomy due to adrenal adenoma. During the night, the nurse should assess the patient for which symptom of hyperaldosteronism?
   a. BP that is difficult to control
   b. Postural hypotension
   c. Cool, clammy skin
   d. Vomiting and diarrhea

*23. The nurse is caring for a patient with Cushing syndrome who is receiving 800 mg of ketoconazole. Which laboratory value should the nurse report to the provider?
   a. Alanine aminotransferase 150 international units/L
   b. Blood urea nitrogen 15 mg/dL
   c. Creatinine 1.5 mg/dL
   d. Glucose 150 mg/dL

24. The nurse is caring for a patient prescribed osilodrostat due to symptoms of Cushing disease which is not well controlled following surgery. Although this drug is generally well tolerated, the nurse knows to monitor the patient for which symptoms? (**Select all that apply.**)
   a. Hyperglycemia
   b. Muscle weakness
   c. Hypokalemia
   d. Peripheral edema
   e. Hypomagnesemia

DOSE CALCULATION QUESTIONS

25. Fludrocortisone acetate is available in 0.1-mg tablets. The patient is prescribed 0.05 mg once a day. How many tablets should the nurse administer for one dose?

26. The recommended dose of hydrocortisone for a patient with adrenal insufficiency is 12–15 mg/m^2. A patient who is 5 feet 11 inches tall and weighs 176 lb has been prescribed 25 mg. Is the dose safe?

CASE STUDY

A young adult has been admitted with severe episodic right upper quadrant (RUQ) pain, anorexia, and nausea. Oral cholecystography reveals acute cholecystitis, and an open cholecystectomy is planned. When gathering data regarding medical history, the patient reveals they have been experiencing extreme fatigue, dizziness when changing position, and muscle weakness. They have felt this way for a long time but thought the symptoms were caused by their stressful job. The patient also states that they love salty food and eat at least one bag of potato chips daily. The nurse notes that the patient has increased pigmentation around the face and hands and decreased body hair. Bloodwork includes fasting glucose 62 mg/dL, sodium 132 mEq/L, potassium 5.3 mEq/L, and blood urea nitrogen (BUN) 28 mg/dL. Synthetic adrenocorticotropic hormone (ACTH) is administered intravenously, and plasma cortisol levels are checked. Levels failed to rise from the ACTH stimulation. The patient is diagnosed with Addison disease. They ask the nurse how this causes their symptoms.

1. Describe how the nurse relates current and possible symptoms to decreased levels of adrenal cortex hormones.

2. The patient is prescribed hydrocortisone 50 mg IV every 8 hours. Texts state that daily doses of hydrocortisone should mimic normal daily secretion (20–30 mg/day). Why is this patient receiving such a high dose?

3. Because the patient is ill with cholecystitis and adrenal insufficiency, what is the most critical concern of the nurse? What should be included in the nursing plan of care to address this concern?

4. The patient is prescribed hydrocortisone 20 mg/day. What administration regimen would be used for the hydrocortisone if the provider wanted to mimic the body's natural basal secretion of glucocorticoids?

5. What teaching should the nurse provide to a patient prescribed oral glucocorticoids?

64 Estrogens and Progestins: Basic Pharmacology and Noncontraceptive Applications

STUDY QUESTIONS

Matching

Match the hormone with its actions during the menstrual cycle.

1. ___ Causes the dominant follicle to swell rapidly, burst, and release its ovum
2. ___ Following menstruation, promotes endometrial restoration
3. ___ Occurs when progesterone levels are insufficient to balance the stimulatory influence of estrogen on the endometrium
4. ___ Converts the endometrium from a proliferative state into a secretory state
5. ___ Acts on the developing ovarian follicles, causing them to mature and secrete estrogens

a. Dysfunctional uterine bleeding
b. Estrogen
c. Follicle-stimulating hormone (FSH)
d. Luteinizing hormone (LH)
e. Progesterone

CRITICAL THINKING, PRIORITIZATION, AND DELEGATION QUESTIONS

6. Which site is not acceptable for application of transdermal formulations of estrogen?
a. Breast
b. Calf
c. Forearm
d. Thigh

7. Which is a function of progesterone during pregnancy? **(Select all that apply.)**
a. Promotes growth of alveolar tubules
b. Prevents immune attack on the fetus
c. Stimulates follicular maturation
d. Suppression of uterine contractions
e. Raises body temperature by 1°F

8. The nurse is teaching a patient with Turner Syndrome and their parent about the adverse effects of estrogen therapy. Which information should be included in teaching?
a. Headache
b. Depression
c. Brown facial discoloration
d. Fluid retention
e. Joint pain

9. The nurse is caring for a patient who is status post–total knee arthroplasty. The patient has been taking estrogen to relieve menopausal symptoms and increase bone mineral density. Which new assessment finding would be of most concern to the nurse?
a. Dizziness with position changes
b. Dyspnea while resting
c. Nausea and vomiting
d. Bloody vaginal discharge

10. Research suggests that hormone therapy does not provide which benefits? **(Select all that apply.)**
a. Cardiovascular protection
b. Increase in bone density
c. Prevention of vaginal atrophy
d. Protection from dementia
e. Relief of insomnia and hot flashes

11. Which symptom, if exhibited by a patient who is receiving estrogen therapy, is most likely to be an effect of this therapy?
a. Constipation
b. Nausea
c. Profuse vaginal drainage
d. Orthostatic hypotension

✳12. The nurse is assessing a female patient who is of status post–total knee arthroplasty. The patient is prescribed raloxifene to treat osteopenia. Which would be of greatest priority to report to the surgeon?
a. Capillary refill 3 seconds
b. Difficulty passing hard stool
c. Dry mucous membranes
d. Pain in the right calf

*13. The nurse is reviewing laboratory test results for a 42-year-old patient who has been taking medroxyprogesterone acetate for dysfunctional uterine bleeding. Which test result would be a priority to report to the provider?
   a. Human chorionic gonadotropin (hCG) 2225 IU/mL
   b. Low-density lipoprotein (LDL) 102 mg/dL
   c. International normalized ratio (INR) 1.1
   d. White blood cell (WBC) 8765/mm^3

14. A patient diagnosed with genitourinary syndrome of menopause has been prescribed an estradiol acetate vaginal ring. Which statement indicates the patient understands the teaching associated with the vaginal ring?
   a. "I need to monitor for pain or tenderness in my legs while on this drug."
   b. "The vaginal ring will need to be replaced every six months."
   c. "This drug will help my vaginal dryness without the risk for blood clots."
   d. "I can use soy with this ring to help control my hot flashes and night sweats."

15. The patient tells their nurse they are frustrated because their interest in sex has declined. The patient states they have been on buspirone, but with no benefit. The nurse facilitates discussion between the patient and their provider, knowing which are approved by the FDA for treatment of female sexual interest-arousal disorder? (**Select all that apply**.)
   a. Cantharidin
   b. Bupropion
   c. Flibanserin
   d. Methylphenidate
   e. Bremelanotide

CASE STUDY

A 46-year-old patient has just received the recommendation that she undergo a total hysterectomy and bilateral salpingo-oophorectomy for uterine fibroids.

1. The patient should be informed which symptoms should be expected postoperatively relating to the removal of both ovaries (surgical menopause)?

2. The provider orders laboratory tests, including a lipid panel, mammogram, and dual-energy X-ray absorptiometry (DEXA) scan, and tells the patient that results are needed before they can discuss options to prevent surgically induced menopausal symptoms. The patient asks the nurse why these tests have been ordered. What information can the nurse provide?

3. Lab results include bone mineral density 1.5 standard deviations below normal, LDL 150 mg/dL, high-density lipoprotein (HDL) 55 mg/dL, and no evidence of lesions on mammogram. The patient is interested in postoperative hormone replacement. What additional information must be obtained before the provider considers ordering hormone replacement?

4. There are no contraindications for estrogen replacement therapy. The patient states that her mother received relief of menopausal symptoms by taking an estrogen-progesterone combination. Why would this drug not be prescribed for this patient?

5. After discussing risks and benefits, the provider orders a transdermal estrogen patch and asks the nurse to teach administration directives. What should the nurse include?

6. What teaching should the nurse provide that can help reduce the risk of cardiovascular events?

65 Birth Control

STUDY QUESTIONS

True or False

For each of the following statements, enter T for true or F for false.

1. ___ Tubal ligation and vasectomy are the most used form of birth control.
2. ___ The most effective pharmacologic forms of birth control have the most adverse effects.
3. ___ Oral contraceptives (OCs) and transdermal contraceptives are the most effective forms of birth control.
4. ___ Most OCs cause spontaneous abortion of a fertilized ovum.
5. ___ Smoking and migraine headache history increases the risk of serious blood clot events when a female uses OCs.
6. ___ Combination OCs are not associated with an increased risk of cancer for most females.
7. ___OCs can speed the growth of existing breast cancer.
8. ___ OCs are contraindicated during pregnancy.
9. ___ Progestin-only OCs are safer and more effective than combination OCs.
10. ___ Newer progestins in combination OCs are not more effective, but they have different adverse effects.
11. ___ Intrauterine devices (IUDs) are only recommended for persons at low risk for sexually transmitted infection (STI).
12. ___ A diaphragm with spermicide is more effective than male condoms with actual and theoretical use.
13. ___ Nonoxynol-9 may increase the risk of HIV transmission through promotion of vaginal, cervical, anal, and rectal lesions that facilitate HIV penetration to cells.

CRITICAL THINKING, PRIORITIZATION, AND DELEGATION QUESTIONS

*14. Which would be the priority teaching when a female is prescribed an OC containing the progestin drospirenone?
   a. "Do not eat too many bananas while you're taking this drug."
   b. "Seek medical care if you have unexplained shortness of breath."
   c. "There should be less bloating with this drug than with other OCs."
   d. "You should have your blood pressure checked at every health visit."

15. Which birth control method is of particular benefit to persons who have multiple partners?
   a. Oral contraceptives
   b. Sterilization
   c. Contraceptive ring
   d. Barrier with spermicide

*16. It would be priority for the patient to report which symptom if she is prescribed an OC containing drospirenone and lisinopril for hypertension?
   a. Spotting
   b. Fatigue
   c. Chest pain
   d. Bruising

17. Which supplement can decrease the effectiveness of OCs?
   a. Echinacea
   b. Garlic
   c. Ginkgo biloba
   d. St. John wort

*18. A patient who has been using OCs has been prescribed warfarin to prevent deep vein thromboses (DVTs) during a period of prolonged impaired mobility. Which is the priority action for this patient?
   a. Intake of adequate calcium in the diet
   b. Adhering to scheduled blood tests
   c. Increasing fluid intake to 2000 mL/day
   d. Using a soft, nonmechanical toothbrush

►19. A patient who has epilepsy that is managed with phenytoin comes to the college health center requesting OCs for birth control and menorrhagia. She has no contraindications for OC use. Which information should the nurse teach the patient concerning breakthrough bleeding or spotting?
   a. Teach the patient to use a barrier in addition to prescribed OCs.
   b. Tell the patient to stop taking phenytoin and see if seizures resume.
   c. Discuss with the patient abstinence as an alternative in this situation.
   d. Talk to the patient about how to predict the times when she is fertile.

►20. Which patient would be at greatest risk for pregnancy when using the contraceptive patch?
   a. 19-year-old with several partners
   b. 25-year-old who weighs 210 lb
   c. 37-year-old who is iron deficient
   d. 40-year-old who smokes two packs per day

✳21. A 19-year-old healthy patient who has been taking a combination OC for 2 years is involved in an automobile accident and undergoes surgical reduction and fixation of multiple fractures of both lower extremities. Which assessment finding is of greatest priority to report to the prescriber?
   a. Capillary refill of 2 seconds
   b. Profuse diaphoresis
   c. Sudden dyspnea
   d. Temperature 100°F (37.8°C)

✳22. The nurse is working in a women's health clinic. Several walk-in patients who take OCs arrive at the same time. Which patient should be given the highest priority for seeing the nurse practitioner?
   a. 17-year-old who is experiencing a migraine headache with aura
   b. 26-year-old who is experiencing breakthrough bleeding
   c. 35-year-old who smokes and needs her prescription refilled
   d. 42-year-old who has had episodes of severe right upper quadrant pain

►23. Which sign suggests that a patient who is prescribed ethinyl estradiol and drospirenone OCs may be experiencing hyperkalemia?
   a. Muscle weakness
   b. Tachycardia
   c. Positive Trousseau sign
   d. Restlessness

►24. Which response should the nurse provide to a patient who is concerned that she has not had a period since starting low-dose OCs 3 months ago?
   a. "Some women do not have periods when taking OCs."
   b. "Talk to the provider to decide if another OC is better."
   c. "You should have a biopsy to test for uterine malignancy."
   d. "You should have a serum pregnancy test drawn immediately."

►25. Because of the effect of OCs on glucose levels of patients with diabetes, it is most important for the nurse to assess for which symptom?
   a. Anorexia
   b. Diaphoresis
   c. Increased thirst
   d. Tachycardia

26. Which is a good choice when adherence could be an issue?
   a. Oral contraceptives
   b. Condom
   c. Diaphragm
   d. Depo-Provera

27. The nurse instructs the patient who is prescribed the transdermal contraceptive patch to apply the patch to which site? (**Select all that apply.**)
   a. Breasts
   b. Buttocks
   c. Lower abdomen
   d. Upper torso
   e. Upper inner arm

28. When a patient has an IUD in place, the nurse should assess for which symptom of a common adverse effect?
   a. Breast tenderness
   b. Dull pelvic pain
   c. Dysmenorrhea
   d. Peripheral edema

29. Which method of birth control is contraindicated when a patient has a pattern of multiple partners?
   a. Subdermal etonogestrel implant
   b. Intramuscular medroxyprogesterone acetate
   c. IUD
   d. Vaginal contraceptive ring

CASE STUDY

A 17-year-old sexually active female patient has used condoms as a form of birth control and prevention of STDs. She is monogamous and has decided to start on an OC. The patient's history includes asthma, dysmenorrhea, and irregular menses. Her last normal menstrual period was 2 months ago, but she says she is not concerned because this is a common occurrence for her. The patient is anxious and asks the nurse about the medical exam and what procedures will be performed.

1. Briefly describe what will be included in the preexam assessment and how frequently the patient will need to have it repeated.

2. The patient asks the nurse, "How do OCs prevent pregnancy?" How does the nurse respond?

3. When educating the patient on the use of OCs, it is important to stress the need to take them every day at the same time as prescribed. The patient is started on a triphasic OC and is concerned that she may forget to take the pills consistently. If she does forget, what procedures should she take to minimize the risk of pregnancy?

4. The patient asks about using an alternative form of contraception. What teaching should the nurse provide about the use of condoms and spermicides?

5. What possible adverse effects warrant discontinuation of the OC, and what symptoms of these conditions should the nurse teach the patient to report to her prescriber?

66 Drug Therapy for Infertility

STUDY QUESTIONS

Matching

Match the drug with its function.

1. ___ Blocks receptors for estrogen in the hypothalamus and pituitary
2. ___ Acts directly on the ovary to promote follicular development
3. ___ Given to induce ovulation
4. ___ Activates dopamine receptors in the pituitary and thereby reduces prolactin secretion
   a. Menotropin
   b. Human chorionic gonadotropin (hCG)
   c. Clomiphene
   d. Bromocriptine

True or False

For each of the following statements, enter T for true or F for false.

5. ___ *Infertility* is defined as being unable to reproduce.
6. ___ Treatment for low sperm count is more successful than treating female causes of infertility.
7. ___ *Nidation* is the medical term for implantation of the products of conception.
8. ___ Menotropins and follitropins act on mature follicles to cause ovulation.
9. ___ hCG stimulates ovarian follicles to mature.
10. ___ Scant or thick mucus produced by the glands at the neck of the uterus can impair the motility of the sperm into the uterus.
11. ___ Symptoms of hyperprolactinemia include secretion of milk when not breastfeeding.
12. ___ Dostinex and choriogonadotropin alfa are drugs used for infertility associated with endometriosis.
13. ___ The priority reason for using drugs to treat polycystic ovary syndrome (PCOS) is to decrease the number of ovarian cysts.
14. ___ Bromocriptine is a highly purified preparation of FSH extracted from the urine of pregnant females.

CRITICAL THINKING, PRIORITIZATION, AND DELEGATION QUESTIONS

*15. The nurse is explaining possible adverse effects of clomiphene. Which adverse effect would be a priority for the patient to report to the provider?
   a. Breast engorgement
   b. Hot flashes
   c. Low abdominal pain
   d. Nausea and vomiting

16. Which laboratory test result would be an absolute contraindication to the administration of clomiphene?
   a. Aspartate aminotransferase (AST) 41 IU/L
   b. Creatinine 1.4 mg/dL
   c. hCG 800 mIU/mL
   d. Sperm motility 70%

17. Patients who are prescribed clomiphene may experience increased viscosity of cervical mucus, hindering sperm motility. Estrogen is a possible treatment to thin the cervical mucus. Estrogen therapy would be of concern if the patient also has which chronic condition?
   a. Asthma
   b. Hypertension
   c. Type 2 diabetes
   d. Thrombophlebitis

*18. The nurse would be most concerned if a patient treated with menotropins reported which symptom?
   a. A fever higher than 100.4°F
   b. A gain of 2 lb in 24 hours
   c. A pulse rate higher than 80 beats/min
   d. Redness across the cheeks and nose

*19. The nurse is caring for a patient undergoing treatment for infertility with hCG. It is a priority to assess for which possible symptom of ovarian hyperstimulation syndrome?
   a. Abdominal pain
   b. Dyspnea
   c. Edema in ankles
   d. Weight gain

20. The nurse is explaining drug therapy to a patient who is prescribed cetrorelix. Which statement, if made by the patient, indicates a need for further teaching?
    a. "I need to inject the drug deep into a muscle using a 1.5-inch needle."
    b. "I should inject the drug into my fat about 2 inches away from my belly button."
    c. "I must stop taking the drug when instructed or I will not ovulate."
    d. "This drug prevents immature eggs from being released."
21. Bromocriptine inhibits prolactin secretion by activating receptors for which neurotransmitter?
    a. Acetylcholine
    b. Dopamine
    c. Nicotine
    d. Norepinephrine

DOSE CALCULATION QUESTIONS

22. Cabergoline is supplied in 0.5-mg tablets. The initial dosage is 0.25 mg. How many tablets should be administered?

23. hCG, 5000 USP units, is prescribed intramuscularly. Available is 10,000 units in 10 mL. How many milliliters should be administered at each site?

CASE STUDY

A couple has been trying to conceive for the past 2 years but has not been successful. During a lengthy diagnostic workup for infertility, the female was found to have no increase in her basal body temperature throughout her menstrual cycle. The male was found to have a normal sperm count and no health issues. The provider diagnoses primary infertility and decides to induce ovulation. Clomiphene and hCG are prescribed to promote ovarian follicular maturation and ovulation.

1. What organ functioning must be present for this drug to work?

2. One year later, the couple has not conceived. Menotropins—specifically, human menopausal gonadotropin (hMG) 1 ampule intramuscularly for days 9–12 of the menstrual cycle, followed by hCG 5000 units—are prescribed for the female. The nurse provides counseling relevant to the need for follow-up and early detection of ovarian hyperstimulation syndrome. What symptoms should the nurse teach the patient to report immediately?

3. What will the nurse teach the patient about the timing of administration of hCG?

4. The couple asks whether a multiple pregnancy (i.e., more than one fetus) is more likely with this drug regimen. How should the nurse respond?

67 Drugs that Affect Uterine Function

STUDY QUESTIONS

True or False

For each of the following statements, enter T for true or F for false.

1. ___ Tocolytic drugs are used to induce and strengthen uterine contractions and to control postpartum bleeding.
2. ___ Magnesium sulfate is the most effective drug available to suppress preterm labor.
3. ___ Ergot alkaloids are not normally used to induce contractions during labor because they can cause prolonged uterine contractions.
4. ___ It is common for patients to have elevated temperature after receiving a dose of carboprost tromethamine to control postpartum hemorrhage.
5. ___ The best way to administer carboprost tromethamine is subcutaneously.

CRITICAL THINKING, PRIORITIZATION, AND DELEGATION QUESTIONS

6. Which is the most common risk factor for preterm labor? **(Select all that apply.)**
   a. Poverty
   b. Inadequate prenatal care
   c. Highly educated
   d. Intrauterine inflammation
   e. Multifetal pregnancy

*7. Which new assessment finding would be a priority to report to the obstetrician when the nurse is caring for a patient who is 35 weeks pregnant and receiving terbutaline to suppress preterm labor?
   a. Diaphoresis
   b. Heart rate of 90 beats/min
   c. Increased thirst
   d. Shortness of breath

*8. The nurse is caring for a neonate whose mother received nifedipine. Which is the priority nursing focus?
   a. Hydration
   b. Nourishment
   c. Ventilation
   d. Warmth

*9. Which laboratory result is most concerning to the nurse caring for a patient receiving magnesium sulfate to suppress preterm labor?
   a. Alanine aminotransferase 50 IU/L
   b. Calcium 11 mg/dL
   c. Creatinine 4 mg/dL
   d. Magnesium 1.2 mEq/L

10. Which nursing outcome best indicates that intravenous (IV) oxytocin therapy has achieved the desired effect during the first hour after delivery of the placenta?
   a. BP is 120/80 mm Hg.
   b. Pulse is 80 beats/min.
   c. Perineal pad saturation >20 minutes.
   d. Skin is warm and dry.

11. Which assessment would be reason to hold the infusion of oxytocin? **(Select all that apply.)**
   a. Contractions lasting longer than 1 minute
   b. Contractions occurring more than every 2 minutes
   c. Late decelerations of fetal heart rate
   d. Intrauterine pressure >20 mm Hg during contractions
   e. Umbilical cord palpable in cervix

*12. The labor and delivery nurse is preparing to administer methylergonovine to a female who has just delivered the placenta. Before administering the medication, it is a priority for the nurse to perform which assessment?
   a. Blood pressure
   b. Lochia flow
   c. Respirations
   d. Uterine firmness

13. Dinoprostone for cervical softening is contraindicated in patients with a history of which condition? **(Select all that apply.)**
   a. Acute pelvic inflammatory disease
   b. Blood sugar higher than 200 mg/dL
   c. Asthmatic bronchitis
   d. Cardiomyopathy
   e. Hypotension
   f. Previous cesarean section
   g. Wheezing

14. Which are the responsibilities relating to dinoprostone gel for obstetric nurses working at most hospitals? **(Select all that apply.)**
    a. Calculating the proper dose of the drug
    b. Determining the number of doses needed
    c. Ordering the correct number of doses for the patient
    d. Positioning the patient during and after administration
    e. Storing the drug at the proper temperature

*15. The dinoprostone vaginal insert pouch has been inserted in a patient's posterior fornix. Monitoring indicates that moderate contractions lasting 15 seconds have begun. Which is the priority nursing intervention?
    a. Immediately begin infusion of oxytocin
    b. Instruct the patient to stay supine for 1 hour
    c. Place the patient on a fetal monitor
    d. Remove the dinoprostone pouch

DOSE CALCULATION QUESTIONS

16. To induce labor, oxytocin is ordered at 1.5 mU/min. Oxytocin is available for IV infusion at a concentration of 10 mU/mL. How many mL/hr will be programmed into the IV pump?

17. Tranexamic acid is ordered 1300 mg three times a day for 5 days each cycle for your patient with heavy menstrual bleeding. Tranexamic acid 650 mg tabs are available. How many tabs are in each dose?

CASE STUDY

A 25-year-old multipara (gravida 2, para 1) is admitted to the labor and delivery unit for induction of labor. She is at 41 weeks gestation. Vital signs and fetal heart rate are stable. Dinoprostone gel is ordered for cervical ripening.

1. What will the nurse teach the patient about this therapy?

2. The cervix has softened and is 50% effaced. The fetal head was at 0 station in a left occiput anterior position. The medication order reads: "Oxytocin 10 mU. May increase 1–2 mU/min every 30 minutes until normal patterns of uterine contractions are established." What is a normal pattern of uterine contractions?

3. When is oxytocin augmentation of labor contraindicated?

4. An IV infusion of 1000 units of oxytocin in 100 mL of 5% dextrose and 0.45% normal saline is infused via a secondary line into a primary infusion line. The oxytocin infusion was regulated by an infusion pump and was initiated at 1 mU/min. Why is the oxytocin infusion piggybacked into the primary infusion line rather than added to the primary infusion solution?

5. The patient has suddenly started having contractions lasting 90 seconds every 2 minutes. What should the nurse do?

6. When reporting the patient's response to oxytocin therapy to the obstetrician, what should the nurse include?

7. The patient has delivered her 6-lb 4-oz baby. She received one dose of carboprost tromethamine 250 mcg intramuscularly (IM) to control postpartum hemorrhage. The next day, she spiked a temperature of 101.6°F. Tylenol 8-Hour Arthritis Pain 650 mg every 6 hours as needed is included in the postpartum orders. Fever is a common adverse effect of carboprost. Why is it important to notify the obstetrician rather than just administer the antipyretic?

68 Androgens

STUDY QUESTIONS

Completion

1. The body responds to increased testosterone levels by suppressing the release of ______________ and ________________ from the anterior pituitary.
2. Androgens may help treat refractory anemia by promoting synthesis of ________________.
3. Because androgens can cause cholestatic hepatitis, the nurse should monitor ________________ tests when a patient is receiving this drug.
4. A weight gain of 2 lb in 24 hours suggests that a patient who is receiving androgen therapy may be experiencing the adverse effect of retention of ________________ and ________________.
5. When taken by females in high doses, androgens can cause clitoral growth, hair loss, and lowering of the voice that may be ________________.

CRITICAL THINKING, PRIORITIZATION, AND DELEGATION QUESTIONS

6. Laboratory test results for a patient who is prescribed androgen therapy include alanine aminotransferase (ALT) 45 mg/dL, calcium 9 mg/dL, fasting blood glucose (FBG) 82 mg/dL, hemoglobin (Hgb) 14.2, hematocrit (Hct) 45%, and high-density lipoprotein (HDL) 22 mg/dL. Which is a priority for patient teaching?
   a. Following a heart-healthy diet
   b. Increasing protein in the diet
   c. Limiting refined carbohydrates in the diet
   d. Performing weight-bearing exercise

*7. When a patient is prescribed an androgen, which adverse effect would be a priority for the nurse to report to the provider?
   a. Breast enlargement
   b. Altered menstruation
   c. Peripheral edema
   d. Increased libido

*8. Which adverse effect of testosterone is a medical emergency?
   a. Closure of epiphyses before age 12 years
   b. Low-density lipoprotein (LDL) 240 mg/dL
   c. 1+ pitting edema of ankles
   d. Erection lasting longer than 4 hours

9. A patient has received instructions regarding administration of testosterone buccal tablets. Which of these statements made by the patient would indicate the need for further teaching?
   a. "I should apply the tablet to my gum above an incisor."
   b. "I should alternate sides of my mouth with each dose."
   c. "I should hold the tablet in place for 30 seconds to ensure adhesion."
   d. "I should remove the tablet when drinking hot fluids."

10. The pediatrician's triage nurse receives a call at 2:00 p.m. from a 14-year-old patient who was recently prescribed testosterone buccal tablets. The patient applied the buccal tablet at 7:00 a.m., and it fell out during lunch. The patient asks what they should do. Which is the appropriate nursing instruction?
    a. Do not replace the tablet until the next dose is due.
    b. Replace the tablet and remove it as scheduled.
    c. Insert a new tablet and remove it in 12 hours.
    d. Place a new tablet and remove it in the morning.

11. Which behavior, if occurring while topical androgen is applied, would be of most concern?
    a. Chewing tobacco
    b. Drinking hot tea
    c. Showering before application
    d. Smoking cigarettes

12. The high school nurse is planning a teaching presentation on the use of anabolic steroids. Developmentally, discussion of which effects of anabolic steroid use would most likely discourage their use by male high school athletes?
    a. Atherosclerosis
    b. Hypertension
    c. Liver damage
    d. Testicular shrinkage

*13. Which assessment findings, if identified in a patient who is receiving oxandrolone for muscle wasting associated with advanced HIV disease, would be a priority to report to the provider?
    a. Acne
    b. Jaundice
    c. Loss of hair
    d. Weight gain

*14. During admission history, a patient who has a history of androgen deficiency describes the symptoms of dark-colored urine and clay-colored stool. Which is the priority nursing action at this time?
   a. Ask the charge nurse for guidance.
   b. Contact the provider immediately.
   c. Review liver function tests.
   d. Notify the pharmacy.

DOSE CALCULATION QUESTIONS

15. Testosterone cypionate 50 mg intramuscular (IM) is prescribed. Two hundred milligrams per milliliter is available. How much should be administered?

16. Testosterone pellets 75 mg are available. Prescribed is 300 mg. How many pellets will the nurse have available for insertion into the patient's abdomen?

CASE STUDY

A 16-year-old male patient has come to the health care provider because of his small testes and penis. The nurse notes that the patient is very tall (6 feet 10 inches) and thin (160 lb). His legs are unusually long for his trunk. He tells the nurse that he has frequently been in trouble in school, and he will finally be a freshman in high school this year. He is considering dropping out of school. Laboratory test results reveal the absence of sperm in the semen and the presence of two more X chromosomes than would be expected for a male. The diagnosis of Klinefelter syndrome is made. The nurse knows that this is not extremely rare, occurring in 1 of every 500 live male births, but is often not discovered until the male patient comes in for an infertility workup. Therapy will be directed toward administration of the male hormone testosterone. The patient is prescribed 1% testosterone transdermal gel. He asks, "Why can't I take a pill?"

1. How should the nurse respond?

2. The patient's mother is 36 years old and may wish to have another child. What precautions does the nurse need to teach the patient's mother and the patient?

3. What teaching should the nurse provide to the patient about administration of the gel?

4. The patient asks if there are any alternative routes of administration of testosterone. How should the nurse respond?

5. What information does the patient need regarding the adverse effects of testosterone?

69 Drugs for Erectile Dysfunction and Benign Prostatic Hyperplasia

STUDY QUESTIONS

True or False

For each of the following statements, enter T for true or F for false.

1. ___ Phosphodiesterase type 5 (PDE-5) inhibitors are contraindicated if the patient has a history of hypertension or diabetes mellitus.
2. ___ PDE-5 inhibitors are most effective if the cause of the erectile dysfunction (ED) is depression.
3. ___ Sexual activity can be more dangerous than the drugs for ED for patients taking nitrates.
4. ___ PDE-5 inhibitors activate the parasympathetic nervous system.
5. ___ Intestinal absorption of PDE-5 inhibitor drugs can be impaired for 3 days if the patient regularly ingests grapefruit juice.
6. ___ Patients who are prescribed sildenafil and vardenafil should be warned of possible loss of vision and/or hearing.
7. ___ Vardenafil works faster, longer, and better than sildenafil.
8. ___ Tadalafil is approved for daily use at lower than an as-needed dose if the patient anticipates sexual activity at least once a week.
9. ___ Finasteride is protective against high-grade prostate cancer.
10. ___ Finasteride can interfere with the laboratory test for prostate cancer.
11. ___ Patients should not donate blood while taking dutasteride.
12. ___ There are no concerns for patients taking PDE-5 inhibitors if they are also prescribed the α_{1a}-blockers silodosin or tamsulosin.
13. ___ Tolterodine, a muscarinic antagonist developed for urge incontinence, is contraindicated in patients with benign prostatic hyperplasia (BPH).
14. ___ The definition of premature ejaculation that is used for research is ejaculation that occurs earlier than a male wants it to occur.

CRITICAL THINKING, PRIORITIZATION, AND DELEGATION QUESTIONS

15. The nurse who works in a reproduction clinic counsels patients who are experiencing ED. Many patients ask if the drugs advertised on television help. The nurse knows these drugs will be effective for which underlying issue? **(Select all that apply.)**
    a. Desire for a more intense experience
    b. Improvement of erection quality
    c. Lack of desire for sexual activity
    d. Improved duration of erection
    e. Premature ejaculation

*16. Which of these findings, occurring 4 hours after sexual activity, would be an emergency for a patient who uses sildenafil?
    a. Blood pressure (BP) 160/80 mm Hg
    b. Diarrhea
    c. Persistent erection (PE)
    d. Headache

*17. It is a priority to determine if a male patient has taken sildenafil within the past 24 hours if the nurse is preparing to administer which medication?
    a. Cimetidine
    b. Doxazosin
    c. Finasteride
    d. Isosorbide

*18. It is a priority for the nurse to immediately report to the provider which of these findings if identified in a patient who has been prescribed sildenafil?
    a. Chest pain with moderate physical activity
    b. Facial flushing within 1 hour of taking the drug
    c. Rhinorrhea in the spring season
    d. Difficulty starting the stream of urine

19. Which sudden change in a patient taking sildenafil should be monitored but does not warrant consulting the provider before continuing to use the drug for ED?
    a. Blurring of vision
    b. Chest pain during sexual activity
    c. Difficulty hearing out of one ear
    d. Dizziness with position changes

*20. A patient who took vardenafil this evening comes to the emergency department complaining of palpitations and dizziness. Assessment findings include a heart rate of 122 beats/min and BP of 80/46 mm Hg. Which is the priority nursing action?
   a. Request echocardiogram.
   b. Request electrocardiogram.
   c. Call for a stress test.
   d. Check serum drug level.

21. Which is the reason tadalafil can be used by males with BPH?
   a. It modestly reduces symptoms of BPH.
   b. It improves urine flow rate in BPH.
   c. It does not increase risk of hypotension.
   d. It provides rapid relief of symptoms.

22. Which is the effect of direct injection of papaverine plus phentolamine that differs from the effects of oral drugs for ED?
   a. Erection occurs without stimulation.
   b. Arterial inflow is increased.
   c. Hypotension will not occur.
   d. Outflow of venous blood is decreased.

23. The nurse is preparing discharge instructions for a male who came to the clinic with reports of inability to ejaculate. Before the nurse can begin talking, he asks why this is happening. Which is the nurse's best response?
   a. "It's probably due to issues between you and your partner."
   b. "You are becoming too excited; you need to relax."
   c. "There are many causes for PE, including physiologic factors."
   d. "It may be caused by alterations in neurotransmitter synthesis."

24. The nurse knows that although no drugs have FDA approval for the treatment of PE, which drugs are prescribed off label in its treatment? **(Select all that apply.)**
   a. Citalopram
   b. Prilocaine
   c. Alprostadil
   d. Tramadol
   e. Finasteride

25. Which is true about BPH? **(Select all that apply.)**
   a. It can cause obstructive nephropathy.
   b. Symptoms may occur with moderate gland enlargement.
   c. Is not associated with risk for prostate cancer.
   d. Symptoms are directly related to the size of the gland.
   e. Treatment is based on the presence of subjective symptoms.

►26. When administering finasteride, which nursing outcome would be expected?
   a. The erection lasts long enough to achieve sexual satisfaction.
   b. The prostate-specific antigen (PSA) level is less than 4 ng/mL.
   c. Postvoid residual urine is less than 50 mL on bladder scan.
   d. The size of the prostate gland is reduced by 50%.

*27. Which action is a priority when a female nurse is administering dutasteride?
   a. Give on an empty stomach.
   b. Administer with food.
   c. Avoid blood donation for 6 months.
   d. Avoid touching the capsule.

*28. Which is the priority assessment before the nurse administers terazosin to a patient who has been diagnosed with BPH?
   a. Bladder scan
   b. BP
   c. Respirations
   d. Temperature

*29. Which is the priority teaching regarding effects of doxazosin prescribed for BPH?
   a. Nasal congestion is possible.
   b. Orthostatic BP precautions must be taken.
   c. Quantity of ejaculate may decrease.
   d. Symptoms may be relieved soon after starting the drug.

30. Which is a disadvantage of the herbal preparation saw palmetto?
   a. It is often toxic in combination with other drugs.
   b. It is available only in specialized stores.
   c. Research suggests that it is not effective.
   d. It has significant adverse effects.

CASE STUDY

The nurse is providing medication teaching for a 45-year-old male patient who was admitted with cellulitis of the left lower leg. The patient has a history of type 2 diabetes mellitus and hypertension. During the discussion, the patient's wife mentions that he has been experiencing "difficulties with sex" since he started taking medication for his high BP.

1. Why is it particularly important to address sensitive adverse effects, such as ED, especially when they occur because of antihypertensive medications?

2. The nurse notifies the provider of the patient's and wife's concerns. After discussing the problem with the patient, the provider orders sildenafil 50 mg as directed and asks the nurse to explain administration of the drug. What should be included in this explanation?

3. Why is it important for the patient to have information on his person stating that he takes sildenafil and to share this information with all providers?

70 Transgender Health

STUDY QUESTIONS

True or False

For each of the following statements, enter T for true or F for false.

1. ____ Transgender is an umbrella term that includes diverse genders beyond the binary man and woman.
2. ____ A multidisciplinary team is recommended for optimal transgender healthcare.
3. ____ A 16-year-old does not need parental consent for gender-affirming hormone therapy (GAHT).
4. ____ Secondary sexual characteristics that come with puberty can cause extreme distress.
5. ____ GAHT that is begun in adolescence does not prevent the development of secondary sex characteristics.
6. ____ Transgender individuals who wish to have biological offspring may elect to continue with endogenous puberty to produce sperm or eggs that can be banked for future use.
7. ____ The therapeutic goal of GAHT is to suppress puberty and promote the desired sex characteristics.
8. ____ The effects of GnRH analogues are irreversible.

Matching

Match the term with its definition.

9. ____ A person whose gender identity aligns with the assigned sex at birth.
10. ____ Attributes and expressions of femininity and masculinity that are shaped by social structures and cultural beliefs, assumptions, and traditions.
11. ____ A sense of distress that an individual experiences when sex assigned at birth is different from one's gender identity.
12. ____ Neither male nor female.
13. ____ A designation of male or female based on genotype.
14. ____ Having changing genders.

   a. Nonbinary
   b. Gender dysphoria
   c. Sex
   d. Gender fluid
   e. Cisgender
   f. Gender

CRITICAL THINKING, PRIORITIZATION, AND DELEGATION QUESTIONS

15. Which assessment is recommended every 3 to 6 months for adolescents undergoing puberty suppression? (**Select all that apply.**)
   a. Tanner staging
   b. Heart rate
   c. Blood pressure
   d. Height sitting
   e. Body mass index

16. Which is the most used antiandrogen?
   a. Enzalutamide
   b. Cyproterone
   c. Spironolactone
   d. Bicalutamide

17. It is important to teach transgender women that they will remain at risk for which condition regardless of gender-confirming surgery?
   a. Colorectal cancer
   b. Bladder cancer
   c. Prostate cancer
   d. Lung cancer

18. The nurse is caring for a transgender man who is being treated with intramuscular (IM) testosterone. The patient reports they are still having menses. Which medication does the nurse anticipate will be prescribed? (**Select all that apply.**)
   a. Medroxyprogesterone
   b. Low-dose estradiol
   c. Levonorgestrel intrauterine device (IUD)
   d. Enzalutamide
   e. Conjugated estrogen

19. The nurse is caring for a transgender man beginning GAHT. It is important to counsel the patient to continue to follow screening recommendations for which condition even after gender-affirming surgery? (**Select all that apply.**)
    a. Cervical cancer
    b. Endometrial cancer
    c. Breast cancer
    d. Prostate cancer
    e. Bladder cancer

20. The nurse is teaching an adolescent and their parents about leuprolide. Which statement by the parents indicates they understand how leuprolide suppresses puberty?
    a. "The drug suppresses the pituitary gland, so it does not secrete hormones."
    b. "Receptors for follicle-stimulating hormone become hypersensitive."
    c. "They cause a surge in luteinizing hormone that desensitizes receptors."
    d. "It only requires two doses to keep the pituitary hormones suppressed."

21. As part of the teaching for an adult patient beginning leuprolide, the nurse includes information about which side effect? (**Select all that apply.**)
    a. Hypoglycemia
    b. Fluid retention
    c. Hypertension
    d. Increased lipids
    e. Vaginal bleeding

22. Which is the recommended estrogen for use in feminizing therapy?
    a. Conjugated estrogens
    b. 17-Beta estradiol
    c. Ethinyl estradiol
    d. Norethindrone

23. When caring for a patient undergoing masculinizing therapy with testosterone, which side effect should be included when teaching about the drug? (**Select all that apply.**)
    a. Polycythemia
    b. Hyperlipidemia
    c. Endometriosis
    d. Prostate cancer
    e. Fluid retention

24. Teaching about testosterone therapy should include information about monitoring which laboratory value closely during the first year?
    a. Total testosterone
    b. Hemoglobin A1c
    c. Hematocrit
    d. Lipid profile

SINGLE-EPISODE CASE STUDY

The nurse meets with a patient and their family prior to beginning GAHT. The nurse is part of the interdisciplinary team providing care.

HEALTH HISTORY	NURSE'S NOTES	PHYSICIAN'S ORDERS	LABORATORY PROFILE

Time: 1040 hrs

A 13-year-old female accompanied by parents, wishing to begin GAHT to promote development of male sexual characteristics. Parents supportive, recognizing the patient has not felt comfortable "in her skin" for several years and does not "dress or play like a girl." When the patient began menses this year, they completely broke down, stating, "boys don't have a period." At the patient's request, the parents have been referring to the patient by their chosen masculine name, Aaron.

Father works full time as a roughneck, spending 2 weeks on an oil rig in the Gulf of Mexico and then 2 weeks at home. Mother works full time as a store manager for a well-known coffee chain. The patient has full insurance coverage from father's job. The patient has no siblings.

The patient attends school full time. They do not participate in any extracurricular activities or clubs. They began individual and family counseling a year ago due to the patient's anxiety and depression. The patient experiences insomnia and frequently misses school due to nausea and vomiting. Has frequent headaches. Has generally done well in school, although this last year, grades have begun to drop from As to Bs.

The family has been attending support group meetings as well. The patient's social circle involves other members of the support group but no one from the school or neighborhood where they live.

Medications include escitalopram 20 mg daily, hydroxyzine 25 mg every 8 hours as needed for anxiety/nausea, and acetaminophen 325 ii tabs every 8 hours as needed for headache.

Weight: 35.45 kg; height 61 inches (body mass index [BMI] 14.7)

Blood pressure 95/58; heart rate 65; respirations 12; temperature 97.4°F; O_2 sat 99% on room air.

1. Highlight the factors that meet criteria for gender dysphoria.

71 Review of the Immune System

STUDY QUESTIONS

Matching

Match the term with its primary action.

1. ___ Antigen-presenting cells found in lymph nodes and other lymphoid tissues
2. ___ Attack and kill target cells directly
3. ___ Attack and destroy foreign particles that have been coated with antibodies of the immunoglobulin E (IgE) class
4. ___ Devour cells that have been tagged with antibodies of the IgG class
5. ___ Mediate immediate hypersensitivity reactions
6. ___ The principal scavengers of the body
7. ___ Make antibodies
8. ___ Promote delayed-type hypersensitivity
9. ___ Molecule that binds to a bacterium, thereby promoting phagocytosis
10. ___ Provide the basis for distinguishing between self and nonself

    a. B lymphocytes (B cells)
    b. Basophils and mast cells
    c. Cytotoxic T cell (CD8)
    d. Dendritic cells
    e. Eosinophils
    f. Helper T cells (CD4 cells)
    g. Macrophages
    h. Major histocompatibility complex (MHC)
    i. Neutrophils
    j. Opsonin

Match the immunoglobulin with its descriptor.

11. ___ Stimulates release of histamine, heparin, and other mediators from mast cells
12. ___ First class of antibody produced in response to an antigen
13. ___ First line of defense against microbes entering the body via the gastrointestinal (GI) tract and lungs
14. ___ The major antibody in blood
15. ___ Found only on the surface of mature B cells

    a. IgA
    b. IgD
    c. IgE
    d. IgG
    e. IgM

Completion

16. Antibodies are also known as ______________ __________ and ______________________.
17. Specific immune responses are possible because __________________ and __________________ possess receptors that can recognize individual antigens.

CRITICAL THINKING, PRIORITIZATION, AND DELEGATION QUESTIONS

18. Which is true about natural immunity?
    a. It intensifies with each exposure to an antigen.
    b. Lymphocyte receptors recognize antigens.
    c. Immunity is specific to a particular antigen.
    d. Skin, as a barrier, confers natural immunity.

►19. The nurse assesses for the declining immune status of patients who are infected with human immunodeficiency virus (HIV) by monitoring for declining levels of which cell type?
    a. Basophils
    b. CD4 cells
    c. CD8 cells
    d. Macrophages

20. Which is true about breastfeeding?
    a. There is no effect on the infant's immunity.
    b. It transfers lifelong immunity from the mother.
    c. It transfers maternal IgA to the infant's GI tract.
    d. It triggers the release of mediators from mast cells.

21. Autoimmune diseases occur under which circumstances?
   a. With introduction of an antigen that is new to the body.
   b. A person has an inflammatory reaction to an antigen.
   c. After antigen introduction, the immune response fades.
   d. There is a failure in MHC molecules' ability to identify self.

22. Which is the reason a person who is allergic to penicillin can expect a more severe reaction with exposure to penicillin in the future?
   a. Helper T cells attack the penicillin molecule.
   b. Higher doses of penicillin would have to be used.
   c. Memory cells allow for a more intense response.
   d. The immune system cannot eliminate the penicillin.

23. The nurse is reviewing the laboratory tests for a patient who is jaundiced. Laboratory results include an elevated tumor necrosis factor (TNF). This suggests the patient has which condition?
   a. Cirrhosis
   b. Diabetes
   c. Tumor
   d. Kidney failure

24. Which is a mediator molecule released by any immune system cell?
   a. Antigen-presenting cell
   b. Cytokine
   c. MHC molecule
   d. Opsonin

25. Which activates the classical complement pathway?
   a. Free antibody
   b. Free antigen
   c. Antibody-antigen complex
   d. Phagocytic cell

CASE STUDY

The nurse is preparing to perform allergy testing by intradermal injection of house dust, molds, foods, and other common allergens.

1. Why are injected extracts called *antigens*?

2. The allergic reaction causes degranulation of mast cells. What cells respond in the skin, what do they release, and what dermal symptoms will the patient have if allergic to the antigen?

3. The patient is required to remain in the office for 20 minutes after injection of any antigen because that is the usual time frame for an immediate hypersensitivity reaction. Describe what the nurse should do if the following reactions occur.
   a. Itching and redness at the site of injection

   b. Tingling around the mouth

4. Why is it important to teach this patient about possible anaphylaxis?

72 Childhood Immunization

STUDY QUESTIONS

Matching

Match the term with its description.

1. ___ Refers to the production of both active immunity and passive immunity
2. ___ Giving a patient preformed antibodies
3. ___ Composed of isolated microbial components.
4. ___ Not pathogenic
5. ___ Documents that describe the benefits and risks of specific vaccines
6. ___ A mercury-based preservative found in some vaccines
7. ___ Preparations that contain a high concentration of antibodies directed against a specific antigen
8. ___ Preparation containing whole or fractionated microorganisms
9. ___ Giving any vaccine or toxoid
10. ___ Microbes that have been weakened or rendered completely avirulent
11. ___ Develops in response to infection or administration of a vaccine or toxoid
12. ___ Bacterial toxin that has been changed to a nontoxic form
13. ___ Carries the code for the COVID-19 spike glycoprotein

a. Active immunity
b. Live vaccine
c. Killed vaccine
d. Avirulent
e. Immune globulin
f. Immunization
g. Passive immunity
h. Modified messenger ribonucleic acid technology
i. Thimerosal
j. Toxoid
k. Vaccine
l. Vaccination
m. Vaccine information statements (VIS)

CRITICAL THINKING, PRIORITIZATION, AND DELEGATION QUESTIONS

14. Because cases of anaphylaxis associated with mumps, measles, and rubella (MMR) vaccine can be severe, the nurse should ensure immediate access to which drug before administering any immunization?
   a. Albuterol
   b. Cetirizine
   c. Diphenhydramine
   d. Epinephrine

►15. Which is the appropriate immunization strategy for a child who is behind in getting immunizations and is being seen at the pediatric office for a temperature of 100.6°F (38.1°C) and uncomplicated acute otitis media that is treated with amoxicillin?
   a. Give needed immunizations at the next well-child visit.
   b. Administer needed immunizations during this visit.
   c. Do not administer immunizations until the child is afebrile.
   d. Wait until antibiotics are complete to administer immunizations.

✳16. It would be priority for the parent to contact the provider if a child experienced which symptom after administration of a diphtheria and tetanus toxoids and acellular pertussis (DTaP) immunization?
   a. Drowsiness
   b. Refusal to eat
   c. Confusion
   d. Fever of 100.4°F (38°C)

17. When should the nurse provide parents or legal guardians with vaccine information sheets?
   a. Before the first dose in a series of vaccines
   b. Before each dose of each vaccine
   c. Once, before the very first vaccines
   d. Only when requested

►18. The nurse would consult with the provider if which immunization was prescribed for a child who is receiving long-term high doses of prednisolone? (**Select all that apply.**)
   a. Diphtheria
   b. *Haemophilus influenzae*
   c. Poliovirus
   d. Rotavirus
   e. Varicella

19. Foster parents bring a 14-month-old child in for the first visit to the pediatrician's office. The Child Protective Agency is unable to obtain any immunization records. The child has no contraindications to vaccination. Which approach to immunizations is appropriate?
   a. Administer immunizations as if the child has not received any vaccines.
   b. Administer the immunizations regularly scheduled for 12–14 months of age.
   c. Delay immunizations until the previous vaccination records can be found.
   d. Immunize the child with the immunizations scheduled for 2 months of age.

20. Which are appropriate measures to decrease discomfort associated with immunizations? **(Select all that apply.)**
   a. Administer acetaminophen 30–60 minutes before the immunization.
   b. Apply topical anesthetic to the injection site prior to injection.
   c. Hold the child still on their parent's lap in the supine position.
   d. Perform intramuscular (IM) injections rapidly without aspiration.
   e. Use microneedles when administering the injection.

✳21. It would be priority to consult the provider if MMR was ordered in which situation?
   a. The mother is receiving chemotherapy for breast cancer.
   b. A monospot test for the child is positive.
   c. Chemotherapy for leukemia has begun in the child.
   d. The child is asymptomatic but HIV positive.

22. Which information should be included when providing teaching about a scheduled MMR vaccination with the parents of a 12-month-old? **(Select all that apply.)**
   a. Does the child have any allergies to gelatin?
   b. Adverse effects will usually occur within 48 hours.
   c. Has the child has received blood products in the past 6 months?
   d. Contact the office for any unusual bleeding.
   e. Avoid the child having close contact with anyone pregnant for 3 weeks.

23. Which information is a reason to consult the provider before administering the varicella vaccine to a 15-month-old child?
   a. The child had a severe reaction to the MMR vaccine.
   b. An allergy to eggs is documented in the records.
   c. An aunt and newborn cousin are staying with the family.
   d. The 15-month-old is screaming uncontrollably.

►24. The triage office nurse receives a call from the parent of a 6-year-old who received the varicella vaccine 10 days prior. Yesterday the child stayed home from school with the stomach flu. The parent gave the child Pepto Bismol for nausea and diarrhea, and they have not had diarrhea today, but the parent is having difficulty awakening the child. Which directions should the nurse provide the parent?
   a. Allow the child to rest and encourage fluid intake.
   b. Make an appointment for the child to be seen in the office.
   c. Reassess the child after administering acetaminophen.
   d. Seek emergency medical care for the child immediately.

25. Which child should return for a booster dose of varicella vaccine 1 month after the first dose?
   a. Did not experience vesicular rash after the first dose
   b. A 14-year-old who has not had chickenpox
   c. The child had a kidney transplant a year ago
   d. A child less than 18 months old

26. The nursery nurse would expect to administer which vaccination to the neonate within 12 hours of birth if the neonate's mother is HBsAg positive? **(Select all that apply.)**
   a. Hepatitis B immunoglobulin
   b. Combined hepatitis A and B
   c. Influenza vaccine
   d. Pneumovax
   e. Monovalent hepatitis B

27. Which is an indication for hepatitis A vaccine? **(Select all that apply.)**
   a. All children aged 1–12 years
   b. A child with factor VIII deficiency
   c. Diagnosed with chronic kidney disease
   d. Person who is traveling to the Caribbean
   e. Individual who is planning a trip to Japan

►28. Parents of a child with asthma were reluctant to have their 3-year-old receive the flu vaccine because they were afraid that they would get the disease from the injection. The pediatrician convinced them to allow immunization in January of this year. Then next flu vaccine should be administered at which time?
   a. When the vaccine is available
   b. September of this year
   c. November of this year
   d. January of next year

*29. The nurse administers rotavirus vaccine to an infant at a medical clinic in the Dominican Republic. It is priority for the nurse to teach the child's caregivers to seek immediate emergency care if, within the next month, the infant exhibits which symptom?
   a. Loose stool × 2 in 24 hours
   b. Runny nose for 3 days
   c. Sore throat and cough
   d. Mucous and blood in stool

30. The nurse is teaching a patient about the Johnson & Johnson COVID vaccine. The patient is hesitant to receive the vaccine, stating they are afraid they will have a stroke. Which is the appropriate response by the nurse?
   a. "You do not need to worry; it is a rare complication that you are unlikely to have."
   b. "The risk of a stroke from COVID is higher than the risk of stroke from the vaccine."
   c. "If you develop symptoms of a stroke, it can be treated with an oral anticoagulant."
   d. "The most common adverse effect from the vaccine is injection site soreness."

CASE STUDIES

Case Study 1

Parents bring their 7-month-old child to the clinic. They state that they were told by an emergency department (ED) physician of the local hospital to bring their child in for "baby shots." The parents are concerned, stating that they have heard that children can die from these shots.

1. What teaching can the nurse provide about the safety and benefits of the immunizations?

2. The parents have difficulty understanding complex concepts. How can the nurse explain reactions to immunizations?

3. How would the nurse explain the laws requiring children to have immunizations before they can attend school and, in some cases, daycare?

4. What subjective data and medical history does the nurse need to review before administering an immunization?

Case Study 2

Parents of an elementary school child in Lancaster, Pennsylvania, have verbalized to the school nurse that their children have never been "contaminated" with immunizations. The parents state that their unimmunized child has not contracted measles, mumps, diphtheria, or other illness for which immunizations are routinely administered.

5. How should the school nurse respond?

6. The parents state that they are particularly concerned about MMR because of its association with autism. What has research suggested about the association between MMR and autism?

7. The school nurse is aware that exposure to certain populations or situations puts unvaccinated children at risk for contracting vaccine-preventable disease. What are possible populations and situations that would put children at risk in this school and geographic area?

Case Study 3

During pharmacology class, a nursing student remarks that they would not have their 11-year-old daughter receive human papillomavirus (HPV) vaccine because "she is a good girl."

8. What should be included in the discussion about this parent's reaction?

9. The concerned parent/nursing student agrees with the explanation but states that their daughter has heard that the injection is painful. What might the parent discuss with the pediatrician about this concern?

10. The literature reports a number of adolescent patients fainting when given the HPV vaccine. What might contribute to this reaction, and what can the office nurse do to prepare for this possible reaction?

11. Another nursing student states that they will have their daughter vaccinated because the adolescent will not have to have Pap smears and pelvic examinations until they are ready to get pregnant. What should be included in response to this statement?

73 Immunosuppressants

STUDY QUESTIONS

Completion

1. The large doses of glucocorticoids used to suppress immune responses can be expected to increase the risk for infection, thin the skin, cause osteoporosis, impair growth in children, and suppress the ________________________________ ____________________.
2. Unexplained bleeding is a possible adverse effect of ________________________.
3. Twice as many patients discontinue tacrolimus because of ________________________.
4. Immunosuppressant drugs, given at doses to prevent allograft rejection, have two toxic outcomes: increased risk for ________________________ and ____________________.
5. The nurse should teach patients who take sirolimus to take the medication consistently either without food or with consistent amounts of ________________________ in foods.
6. The nurse should teach a patient who is prescribed mycophenolate mofetil not to take over-the-counter (OTC) ________________________.

CRITICAL THINKING, PRIORITIZATION, AND DELEGATION QUESTIONS

*7. The nurse is providing postoperative teaching for a patient who has had carpal tunnel release surgery and who is on immunosuppressant therapy following kidney transplant. Which is the priority patient problem?
   a. Airway obstruction
   b. Tissue perfusion
   c. Wound infection
   d. Acute pain

8. A patient who has been prescribed immunosuppressant drugs should be taught to report which early sign of infection?
   a. Chills
   b. Cough
   c. Rash
   d. Sore throat

9. A 16-month-old child receives a heart-lung transplant. Which teaching should the nurse provide about immunizations?
   a. Increased doses of vaccines may be needed.
   b. Inactivated vaccines should not be given.
   c. Live vaccines should be given in lower doses.
   d. Immune response to all vaccines is reduced.

10. Which side effect of cyclosporine can alter a female patient's self-concept?
   a. Acne
   b. Facial hair
   c. Rash
   d. Weight gain

*11. Which is a priority nursing assessment in a patient receiving cyclosporine?
   a. Intake and output
   b. Pulse
   c. Temperature
   d. Weight

*12. The nurse is administering IV cyclosporine. Within 15 minutes after beginning the infusion, the patient complains of feeling hot and says their chest feels tight. Which is the priority nursing action?
   a. Administer epinephrine
   b. Check vital signs
   c. Assess lung sounds
   d. Stop the infusion

13. When reviewing the laboratory results of a patient receiving tacrolimus, which result would be a reason to contact the provider? (**Select all that apply.**)
   a. Platelet count 300 × 109/L
   b. Blood urea nitrogen 17 mg/dL
   c. Creatinine 3.2 mg/dL
   d. Potassium 5.4 mEq/L
   e. White blood cell 3800/mm^3

14. The nurse is providing discharge teaching regarding cyclosporine. Which statement suggests understanding of the teaching? **(Select all that apply.)**
   a. "I should call the provider if my stool changes color."
   b. "All of my prescriptions should come from the same pharmacy."
   c. "If I develop hot flashes, I should take a soy supplement."
   d. "Brushing my teeth and seeing my dentist are important."
   e. "Cyclosporine is best if taken with grapefruit juice."

▶15. A liver transplant recipient who is prescribed tacrolimus reveals that they have been drinking grapefruit juice, but the patient has made sure it has been at least 4 hours between the juice and the medication. Which lab result suggests a drug-food interaction?
   a. Blood pressure 88/47 mm Hg
   b. Estimated glomerular filtration rate (eGFR) 50 mL/hour
   c. Blood glucose 235 mg/dL
   d. Temperature 102°F

✳16. Which OTC drugs should a patient taking tacrolimus avoid?
   a. Acetaminophen
   b. Acetylsalicylic acid
   c. Diphenhydramine
   d. Ibuprofen

17. A kidney transplant recipient has trough levels of cyclosporine at 125 ng/mL. Which is the appropriate nursing action?
   a. Repeat the trough level
   b. Consult the provider
   c. Administer the drug
   d. Withhold the drug

✳18. Which symptom, if reported by a patient receiving sirolimus, would be a priority to report to the provider?
   a. Cough
   b. Fatigue
   c. Joint pain
   d. Tinnitus

19. Which drug, if taken with everolimus, is most likely to cause toxicity?
   a. Erythromycin
   b. Phenobarbital
   c. Phenytoin
   d. Rifamycin

✳20. Due to the adverse effect on bone density, it would be a priority for a patient to avoid falls when taking which drug?
   a. Azathioprine
   b. Prednisone
   c. Sirolimus
   d. Tacrolimus

21. Which laboratory results should be immediately reported to the provider when a patient is administered azathioprine?
   a. Alanine aminotransferase (ALT) 65 IU/L
   b. hCG 328 mIU/mL
   c. Platelets 145,000/mm3
   d. WBC 4900/mm^3

22. When administering antithymocyte globulin, the patient should be premedicated with which drug 1 hour before administration **(Select all that apply.)**
   a. Acetaminophen
   b. Epinephrine
   c. Glucocorticoid
   d. Diphenhydramine
   e. Ibuprofen

23. Which drug should be used in combination with mycophenolate mofetil? (**Select all that apply**.)
   a. Azathioprine
   b. Tacrolimus
   c. Glucocorticoids
   d. Cyclophosphamide
   e. Cyclosporine

24. Which drug is approved for prophylaxis of acute renal transplant rejection for the first 6 months following surgery?
   a. Muromonab-CD3
   b. Basiliximab
   c. Ruxolitinib
   d. Leflunomide

25. In addition to hepatotoxicity, which drug remains teratogenic for up to 2 years after discontinuation?
   a. Cyclophosphamide
   b. Leflunomide
   c. Methotrexate
   d. Mitoxantrone

DOSE CALCULATION QUESTIONS

26. A patient is prescribed oral cyclosporine 9 mg/kg per day divided into two doses 12 hours apart. The patient weighs 132 lb, and the medication is available as a solution of 100 mg/mL. How much medication should the nurse administer per dose?

27. Antithymocyte globulin 50 mg/mL solution is ordered at 15 mg/kg per day for 14 days to prevent renal allograft rejection. Your patient weighs 240 lb. How many mg of antithymocyte globulin will be administered?

CASE STUDIES

Case Study 1

A 4-year-old received an allogeneic heart transplant at age 16 months for heart failure secondary to transposition of the great vessels and only one ventricle.

1. What is an allogeneic transplant?

The patient was discharged on cyclosporine, azathioprine, and prednisone. They are brought back to the transplant hospital monthly for bloodwork to monitor rejection status and performance of the new heart. During the past year, the patient has shown no sign of rejection or limitation of activities. Growth has closely followed normal growth charts, and outwardly they appear to be a healthy 4-year-old. Recently, following a trip to a national park, the patient developed fatigue and appeared tired. Bloodwork indicated evidence of macrophages and monocytes beginning the rejection process. The patient was hospitalized and diagnosed with evidence of transplant rejection.

2. What are the priority patient problems for this patient?

3. IV muromonab-CD3 is added to the patient's medication regimen to prevent rejection of the transplanted heart. What actions should the nurse take in the hospital to prevent the patient from contracting an infection?

4. What special steps must be taken when administering this drug IV?

Case Study 2

A 38-year-old kidney transplant recipient is prescribed immunosuppressant therapy with IV cyclosporine, prednisone, and ketoconazole.

5. The patient asks why they are prescribed ketoconazole in addition to cyclosporine. What should the nurse explain is the main reason these two drugs are administered concurrently?

6. It is important for the nurse to teach the patient about cyclosporine's possible effects on a developing fetus and that current contraceptive recommendations include use of which type of birth control?

7. What teaching should the nurse provide relating to the adverse effect of increased risk of neoplasms from taking cyclosporine?

8. The provider of cyclosporine has ordered a trough level after the fourth dose. When should the trough level be drawn?

9. The patient's cyclosporine is changed to cyclosporine capsules. The hospital pharmacy sends the cyclosporine oral solution. What should the nurse do?

10. The patient has a history of osteoarthritis and a seizure disorder. What should be included in the plan of nursing care relating to immunosuppressant therapy that they are receiving and their medical history?

74 Antihistamines

STUDY QUESTIONS

True or False

For each of the following statements, enter T for true or F for false.

H_1-blocking drugs

1. ___ are the active ingredient in most over-the-counter (OTC) drugs to induce sleep.
2. ___ can cause excitement, nervousness, and tremors.
3. ___ can cause urinary retention.
4. ___ cause the skin to become red and warm.
5. ___ decrease release of histamine present in high levels in the skin.
6. ___ decrease pruritus.
7. ___ elevate the pH of stomach secretions.
8. ___ have sedation as the most common adverse effect.
9. ___ prevent local edema.
10. ___ prevent the release of histamine from mast cells and basophils.

CRITICAL THINKING, PRIORITIZATION, AND DELEGATION QUESTIONS

11. A patient is scheduled to receive radiocontrast media for a computerized axial tomography (CAT) scan. The patient has never received any radiocontrast media. What is the reason the nurse should carefully assess for an allergic reaction?
    a. Patients may not know if they have had radiocontrast media in the past.
    b. The reaction can occur in patients even without prior exposure to radiocontrast media.
    c. The reaction occurs in more than 30% of patients receiving radiocontrast media.
    d. Reactions to contrast media are usually asymptomatic until anaphylaxis occurs.

12. The parent of a 3-year-old child who was recently diagnosed with asthma calls the pediatrician's office. The child has a cold, which often triggers an asthma attack. The parent has forgotten which drug the child should be given when they start wheezing. Which drug would be safe and effective?
    a. Diphenhydramine
    b. Loratadine
    c. Fexofenadine
    d. None of the above

13. On admission, the nurse is reviewing drugs that a 78-year-old patient takes at home. The patient has a history of hypertension and diabetes. The patient takes OTC diphenhydramine when they have a cold. That nurse explains the effect of first-generation histamine blockers on the body and on a cold. Which statement, if made by the patient after the teaching, suggests a need for additional teaching?
    a. "It can make my cold go away faster."
    b. "The drug can dry up my nasal drainage."
    c. "Constipation is worse with antihistamines."
    d. "I need to keep it away from my grandkids."

14. Which is true about first-generation antihistamines?
    a. The drugs are highly sedating.
    b. They block H_2 receptors.
    c. Localized flushing occurs with use.
    d. CNS depression is negligible.

15. What is the reason second-generation H_1 blockers cause less sedation than first-generation H_1 blockers?
    a. First-generation H_1 blockers are more potent.
    b. Second-generation blockers bind reversibly to histamine receptors.
    c. Second-generation blockers cross the blood-brain barrier poorly.
    d. Second-generation drugs are rapidly metabolized.

✳16. Which of these assessment findings, if identified by the delivery room nurse in a full-term neonate whose mother has taken diphenhydramine just before going into labor, would be a priority to immediately report to the pediatrician?
    a. Systolic blood pressure (BP) 60 mm Hg
    b. Temperature 37.2°C (99°F)
    c. Pulse 180 beats/min
    d. Respirations 25 breaths/min

17. The nurse is teaching a patient who has a history of benign prostatic hyperplasia (BPH) and allergic rhinitis about taking desloratadine. Which teaching should be included?
    a. Avoid CNS depressants.
    b. Do not perform any activity that requires alertness.
    c. The drug may aggravate urinary retention.
    d. Take the drug with food or milk.

▶18. The nurse is administering 6:00 a.m. medications, including chlorpheniramine 4 mg every 6 hours for urticaria. The patient complains of nausea associated with the medication. Which is the appropriate nursing action?
    a. Change the timing of the medication.
    b. Decrease the dose of the medication.
    c. Consult the provider about dose timing.
    d. Provide a snack with each dose of medication.

DOSE CALCULATION QUESTIONS

19. Fexofenadine, 30 mg twice a day, is prescribed for a 4-year-old with allergy-induced asthma. It is available as a suspension containing 6 mg/mL. How many milliliters should be administered at each dose?

20. Promethazine 12.5 mg IV is prescribed for a patient with nausea and vomiting. The drug is available as 25 mg/mL. How much promethazine is to be administered? What is the recommended time over which it should administered?

SINGLE-EPISODE NEXTGEN CASE STUDY

HEALTH HISTORY	NURSE'S NOTES	PROVIDER NOTES	LABORATORY PROFILE

Time: 10:00 hrs

A 25-year-old taxi driver comes to the clinic with reports of "hay fever." The patient has tried diphenhydramine 25 mg, but it makes them too sleepy to work. They have also tried sinus spray, but it burns and tastes bad, so they stopped taking it. Tylenol 8-Hour Arthritis Pain 650 mg has been great for the headaches. They do not know what to take anymore because "OTC drugs seem so confusing."

Patient diagnosed with persistent allergic rhinitis, with acute reactions lasting from November until the end of April each year, when Mountain Cedar releases pollen. However, the patient also says they are occasionally bothered by pollen year-round, as well as by cat dander. Symptoms have been present for the past 2 years and have progressively gotten worse.

Review of symptoms: headache, congestion, sneezing, rhinorrhea, and itchy, burning, watery eyes.

Physical exam: Alert, oriented. Cleanly dressed. Appears fatigued. Patient breathes through their mouth and frequently rubs their nose, sniffs, and clears their throat. There are dark circles under their eyes. Nasal mucosa is pale and boggy with thin, watery secretions and inferior turbinate swelling. The nasal septum is midline. Eyes with scleral injection and conjunctival swelling. Tearing present. Posterior pharynx with cobble-stoning. Lungs clear to auscultation throughout; heart with normal S_1S_2; no peripheral edema. Abdomen soft and nontender with normoactive bowel sounds.

Vital signs: BP 122/84, heart rate (HR) 88, respiration 18, temperature 99.0°F, O_2 sat on room air 98%.
Provider started the patient on cetirizine 10 mg daily; drug teaching provided. Patient verbalizes understanding and provided teach back.

Which findings indicate improvement, no change, or a worsening of symptoms? Each finding is consistent with only one outcome.

ASSESSMENT FINDING	IMPROVED	NO CHANGE	WORSENING
Erythematous posterior pharynx			
Clear sclera			
Turbinate swelling present			
Thick nasal discharge			
Temperature 98.2°F			

75 Cyclooxygenase Inhibitors: Nonsteroidal Antiinflammatory Drugs and Acetaminophen

STUDY QUESTIONS

Completion

1. The half-life of aspirin is 15–20 minutes, but the antiplatelet effects last _________ ____________.
2. Preoperative teaching for knee replacement surgery should include that the patient should discontinue high-dose aspirin therapy for ___________________ before surgery.
3. When taking aspirin for its antiplatelet action, other nonsteroidal antiinflammatory drugs (NSAIDs) should be given at least _______ hours after aspirin.
4. Aspirin should not be taken by children, especially for symptoms of viral illness, because of the risk of ________________ ________________.
5. The nurse should instruct patients to dispose of aspirin tablets if they develop an odor that smells like ___________________.
6. Chronic alcohol use interferes with the metabolism of excessive doses of __________________.
7. __________________________ is the antidote for acetaminophen overdose.
8. The recommended maximum dose of acetaminophen for individuals who regularly consume alcohol is ____________.

CRITICAL THINKING, PRIORITIZATION, AND DELEGATION QUESTIONS

*9. The nurse is caring for a patient who is prescribed aspirin for its antiplatelet effects. Which symptom would be a priority to report to the provider?
   a. Abdominal bloating
   b. Emesis of black/brown particles
   c. Heartburn when recumbent
   d. Two liquid stools in 24 hours

▶10. In which situation would the nurse hold as-needed (PRN) ibuprofen and notify the provider?
   a. Hand stiffness when arising
   b. Knee pain with ambulation
   c. Right temporal headache
   d. Stomach pain with bloating

11. Which action should the nurse take to prevent the most common adverse effect of long-term aspirin therapy?
   a. Administer the drug with fluids and food.
   b. Assess lung sounds for wheezing.
   c. Monitor urine output on a daily basis.
   d. Teach the patient to report tarry stool.

12. Which statement, if made by a patient who is receiving aspirin therapy for rheumatoid arthritis, suggests that the patient needs further teaching?
   a. "It is important to drink at least a full glass of water when I take aspirin."
   b. "I will know if aspirin is causing ulcers because it will cause abdominal pain."
   c. "If I drink alcohol, it can make it easier for aspirin to cause it to bleed."
   d. "I should consult my provider if I experience a sudden watery runny nose."

13. Which diagnostic test is performed before starting long-term aspirin therapy to identify an increased risk for gastric ulceration?
   a. Colonoscopy
   b. pH monitoring
   c. Gastroscopy
   d. *Helicobacter pylori*

*14. It is priority for the nurse to communicate self-prescribed aspirin use to the provider if the patient has which history?
   a. Coronary artery disease
   b. Obstructive sleep apnea
   c. Smokes two packs per day
   d. Type 2 diabetes mellitus

*15. A patient brought to the emergency department (ED) exhibits the following symptoms after taking aspirin for a headache. Which symptom would be priority for the nurse to address?
   a. Bronchospasm
   b. Watery nasal discharge
   c. Tachycardia
   d. Urticaria

16. Which symptom suggests that blood levels of salicylate are too high?
   a. Fatigue
   b. Heartburn
   c. Tinnitus
   d. Vomiting

17. A patient has been prescribed enteric-coated aspirin 81 mg once a day following angioplasty. It is important for the nurse to teach this patient to avoid using which over-the-counter (OTC) medication?
   a. Acetaminophen
   b. Calcium carbonate
   c. Guaifenesin
   d. Ibuprofen

18. Which aspirin preparation is the least irritating to the stomach?
   a. Buffered aspirin solution
   b. Enteric-coated aspirin
   c. Chewable children's aspirin
   d. Timed-release aspirin

✳19. It is a priority to assess for which symptom if a patient has taken aspirin before delivery of a neonate?
   a. Boggy uterus
   b. Fatigue
   c. Perineal pain
   d. Sedation

►20. Which condition would be of concern when a patient reports regular use of sodium salicylate for joint pain?
   a. Asthma
   b. Heart failure
   c. Diabetes mellitus
   d. Chronic anemia

21. A patient has been prescribed naproxen-esomeprazole. Which statement suggests that patient teaching regarding administration of this drug has been successful?
   a. "Taking one drug is better than taking the drugs separately."
   b. "This drug combination will protect my kidney function."
   c. "Esomeprazole decreases acid production in my stomach."
   d. "The second drug will make the naproxen more effective."

22. Indomethacin is prescribed for premature neonates to promote duct closure in which location?
   a. Inner ear and cochlea
   b. Liver and the duodenum
   c. Ductus arteriosus
   d. Umbilical vein and abdomen

►23. The provider orders celecoxib 100 mg to be administered twice a day. The nurse would consult the provider before administering the drug if the patient is allergic to which drug?
   a. Amoxicillin
   b. Sulfamethoxazole
   c. Cefuroxime axetil
   d. Azithromycin

✳24. Which assessment finding would be a priority for the nurse to report if a patient was receiving celecoxib?
   a. Bruising of arms and shins
   b. A daily weight gain of 2 lb
   c. Heartburn at night
   d. Inadequate joint pain relief

✳25. It is priority to report which change when a 65-year-old female patient is prescribed celecoxib?
   a. Belching
   b. Bruise on left arm
   c. Difficulty speaking
   d. Headache

►26. Which nursing action is appropriate when a parent calls the pediatrician's office stating that their 15-month-old child just ingested an unknown quantity of children's chewable acetaminophen tablets?
   a. Assess for the presence of nausea, vomiting, and abdominal pain.
   b. Direct the parent to seek immediate medical care for the child.
   c. Make an appointment for the child to be seen as soon as possible.
   d. Take the opportunity to teach the parent about childproofing their home.

✳27. While caring for a patient taking Tylenol 8-Hour Arthritis Pain 650 mg around the clock for arthritis pain, the nurse notes that the patient is scratching their arms and states they hurt. On exam, a rash is noted. Which is the appropriate nursing action?
   a. Assess for petechiae.
   b. Consult the provider STAT.
   c. Give diphenhydramine.
   d. Discontinue the drug.

►28. A 3-year-old child is brought to the ED. The child's parent states that they had a rash and fever over a week ago. The child vomited several times last night. This morning they were so drowsy that the parent could not rouse them. The child is lethargic and does not resist examination. It is priority to ask the mother if they administered which drug to their child during their illness?
   a. Children's aspirin
   b. Dextromethorphan
   c. Pseudoephedrine
   d. Acetaminophen elixir

DOSE CALCULATION QUESTIONS

29. Acetylcysteine 9000 mg intravenous is to be infused over 60 minutes in the first bag of a 3 bag regimen. The drug is diluted in 200 mL of 5% dextrose. The infusion pump is calibrated in milliliters per hour. What rate should the nurse enter on the pump?

30. The nurse is teaching parents about use of infant acetaminophen drops (80 mg/0.8 mL) and age-appropriate dose. How many milliliters should be administered per dose if 150 mg is an appropriate dose for a 13-month-old child?

CASE STUDIES

Case Study 1

The nurse is assisting a science teacher who is postoperative total abdominal hysterectomy and bilateral salpingo-oophorectomy (TAH-BSO) with ambulation in the hallway when the patient complains of knee pain and stiffness. The patient has a history of hypertension and osteoarthritis. The patient states she was prescribed celecoxib for a short period of time several years ago. She tells the nurse that the drug really helped her knee pain and did not cause stomach distress like other drugs. She asks the nurse if she could have the medication again.

1. What could the nurse tell the patient?

2. The patient says, "I am glad there is still one drug that I can take for my arthritis that does not cause side effects." How should the nurse respond?

3. What nonpharmacologic teaching can the nurse provide this patient?

Case Study 2

A young adult patient comes to the family planning clinic to determine what she can do for relief of moderate dysmenorrhea. She states that the pain is not incapacitating but creates discomfort during the first day of her menses. She says she does not want anything that makes her sleepy and that she has tried Tylenol 8-Hour Arthritis Pain 650 mg without relief. After further assessment, the nurse practitioner suggests that she try ibuprofen as a beginning drug to see how she responds. She is told to take two ibuprofen (200-mg tablets) every 4 hours for the first 2–3 days of her menstrual period, starting with the first symptom of menses or cramping.

4. Why is this schedule appropriate in this situation?

5. What information should be provided to this patient about possible adverse effects of this drug therapy?

6. Based on the developmental stage of this patient, what teaching should the nurse provide about use of ibuprofen and other OTC NSAID drugs?

76 Glucocorticoids in Nonendocrine Disorders

STUDY QUESTIONS

Matching

Match the drug to the possible glucocorticoid-drug interactions or glucocorticoid-induced condition.

1. ___ May require increased dose
2. ___ Increased risk of hypokalemia
3. ___ Can decrease antibody response
4. ___ Increased risk of gastric ulceration
5. ___ Can help prevent osteoporosis

   a. Bisphosphonates
   b. Insulin
   c. Loop diuretics
   d. Nonsteroidal antiinflammatory drugs (NSAIDs)
   e. Vaccines

CRITICAL THINKING, PRIORITIZATION, AND DELEGATION QUESTIONS

✳6. Which possible effect of glucocorticoid therapy would be a priority to report to the provider?
   a. Calcium 9 mg/dL
   b. Chloride 95 mg/dL
   c. Potassium 3.1 mg/dL
   d. Sodium 145 mg/dL

✳7. It would be a priority to report which laboratory result to the provider if a patient is receiving therapeutic doses of glucocorticoids?
   a. Platelet count 250 × 10^9/L
   b. Blood urea nitrogen (BUN) 20 mg/dL
   c. Hemoglobin A1c 5.9%
   d. White blood cell (WBC) 2000/mm^3

►8. The school nurse would notify the parents of a fourth-grade child who is receiving oral glucocorticoids to control asthma symptoms if height and weight screening findings included which change?
   a. Increase to the 75th percentile in height
   b. Decrease to the 35th percentile in height
   c. Weight gain of 2 lb in the last year
   d. In the last year, a weight gain of 5 lb

►9. A patient would be at risk for contracting the disease if which immunization was administered while receiving glucocorticoid therapy? (**Select all that apply.**)
   a. Nasal influenza
   b. Injected influenza
   c. Yellow fever
   d. Pneumococcal
   e. Varicella

►10. Patients on long-term glucocorticoid therapy may minimize a common complication of therapy by having adequate servings of which foods in their diet?
   a. Broccoli
   b. Citrus fruits
   c. Legumes
   d. Whole grains

11. Which are common symptoms of hypokalemia caused by glucocorticoids with high mineralocorticoid activity?
   a. Flushed skin
   b. Hypotension
   c. Fatigue
   d. Tingling

12. Alternate-day glucocorticoid therapy is most appropriate for which patient?
   a. 9 years old
   b. 29 years old
   c. 45 years old
   d. 65 years old

►13. A patient who has been receiving glucocorticoid therapy for 2 months is being tapered off the glucocorticoids. Which symptom suggests a withdrawal syndrome?
   a. Blood pressure 84/47 mm Hg
   b. Fasting glucose 255 mg/dL
   c. Potassium 3.5 mEq/L
   d. Heart rate 55 beats/min

►14. A patient is taking dexamethasone for chronic obstructive pulmonary disease (COPD) and digoxin for heart failure (HF). Because of the increased risk for digoxin toxicity, the nurse should assess for which effect? (**Select all that apply.**)
   a. Loss of appetite
   b. Positive Chvostek sign
   c. Flushed skin
   d. Confusion
   e. Visual changes

DOSE CALCULATION QUESTIONS

15. A patient with osteoarthritis is to have methylprednisolone acetate 60 mg intraarticular injection on the right knee. On hand is methylprednisolone acetate 80 mg/mL. How many milliliters will be injected?

16. Dexamethasone 5 mg orally every 12 hours is prescribed for a 10-year-old child who weighs 82.5 lb. The recommended maximum safe dose for children is 0.3 mg/kg per day. Is the dose safe?

CASE STUDY

A young adult with severe persistent asthma is admitted with an acute exacerbation. After the crisis is averted, the patient is prescribed dexamethasone sodium succinate 4 mg intravenous (IV) push. The pharmacy sends dexamethasone acetate 16 mg/mL.

1. How much should the nurse administer?

2. The patient is switched to oral glucocorticoid therapy. Because of the severity of the patient's asthma, the provider explains that long-term oral glucocorticoids will probably be necessary in addition to an inhaled glucocorticoid and bronchodilator. What instructions should the nurse provide this patient regarding minimizing the following adverse effects of glucocorticoid therapy?
   a. Adrenal insufficiency
   b. Osteoporosis
   c. Infection
   d. Glucose intolerance
   e. Myopathy
   f. Edema, hypernatremia, and hypokalemia
   g. Mood
   h. Cataracts and glaucoma
   i. Peptic ulcer disease

77 Drug Therapy for Rheumatoid Arthritis

STUDY QUESTIONS

Matching

Match the drug to its action.

1. ___ Provide rapid relief of symptoms and can slow disease progression; with long-term use, they can cause serious toxicity.
2. ___ Provide rapid relief of symptoms but do not prevent joint damage and do not slow disease progression.
3. ___ Reduce the immune and inflammatory responses that underly rheumatoid arthritis (RA).
4. ___ Drugs that reduce joint destruction and slow disease progression; benefits develop slowly.
5. ___ Target specific components of the immune response.
   a. Targeted disease-modifying antirheumatic drugs (DMARDs)
   b. Conventional DMARDs
   c. Glucocorticoids
   d. Biologic DMARDs
   e. Nonsteroidal antiinflammatory drugs (NSAIDs)

CRITICAL THINKING, PRIORITIZATION, AND DELEGATION QUESTIONS

6. Which are nondrug measures to manage RA? **(Select all that apply.)**
   a. Hot oil baths
   b. Heat therapy
   c. Joint replacement
   d. Light exercise
   e. Acupuncture

*7. Which teaching is priority if a patient has taken prednisone 10 mg twice a day for 6 weeks for an RA flare and the flare has subsided?
   a. Avoid people with infection.
   b. Be sure to get enough rest.
   c. Follow tapering instructions.
   d. Take steps to manage stress.

8. A patient has been prescribed methotrexate (DMARD) immediately after being diagnosed with RA. The patient has heard that these drugs can be dangerous and asks the nurse why the provider has not ordered a prescription-strength NSAID. Which is the best response by the nurse?
   a. "Methotrexate can delay your joint degeneration."
   b. "This drug has fewer adverse effects than NSAIDs."
   c. "Onset of action of NSAIDs isn't as quick as methotrexate."
   d. "There isn't the risk of peptic ulcers with methotrexate."

9. A patient who is unwilling to take other drugs for their RA has been prescribed gold salts for years. Which symptom suggests gold toxicity?
   a. Extremity Bruising
   b. Epigastric pain
   c. Scleral jaundice
   d. Profuse diarrhea

*10. A 16-year-old female patient takes methotrexate once a week for juvenile RA (JRA). Which laboratory test result for this patient would be of concern for the nurse?
   a. Blood urea nitrogen (BUN) 20 mg/dL
   b. Erythrocyte sedimentation rate (ESR) 30 mm/hour
   c. Urine human chorionic gonadotropin (hCG) positive
   d. White blood cell count 11,000/mm^3

11. Which laboratory test result should be monitored when a patient is receiving sulfasalazine?
   a. Complete blood count (CBC)
   b. Electrolytes
   c. Fasting blood glucose
   d. Urine specific gravity

12. When performing a nursing assessment on a patient receiving tocilizumab, which observations would be a reason for the nurse to hold the medication and contact the provider?
   a. Abdominal pain
   b. Skin rash
   c. Diarrhea
   d. Rhinorrhea

✳13. When a patient is prescribed hydroxychloroquine for RA, it is priority for the nurse to determine if the patient has adhered to recommended follow-up care with which specialist?
   a. Endocrinologist
   b. Gastroenterologist
   c. Audiologist
   d. Ophthalmologist

►14. Which assessment finding, if identified in a patient who is receiving a biologic DMARD, should the nurse report to the provider immediately?
   a. Dizziness
   b. Fever
   c. Headache
   d. Injection-site erythema

15. Which symptom suggests that a patient who is prescribed etanercept may be experiencing the adverse effect of Stevens-Johnson syndrome?
   a. Wheezing
   b. Constipation
   c. Painful red rash
   d. Perioral edema

►16. The pediatric office nurse is preparing a referral to a rheumatologist for a child with JRA who has been unresponsive to methotrexate. It would be most important for the nurse to identify whether the child has received or is scheduled to receive which immunization before the child sees the specialist?
   a. DTaP
   b. Polio
   c. Hepatitis A
   d. Varicella

✳17. It would be priority to report which test result to the provider if a patient is prescribed infliximab?
   a. Absolute neutrophil count (ANC) 3500/mm^3
   b. Aspartate aminotransferase (AST) 45 IU/L
   c. Brain natriuretic peptide (BNP) 2875 pg/mL
   d. Thyroid-stimulating hormone 2.8 mIU/L

►18. A patient has returned to the office for reading of the purified protein derivative (PPD) tuberculin test administered 50 hours ago before initiation of treatment for RA with adalimumab. The nurse would document the test results as positive and consult the provider for which reaction?
   a. 5 mm of erythema
   b. 5 mm of induration
   c. 2.5 mm of erythema
   d. 2.5 mm of induration

19. A male patient who has been taking a DMARD is planning to try to conceive a child with his wife. The nurse must counsel him about the need for a specific protocol to be followed to clear his body of the drug if the patient has been taking which DMARD?
   a. Adalimumab
   b. Anakinra
   c. Infliximab
   d. Leflunomide

✳20. Which is the priority patient problem when administering intravenous rituximab?
   a. Airway obstruction
   b. Dehydration
   c. Infection
   d. Tissue injury

►21. Which should be reported to the provider as soon as possible when a patient has been receiving tocilizumab once a month for the past 2 years? (**Select all that apply.**)
   a. BUN 22 IU/L
   b. ANC 480/mm^3
   c. Blood pressure (BP) 120/72 mm Hg
   d. Abdominal pain
   e. Peripheral edema

22. The nurse is caring for a patient with RA, which has not responded to other DMARDs. The nurse knows which are new drugs approved by the US Food and Drug Administration (FDA) for this population? (**Select all that apply.**)
   a. Rituximab
   b. Sarilumab
   c. Etanercept
   d. Tofacitinib
   e. Baricitinib

DOSE CALCULATION QUESTIONS

23. Etanercept 25 mg is prescribed for a 55-lb 10-year-old with JRA. Is the dose safe?

24. Etanercept 15 mg is prescribed subcutaneously for a child. Available is 25 mg/mL. What amount should the nurse administer?

CASE STUDY

A 28-year-old female who works as a grocery store clerk has been diagnosed with RA after seeking care for carpal tunnel syndrome.

1. The patient asks how the disease developed from carpal tunnel syndrome. How should the nurse respond?

2. The patient's physician has recommended that the patient see a vocational rehabilitation counselor. The patient asks the nurse, "What type of job should I be thinking about?" What guidance can the nurse provide?

3. When developing a long-range plan of care for this patient, what interventions might the nurse include to address the four goals of RA therapy?

   a. Relieving symptoms

   b. Maintaining joint function

   c. Minimizing systemic joint involvement

   d. Delaying disease progression

4. The rheumatologist has recommended that the patient start a drug regimen that includes NSAIDs and methotrexate. Based on the developmental stage of this patient, what teaching would be especially important for the nurse to provide to this patient?

5. What symptoms of methotrexate toxicity to these organs should the nurse teach the patient to report to her provider?

   a. Liver

   b. Kidney

   c. Bone marrow

   d. Gastrointestinal (GI)

78 Drug Therapy for Gout

STUDY QUESTIONS

True or False

For each of the following statements, enter T for true or F for false.

1. ___ Colchicine is the most common drug used to prevent gout flares.
2. ___ Chemotherapy for cancer can cause gout.
3. ___ Gout can be acute or chronic.
4. ___ Gout is a systemic disease.
5. ___ In patients with gout, enzymes released when white blood cells break down damage the joints.
6. ___ Urate crystals can damage kidneys.

CRITICAL THINKING, PRIORITIZATION, AND DELEGATION QUESTIONS

►7. A patient who experiences gout flares once every 1 or 2 years has been self-treating with over-the-counter (OTC) drugs. Which drug would the nurse expect to provide the least relief of gout pain?
   a. Acetaminophen
   b. Acetylsalicylic acid
   c. Ibuprofen
   d. Naproxen

8. A patient develops a gout flare of the left first toe. They are prescribed colchicine and can return to work in 48 hours. The patient calls the provider stating that they are experiencing nausea and abdominal pain. They want to know what they should do. Which advice should the telephone triage nurse provide?
   a. Stop taking the medication.
   b. Take the medication at bedtime.
   c. Take the medication with food.
   d. Take the medication with milk.

*9. A patient has been prescribed allopurinol for chronic tophaceous gout. Which laboratory test result would be a priority to report to the provider?
   a. Blood urea nitrogen (BUN) 22 mg/dL
   b. Creatinine 3.8 mg/dL
   c. White blood cells (WBC) 4.2/μL
   d. Uric acid 9 mg/dL

10. The nurse teaches the patient to stop taking allopurinol and contact the provider if they experience which adverse effect?
   a. Diarrhea
   b. Drowsiness
   c. Fever
   d. Headache

*11. The nurse administers allopurinol to a patient who also receives warfarin. Which laboratory test result would be a priority to report to the provider?
   a. BUN 15 mg/dL
   b. Estimated glomerular filtration rate (eGFR) 90 mL/min
   c. International normalized ratio (INR) 4.6
   d. WBC 9.200/μL

12. Which is an appropriate nursing action to prevent side effects of therapy with probenecid?
   a. Avoid drawing blood from the affected extremity.
   b. Take with food to reduce GI effects.
   c. Elevate the affected extremity.
   d. Measure intake and output each day.

*13. It is priority to assess for which possible adverse reaction to pegloticase?
   a. Dyspnea
   b. Injection site pain
   c. Itching
   d. Flare of pain

14. A patient undergoing chemotherapy for lymphoma has a uric acid level of 7.4 mg/dL. They are unable to take allopurinol due to previous development of eosinophilia when on the drug. Which alternative drug does the nurse anticipate will be ordered for this patient?
   a. Pegloticase
   b. Rasburicase
   c. Febuxostat
   d. Colchicine

DOSE CALCULATION QUESTIONS

15. A patient is prescribed allopurinol 150 mg once a day. Available are 100-mg tablets. How many tablets should be administered per dose?

16. Pegloticase 8 mg is available mixed in a 250-mL bag of normal saline solution. The drug is to be administered over 120 minutes. What is the rate of infusion in milliliters per hour?

CASE STUDY

A pediatric patient who is scheduled to start chemotherapy in 2 weeks for acute leukemia is prescribed allopurinol 150 mg once a day. The patient's parent researches the drug on the internet and asks the nurse why it is being prescribed when the patient does not have gout.

1. How should the nurse respond?

2. The patient's parent does not like to give drugs to their children. What protective effects of allopurinol would be most important for the nurse to include in an explanation of why this drug is prescribed?

79 Drugs Affecting Calcium Levels and Bone Mineralization

STUDY QUESTIONS

Completion

1. The three factors that regulate serum calcium levels are ______________, ______________, and ________________.

2. Because free calcium is the active form of calcium, a patient with low protein levels can exhibit symptoms of ____________________________.

3. An inadequate level of free, ionized calcium may result in blood taking longer to ____________________.

4. Central nervous system symptoms of hypercalcemia include ______________________ and ______________________.

5. Hypocalcemia increases neuromuscular excitability, which, in addition to spasms of the pharynx and other muscles, can cause symptoms such as ____________________ and ____________________.

6. Parathyroid hormone secretion _____________ calcium absorption in the small intestine.

7. Patients should not take calcium supplements with ______________ or ________________ because they interfere with calcium absorption.

8. Patients should take calcium supplements that also contain _____________________ because this increases absorption of the calcium.

9. In addition to tetracycline, fluoroquinolones, and phenytoin, calcium supplements decrease the absorption of ____________________ and ____________________.

CRITICAL THINKING, PRIORITIZATION, AND DELEGATION QUESTIONS

*10. The priority goal of the body's regulation of calcium is maintaining normal calcium levels in which body system?
   a. Cardiovascular
   b. Muscular
   c. Nervous
   d. Skeletal

11. An older adult with vitamin D deficiency is prescribed cholecalciferol. Which is the recommended dosage?
   a. 10,000 IU/day
   b. 4,000 IU/day
   c. 2,000 IU/day
   d. 1,000 IU/day

12. Which is a known adverse effect of excessive calcium supplementation?
   a. Bleeding
   b. Diarrhea
   c. Dysrhythmias
   d. Euphoria

*13. The nurse is caring for a patient whose lab results include calcium 12 mg/dL. Which is the priority nursing intervention?
   a. Administering medications on time
   b. Ensuring adequate hydration
   c. Preventing patient falls
   d. Supporting respirations

*14. The nurse is caring for a patient whose lab results include calcium 6.8 mg/dL. Which is the priority nursing intervention?
   a. Administering medications on time
   b. Ensuring adequate hydration
   c. Preventing patient falls
   d. Supporting respirations

►15. A 62-year-old female is receiving chemotherapy for metastatic breast cancer. Which laboratory result suggests the patient is at increased risk for hypercalcemia?
   a. Creatinine 3.2 mg/dL
   b. Hemoglobin 11 g/dL
   c. Potassium 3.8 mEq/L
   d. Glucose 145 mg/dL

16. You are teaching a patient with bone cancer about the risk for hypercalcemia. You tell your patient to avoid which food that is highest in calcium?
   a. Bran
   b. Sardines
   c. Spinach
   d. Oatmeal

17. Which question would provide the most useful information when taking the history of a child diagnosed with rickets?
    a. "Does your child have any trouble with schoolwork?"
    b. "Has your child ever had a bacterial kidney infection?"
    c. "Have you noticed a change in your child's energy level?"
    d. "How many hours a day does your child watch television?"

18. The nurse is assessing a postoperative thyroidectomy patient. Which assessment suggests that the parathyroid glands may have been damaged or removed during surgery? (**Select all that apply.**)
    a. Dorsiflexion of first toe when sole of the foot is stroked
    b. BP cuff inflation for 3 minutes produces wrist spasms
    c. Loss of balance when standing with the eyes closed
    d. Sharp calf pain with dorsiflexion of the foot
    e. Facial muscles twitch when the facial nerve is tapped

19. A 58-year-old female is at risk for osteoporosis caused by hypothyroidism treated with levothyroxine 0.15 mg every morning. She has been instructed to take supplemental calcium. She is considering taking calcium carbonate (TUMS) with 400 mg of elemental calcium. Which statement, if made by the patient, would indicate a need for further teaching?
    a. "Calcium will not be as well absorbed if taken with eating bran cereal."
    b. "I should take the calcium with a large glass of water."
    c. "Calcium should be taken at separate times throughout the day."
    d. "TUMS are not as good a source of calcium as oyster shell calcium."

✳20. It is priority for the nurse to monitor for which symptom when administering parenteral calcium to a patient who is prescribed digoxin?
    a. Hypertension
    b. Anuria
    c. Dehydration
    d. Bradycardia

21. The pediatric nurse is explaining why vitamins should be kept out of the reach of children. Which is a possible effect of vitamin D toxicity? (**Select all that apply.**)
    a. Diarrhea
    b. Constipation
    c. Weakness
    d. Tetany
    e. Vomiting

►22. Patients with which chronic disorders are less able to activate vitamin D from sunlight? (**Select all that apply.**)
    a. Chronic kidney disease
    b. Asthmatic bronchitis
    c. Hepatic dysfunction
    d. Osteoarthritis
    e. Type 2 diabetes

23. A 3-year-old child is admitted after ingesting an unknown number of chewable multiple vitamins, including vitamin D. Which assessment finding would be of most concern to the nurse?
    a. BP 80/50 mm Hg
    b. Watery stools
    c. Pulse 102 beats/min
    d. Confusion and ataxia

24. Which statement is true regarding calcitonin?
    a. It is usually administered once a week.
    b. The drug is the more effective in males.
    c. Prime the metered-dose pump before first use.
    d. The drug promotes bone formation.

✳25. Which assessment finding, if identified in a patient who is receiving alendronate, would be priority for the nurse to report to the provider?
    a. Dysphagia
    b. Dysphasia
    c. Headache
    d. Muscular pain

26. Taking calcium supplements at the same time as a dose of a bisphosphonate for osteoporosis results in which action?
    a. Increases bone building
    b. Interferes with drug absorption
    c. Potentiates the drug action
    d. Prevents adverse effects

27. A patient who has just started taking enteric-coated delayed-release risedronate for Paget disease calls the provider's office and reports that they have been experiencing nausea since starting the drug. Which is the priority nursing action?
    a. Advise the patient to stop taking the drug.
    b. Determine if the patient is taking the drug with food.
    c. Teach the patient to take the drug with an antacid.
    d. Instruct the patient to take the drug at bedtime.

28. A patient with hypercalcemia of malignancy (HCM) receives zoledronate. Which symptom suggests the patient may be experiencing drug-induced hypomagnesemia? (**Select all that apply.**)
    a. Anorexia
    b. Dry mucous membranes
    c. Muscle weakness
    d. Muscle spasms
    e. Constipation

►29. When a patient is prescribed a bisphosphonate, which patient teaching would be most effective in preventing osteonecrosis of the jaw?
a. Emphasize excellent oral hygiene.
b. Take calcium supplements with the drug.
c. Teach the importance of exercise.
d. Avoid taking alcohol with the drug.

30. Which represents the cause of osteonecrosis when a patient is prescribed bisphosphonates?
a. Decreased bone breakdown
b. Increased bone deposition
c. Impaired blood perfusion
d. Reduction in blood calcium

31. Which is true of raloxifene?
a. It may damage the eyes.
b. Hot flashes are a side effect.
c. It reduces the risk of hip fractures.
d. It must be avoided in those with breast cancer.

*32. Which information, if elicited from a patient who is receiving raloxifene, would be priority for the nurse to communicate to the provider?
a. Has family history of breast cancer
b. History of total hysterectomy
c. Is experiencing hot flashes
d. Work requires long airplane trips

*33. Which laboratory result, if found in a female who has just been prescribed raloxifene, would be the priority concern to the nurse?
a. Calcium 11.1 mg/dL
b. Hemoglobin (Hgb) 11.6 g/dL
c. Hemoglobin A1c 6.8%
d. hCG 330 mIU/mL

34. To increase bone mineral density, which is the proper way to administer teriparatide?
a. Continually
b. Injection
c. Intravenously (IV)
d. Orally

35. Which is the appropriate nursing action when administering teriparatide?
a. Administer in the deltoid with a 1-inch needle.
b. Inject intradermally in the forearm.
c. Discard the prefilled pen after 28 days.
d. Warm for 20 minutes before administration.

*36. Which symptom would be a priority to report to the provider if a patient who is receiving chemotherapy is scheduled to receive denosumab?
a. Fatigue and anorexia
b. Flank pain and fever
c. Nausea and vomiting
d. Injection site redness

37. Which is the appropriate nursing action when administering denosumab to a patient with osteoporosis? (**Select all that apply.**)
a. Give in posterior gluteal muscle.
b. Assess current dental needs.
c. Inspect solution for clarity.
d. Discard if cloudy solution.
e. Warm to room temperature.

►38. The nurse would withhold cinacalcet and consult the provider if which new finding was discovered during patient assessment?
a. Anorexia
b. Diarrhea
c. Headache
d. Numbness

39. IV furosemide has been prescribed for a patient in a hypercalcemic emergency. The nurse knows which imbalance would be least likely to occur as a result of this therapy?
a. Hypocalcemia
b. Hypoglycemia
c. Hypokalemia
d. Hyponatremia

DOSE CALCULATION QUESTIONS

40. The nurse's drug book recommends that calcium gluconate be infused at a rate of 0.5–2 mL/min. If the nurse infuses 5 mL of 10% calcium gluconate, how long will it take to infuse the entire amount?

41. Denosumab 120-mg subcutaneous injection is prescribed every 4 weeks. Available is 120 mg/1.7 mL. What amount should be administered?

42. Etidronate is prescribed for a 180-pound patient with Paget disease. Initial dosing of the drug is at 10 mg/kg/day PO. The drug is available in 400 mg tablets. How many tablets will the nurse administer?

CASE STUDY

A 50-year-old patient who states they are going through menopause is undergoing a thyroidectomy today. The literature states that the nurse should be sure IV calcium is available postoperatively. The patient has just been admitted to the nursing unit from the postanesthesia care unit (PACU).

1. Knowing the anatomy of the thyroid gland, why would the nurse anticipate a potential need for IV calcium?

2. What is the average normal value for total serum calcium?

3. The patient's calcium level drops to 6.8 mg/dL. Ten percent calcium gluconate 5 mL via IV (push) infusion is prescribed. The patient is sitting in a chair when the nurse prepares to administer the calcium gluconate. Why is it important for the nurse to assist the patient back to bed before the drug is administered?

4. What should be monitored while the nurse is administering the calcium gluconate?

5. The patient's spouse has assumed that calcium is in the bone. The spouse asks how surgery on the neck can cause an imbalance in the calcium in the body. What could the nurse include in the discussion of the functions of calcium and the mechanism for calcium regulation?

80 Drugs for Asthma and Chronic Obstructive Pulmonary Disease

STUDY QUESTIONS

Matching

Match the term with its definition.

1. ___ Adventitious breath sound that occurs with bronchoconstriction of asthma
2. ___ Drug that reduces asthma respiratory symptoms by suppressing inflammation
3. ___ Devices that attach directly to the metered-dose inhaler (MDI) to increase delivery of drug to the lungs and decrease deposition of drug on the oropharyngeal mucosa
4. ___ Hoarseness, speaking difficulty
5. ___ Measures taken to prevent illness
6. ___ Most effective drugs available for relieving acute bronchospasm and preventing exercise-induced bronchospasm
7. ___ A small machine used to convert a drug solution into a mist
8. ___ Used to deliver drugs in the form of a dry, micronized powder directly to the lungs
9. ___ Handheld pressurized devices that deliver a measured dose of drug with each actuation
10. ___ Spasm of bronchial smooth muscle that narrows airways
11. ___ Underlying cause of asthma
    a. β_2-Agonist
    b. Bronchoconstriction
    c. Dry-powder inhaler (DPI)
    d. Dysphonia
    e. Glucocorticoid
    f. Inflammation
    g. MDI
    h. Nebulizer
    i. Prophylaxis
    j. Spacer
    k. Wheezing

CRITICAL THINKING, PRIORITIZATION, AND DELEGATION QUESTIONS

✳12. Which outcome would be priority for most asthma patients?
  a. Avoiding environmental pollution
  b. Increasing exercise tolerance
  c. Preventing airway inflammation
  d. Stimulating release of eosinophils

13. A patient has received instructions from the nurse to administer two puffs of a β_2-agonist drug via an MDI. Which statement by the patient would indicate a need for further teaching?
  a. "I need to inhale slowly and deeply to get the drug deep in my lungs."
  b. "I may need to count the MDI doses so I know when it is empty."
  c. "I should start to inhale 2 seconds after activating the inhaler."
  d. "It is best to wait 1 full minute before I take the second MDI puff."

14. Which are current recommendations for use of inhaled glucocorticoids for persistent asthma?
  a. Administer daily even when there are no symptoms.
  b. Administer first when giving with a bronchodilator.
  c. Only use as a rescue drug for acute flares of wheezing.
  d. Use on a regular basis if acute attacks occur every day.

15. Which symptom suggests that a child with asthma is not rinsing their mouth after using a glucocorticoid inhaler?
  a. Enlarged tonsils
  b. Postnasal drainage
  c. Persistent cough
  d. White patches in mouth

✳16. It is priority to teach which strategies to maintain adequate bone mass if a patient with asthma is prescribed which drug?
  a. Flunisolide MDI
  b. Fluticasone-salmeterol DPI
  c. Nebulized levalbuterol
  d. Prednisolone oral tablets

▶17. A hospitalized patient has orders for budesonide and salmeterol, one inhalation every 12 hours, and albuterol MDI, two puffs every 4 hours as needed. The patient has not required albuterol for the last 24 hours. When preparing to administer the budesonide and salmeterol, the nurse notes audible wheezing and dyspnea. Blood pressure is 134/88, respirations 18, pulse 100, O_2 saturation 94%, and temperature 99.°F. Place the nursing actions in sequential order, 1 through 6.
   a. ____Administer salmeterol.
   b. ____Wait 5 minutes.
   c. ____Administer albuterol.
   d. ____Wait 1 minute.
   e. ____Reassess lung sounds.
   f. ____Administer budesonide.

✳18. The nurse is caring for several patients who receive β-agonist inhalation treatments for asthma. After treatments are administered, it is priority to reassess the patient who also has a history of which condition?
   a. Heart failure
   b. Deep vein thrombosis
   c. Gastroesophageal reflux
   d. Rheumatoid arthritis

✳19. A 42-year-old patient with asthma is admitted for surgery. Which information about the patient would be priority for the nurse to share with the anesthesiologist?
   a. Allergic to tobacco smoke
   b. Degenerative joint disease
   c. Uses albuterol MDI as needed
   d. Finished Medrol dose pack yesterday

20. The nurse administers albuterol via a nebulizer to a patient who experienced acute wheezing while trying to eat lunch. Several minutes after the treatment, the patient is resting quietly with their eyes closed. Which is the appropriate nursing action?
   a. Allow the patient to rest.
   b. Assess the patient's lung sounds.
   c. Ask dietary to deliver a snack later.
   d. Wake the patient to finish lunch.

▶21. Which assessment finding in a patient who is prescribed a β_2-adrenergic agonist would be a reason for the nurse to consult the provider?
   a. Blood pressure 140/90 mm Hg
   b. Blood glucose 165 mg/dL
   c. Unexplained fainting
   d. Tremors bilateral hands

22. Which is the benefit of using of using combination glucocorticoid and long-acting $beta_2$-agonist combination drugs?
   a. Are more convenient than taking either drug separately.
   b. Increased flexibility in dosing both drugs.
   c. Ensure optimal dosing for initial therapy with the drugs.
   d. Decreases the risk for asthma-related death.

23. The nurse is caring for a patient who is prescribed zafirlukast for asthma and warfarin for atrial fibrillation. Which is a possible result of the interaction of these two drugs?
   a. Bradycardia
   b. Hemorrhage
   c. Pulmonary emboli
   d. Myocardial infarction

24. The nurse would be most concerned about drug interactions if a patient were prescribed both zileuton and
   a. Albuterol.
   b. Prednisolone.
   c. Terbutaline.
   d. Theophylline.

25. Zafirlukast is listed on the medication administration record (MAR) to be administered at 7:00 a.m. Breakfast is served at 8:30 a.m. Which is the appropriate nursing action?
   a. Administer the drug as ordered.
   b. Change the drug to 8:30 a.m.
   c. Retime the drug to 10:00 a.m.
   d. Consult the provider ASAP.

26. The nurse is explaining cromolyn therapy to a patient who has asthma. Which statement should **NOT** be included in the teaching?
   a. Cromolyn must be taken on a regular basis to control inflammation.
   b. Rinse the mouth immediately after administration to prevent thrush.
   c. Take 15 minutes before exertional activities to prevent bronchospasm.
   d. The drug is not effective in stopping an episode once it has begun.

✳27. The emergency department nurse is caring for a patient who takes omalizumab for asthma. Which sign warrants immediate intervention?
   a. Fever
   b. Headache
   c. Perioral edema
   d. Severe pharyngitis

✳28. An adolescent patient has controlled their asthma using a drug regimen that includes theophylline. Which new behavior would be priority to report to the provider?
   a. Joining the soccer team
   b. Occasionally skipping school
   c. Becoming sexually active
   d. Smoking marijuana

29. Umeclidinium may cause hypersensitivity reactions in people with which allergy?
   a. Peanuts
   b. Milk
   c. Horses
   d. Eggs

30. Which adverse effect would the patient be most likely to experience when prescribed tiotropium?
    a. Blurred vision
    b. Constipation
    c. Dry mouth
    d. Urinary retention

▶31. A child with moderate asthma is distressed because they have just learned they are allergic to the family dog. Which intervention would most effectively address the physical and psychosocial needs of the child?
    a. There are no interventions to prevent allergies.
    b. Increase the dose of asthma drugs around the dog.
    c. Take the dog to the local shelter and get a cat.
    d. Train the dog to stay out of bedrooms and off furniture.

DOSE CALCULATION QUESTIONS

32. A 4-year-old patient has been taking oral steroids and is now prescribed 0.5 mg budesonide via a nebulizer twice a day. Budesonide is available as 0.25 mg/2 mL. How much budesonide should be administered via a nebulizer at each dose?

33. Omalizumab, once reconstituted, is available as a solution of 150 mg/1.2 mL. Three hundred milligrams subcutaneously is prescribed once every 4 weeks. How much drug should be administered?

CRITICAL JUDGMENT CASE STUDY

A 7-year-old, who was first diagnosed with asthma at age 4 years, has been admitted to a medical unit from intensive care after experiencing a severe acute exacerbation. Based on the frequency, characteristics, and severity of symptoms, the patient is currently classified as having severe persistent asthma. On exam, the patient has expiratory wheezing and diminished breath sounds in bilateral lung bases. Vital signs are blood pressure 100/70 mm Hg, heart rate of 100 bpm, respirations 20 bpm, and temperature 37.5°C. Oxygen saturation is 92%. The provider has ordered oral prednisolone 2 mg/kg/day divided twice daily, budesonide 0.2 mg, and albuterol 1.25 mg via a nebulizer every 6 hours as needed. The child weighs 40 pounds. The child's mother tells the nurse she is overwhelmed and does not understand why her child needs steroids.

1. Which content does the nurse need to teach regarding the steroid therapy for this child? **(Select one, some, or all that apply.)**
    a. Avoid people who have infections.
    b. Do not take any live vaccines.
    c. Ensure adequate intake of vitamin D.
    d. Avoid weight-bearing exercise.
    e. Monitor and record symptoms' frequency.
    f. Give glucocorticoids on a regular schedule.
    g. Glucocorticoids can abort an ongoing attack.

81 Drugs for Allergic Rhinitis, Cough, and Colds

STUDY QUESTIONS

Matching

Match the term with its description.

1. ___ Conjunctivitis
2. ___ Erythema
3. ___ Immunoglobulins
4. ___ Perennial
5. ___ Pruritus
6. ___ Rhinitis
7. ___ Rhinorrhea
8. ___ Seasonal
   a. Protein that functions as antibody
   b. Inflammation of the upper airway
   c. Inflammation of mucous membrane lining the eyelids and eye surface
   d. Itching
   e. Occurs during spring and fall in reaction to outdoor allergens
   f. Nonseasonal, triggered by indoor allergens
   g. Redness because of injury or irritation
   h. Runny nose

Match the drug with its descriptor.

9. ___ Renders cough more productive by stimulating the flow of respiratory tract secretions
10. ___ Decreases the sensitivity of respiratory tract stretch receptors
11. ___ Monoclonal antibody directed against immunoglobulin E (IgE)
12. ___ Blocks cholinergic receptors, thereby decreasing rhinorrhea
13. ___ The most effective over-the-counter (OTC) non-opioid cough medicine and the most widely used of all cough medicines
14. ___ Smells like rotten eggs
15. ___ Cough suppression is achieved only at doses that produce prominent sedation
16. ___ Somewhat more potent than codeine and carries a greater liability for abuse
   a. Acetylcysteine
   b. Benzonatate
   c. Dextromethorphan
   d. Diphenhydramine
   e. Guaifenesin
   f. Hydrocodone
   g. Ipratropium
   h. Omalizumab

CRITICAL THINKING, PRIORITIZATION, AND DELEGATION QUESTIONS

17. A patient exhibits watery nasal discharge and sneezing every winter when the house is closed and the forced-air furnace is running. Which is the classification of these symptoms?
   a. Perennial rhinitis
   b. Seasonal rhinitis
   c. Intolerance
   d. Urticaria

18. Allergic rhinitis involves the release of which acute inflammatory markers? (**Select all that apply.**)
   a. Glucocorticoids
   b. Histamine
   c. Leukocytes
   d. Leukotrienes
   e. Prostaglandins

19. Which are the most effective drugs for the prevention and treatment of symptoms of seasonal and perennial rhinitis?
   a. First-generation antihistamines
   b. Intranasal glucocorticoids
   c. Oral glucocorticoids
   d. Second-generation antihistamines

►20. The school nurse notes that a child is receiving long-term therapy with intranasal glucocorticoids for seasonal rhinitis. Which is the appropriate nursing action?
   a. Check blood sugar.
   b. Evaluate hearing.
   c. Measure height.
   d. Obtain weight.

►21. A patient was prescribed fluticasone two sprays in each nostril 2 weeks ago. They call the nurse to report that the drug has not helped. Which question should the nurse ask to identify a common cause of early treatment failures?
   a. "Does administration cause burning?"
   b. "Do you have nasal congestion?"
   c. "How often are you administering the sprays?"
   d. "What is the expiration date on the bottle?"

22. The nurse teaches a patient with allergic rhinitis that oral antihistamines are not effective in reducing which symptom?
    a. Nasal itching
    b. Runny nose
    c. Nasal congestion
    d. Sneezing

23. A patient has received instructions regarding administration of a second-generation oral antihistamine for seasonal allergic rhinitis. Which of these statements made by the patient would indicate that the patient needs further teaching?
    a. "I should only use the medication when I experience symptoms."
    b. "This drug should be taken as prescribed throughout my allergy season."
    c. "Due to sedation, I need to be careful when driving."
    d. "OTC antihistamines are just as effective."

24. Which is an advantage of intranasal cromolyn in allergic rhinitis?
    a. It can be used prophylactically.
    b. It has once-a-day dosing.
    c. It is more effective than other drugs.
    d. It has fewer adverse reactions.

*25. Which of these assessment findings, if identified in a patient who is taking an oral decongestant, would be a priority to report to the provider?
    a. Agitation
    b. Chest pain
    c. Epistaxis
    d. Sore throat

26. A patient who recently saw a commercial for montelukast asks the office nurse why the provider will not order this drug for their allergic symptoms. The nurse knows that providers may not readily prescribe this drug for allergic rhinitis for which reason?
    a. It can cause nasal irritation.
    b. It has many adverse effects.
    c. Decongestant effects are limited.
    d. The drug only treats sneezing and itching.

27. A patient is prescribed intranasal cromolyn for allergic rhinitis. Which statement suggests a need for further teaching?
    a. "Benefits are less than intranasal glucocorticoids."
    b. "This drug suppresses the release of histamine."
    c. "I can go to the flower show tomorrow and not sneeze."
    d. "Cromolyn has fewer adverse reactions than other drugs."

28. Research suggests that codeine, dextromethorphan, and diphenhydramine are not effective in suppressing coughs induced by which trigger?
    a. Chemical irritation
    b. Common cold
    c. Mechanical irritation
    d. Smoking

29. A patient has received instructions regarding the administration of benzonatate. Which statement would indicate that the patient needs further teaching?
    a. "The drug should not be given to infants."
    b. "I can take the drug three times a day."
    c. "This drug may make me drowsy."
    d. "Benzonatate can be mixed in applesauce."

*30. Despite instruction by the nurse to swallow the benzonatate whole, the patient proceeds to chew the capsule. Which is a priority nursing concern until the effect of this drug has diminished?
    a. Aspiration
    b. Bronchospasms
    c. Respiratory depression
    d. Severe constipation

31. Which statement is true about the common cold? (**Select all that apply.**)
    a. Antibiotics are not effective.
    b. Antihistamines do not help.
    c. Multisymptom drugs work best.
    d. Vitamin C prevents colds.
    e. Zinc can cure a cold.

DOSE CALCULATION QUESTIONS

Diphenhydramine 50 mg orally every 6 hours is prescribed. The patient has purchased 25 mg capsules.

32. How many diphenhydramine capsules should the patient take for each dose?

33. The nurse would teach the patient not to take more than how many diphenhydramine capsules in 24 hours?

CASE STUDIES

Case Study 1

A 19-year-old college student presents to the student health clinic during spring semester with reports of runny and itchy nose, sneezing, and nasal congestion. They are diagnosed with allergic rhinitis. The student states reports using an OTC nasal spray for 2 weeks. It really helps, but the congestion comes back and seems to be getting worse.

1. Explain what is happening and how the drug can be discontinued.

2. The nurse practitioner prescribes loratadine 10 mg daily and triamcinolone two sprays twice a day. What teaching can the nurse provide?

3. If the patient develops a common cold, how should they change their medications?

Case Study 2

A patient asks the nurse why they don't need a prescription but can't buy Sudafed off the shelf. The student says they had to go to the pharmacy counter and sign a paper to get Sudafed but could not buy enough to take on their Peace Corps assignment.

4. What should the nurse include in the response?

5. The patient asks why they can buy Sudafed PE off the shelf if Sudafed can be made into an abused substance. What should the nurse include in the explanation?

82 Drugs for Peptic Ulcer Disease

STUDY QUESTIONS

Matching

Match the drug with its mechanism of action.

1. ___ Can cause a disulfiram-like reaction and, hence, must not be combined with alcohol
2. ___ Works quickly to neutralize acid in the stomach
3. ___ Promotes secretion of cytoprotective mucus
4. ___ Creates a protective barrier in the stomach against hydrogen ions and pepsin
5. ___ Disrupts the cell wall of *Helicobacter pylori*, thereby causing lysis and death
6. ___ Causes irreversible inhibition of H^+, K^+-ATPase, the enzyme that generates gastric acid
7. ___ Suppresses the growth of *H. pylori* by inhibiting protein synthesis
8. ___ Blocks H_2 receptors, thereby reducing both the volume of gastric juice and its hydrogen ion concentration

a. Magnesium hydroxide
b. Bismuth
c. Clarithromycin
d. Cimetidine
e. Misoprostol
f. Omeprazole
g. Sucralfate
h. Tinidazole

True or False

For each of the following statements, enter T for true or F for false.

9. ___ Cimetidine inhibits the drug-metabolizing enzymes that affect warfarin, phenytoin, and theophylline.
10. ___ Aluminum hydroxide antacids frequently cause diarrhea.
11. ___ Sodium bicarbonate should be avoided by patients with heart failure.
12. ___ Calcium carbonate forms a barrier over the ulcer crater that protects against acid, and pepsin.
13. ___ Bismuth can impart a harmless black coloration to the tongue and stool.
14. ___ Magnesium hydroxide antacids are used to help diagnose abdominal pain.
15. ___ Magnesium hydroxide antacids should not be used in severe renal impairment.
16. ___ Sodium bicarbonate antacids can be absorbed into systemic circulation.
17. ___ Sodium bicarbonate decreases blood pH.

CRITICAL THINKING, PRIORITIZATION, AND DELEGATION QUESTIONS

*18. Which should be included in teaching for a person with peptic ulcer disease (PUD)?
a. Avoiding use of alcohol
b. Consuming more dairy products
c. Not using tobacco products
d. Using ibuprofen for headaches

19. Hypersecretion of gastric acid is the etiology of which condition?
a. Duodenal ulcers
b. Gastric ulcers
c. Peptic ulcers
d. Zollinger-Ellison syndrome ulcers

20. A drug from which class, prescribed to prevent recurrence of PUD, is included in the treatment of *H. pylori*?
a. Antacids
b. Antibiotics
c. Antisecretory agents
d. Mucosal protectants

21. Which dietary alteration may facilitate recovery from ulcers?
a. Avoiding caffeine intake
b. Eating only bland foods
c. Six small meals a day
d. Frequent intake of milk

✳22. A patient taking bismuth subsalicylate, tetracycline, and metronidazole experiences black-colored stool. Which is the priority nursing action?
   a. Perform an abdominal assessment.
   b. Consult the provider.
   c. Continue with nursing care.
   d. Obtain stool for occult blood.

►23. A patient is prescribed drug therapy that includes bismuth subsalicylate, metronidazole, tetracycline, and omeprazole. The patient reveals to the nurse that they do not like taking so many medications. The nurse should explain that it is important for the patient to take the therapy as prescribed because failure to take the medications as prescribed may lead to which condition?
   a. Drug-resistant *H. pylori*
   b. Increased adverse effects
   c. Risk of cancer is increased
   d. Nausea and diarrhea

24. A patient with gastroesophageal reflux disease (GERD), who has difficulty following drug regimens with multiple doses, has been prescribed cimetidine 800 mg once a day at bedtime. The patient reports that the medication effects wear off before taking the next dose. The nurse provides which instructions to prolong the beneficial effects of the drug?
   a. Take the drug twice a day.
   b. Try taking it with food.
   c. Swallow with a glass of water.
   d. Follow it with an antacid.

25. The nurse must be particularly cautious for toxic effects of which drug when administered with cimetidine? (**Select all that apply.**)
   a. Nateglinide
   b. Phenytoin
   c. Prednisone
   d. Theophylline
   e. Warfarin

26. The generic names of histamine$_2$ receptor antagonists (H_2RAs) share which common suffix?
   a. -azole
   b. -lol
   c. -dine
   d. -sartan

27. A patient with Zollinger-Ellison syndrome asks why they were prescribed omeprazole, since their partner takes cimetidine for GERD. The nurse will base their response on which fact? (**Select all that apply.**)
   a. Too high of a dose of cimetidine would be required.
   b. Gastric acid secretion is suppressed better with omeprazole.
   c. Cimetidine can cause severe diarrhea and vomiting.
   d. Omeprazole has fewer side effects than cimetidine.
   e. Omeprazole relieves symptoms faster than cimetidine.

28. The generic names of proton pump inhibitors (PPIs) share which common suffix?
   a. -azole
   b. -lol
   c. -dine
   d. -sartan

✳29. Which action by the nurse would be priority when a patient experiences five watery stools in 24 hours while taking a PPI?
   a. Send the patient's stool for ova and parasites.
   b. Increase fluids to 2000 mL in 24 hours.
   c. Place the patient on contact isolation.
   d. Wash hands with soap and water after patient care.

►30. A patient had been prescribed omeprazole capsules for GERD. Which is the reason PPIs increase the risk for hospital and community acquired pneumonia in the first few days of treatment? (**Select all that apply.**)
   a. Aspiration due to confusion
   b. Altered upper GI flora
   c. Impairment of WBC function
   d. Due to acid rebound
   e. Stimulates secretion of mucous

31. The nurse is preparing to administer clarithromycin-based triple therapy 1 for eradicating H. pylori. Which is included in this regimen? **(Select all that apply.)**
   a. Metronidazole 500 mg twice daily.
   b. Omeprazole 40 mg twice daily.
   c. Clarithromycing 500 mg twice daily.
   d. Amoxicillin 1 gm daily.
   e. Tetracycline 500 mg 4 times daily.

►32. The nurse is caring for a patient on long-term warfarin for mechanical valve replacement. They were started on sucralfate on admission to the hospital for treatment of ulcers. Which laboratory result would be a reason for the nurse to consult the provider?
   a. Hematocrit 42%
   b. International normalized ratio (INR) 1
   c. Hemoglobin 13.8 g/dL
   d. White blood cell (WBC) 10,000/mm^3

▶33. A 47-year-old female who has been taking a nonsteroidal antiinflammatory drug (NSAID) for rheumatoid arthritis and an oral contraceptive is prescribed misoprostol to treat gastrointestinal (GI) distress relating to NSAID use. She informs the nurse that she has stopped taking her oral contraceptives because she has not had a period for 2 months and thinks she could be in menopause. Which is the appropriate nursing action?
a. Request tests for menopause.
b. Administer the misoprostol.
c. Only administer the NSAID.
d. Call for a pregnancy test.

DOSE CALCULATION QUESTIONS

34. Sucralfate is available in a suspension (1 g/10 mL) for oral dosing. The patient is prescribed 2 g a day in two divided doses. How many milliliters should be administered at each dose?

35. Cimetidine IV infusion is diluted in 100 mL of normal saline solution and is to be administered over 15 minutes. The IV tubing has a drip factor of 10 drops/mL. What is the drip rate per 15 seconds?

CASE STUDY

An adult with a history of type 2 diabetes mellitus (T2DM) and osteoarthritis has recently been experiencing GI distress attributed to use of NSAIDs for joint pain. Eating small, frequent meals has helped, but not relieved, the GI distress. The patient asks how arthritis medication can cause stomach distress.

1. How should the nurse respond?

2. Cimetidine, an H_2RA, is prescribed. To promote adherence, which side effects must be discussed with the patient?

3. Why do patients prescribed cimetidine have an increased relative risk of acquiring pneumonia?

83 Laxatives

STUDY QUESTIONS

Matching

Match the type of laxative to its mechanism of action.

1. ___ Increase secretion of water and ions into the intestine and reduce water and electrolyte absorption
2. ___ Lower surface tension, which facilitates penetration of water into the feces
3. ___ Swell in water to form a viscous solution or gel, thereby softening the fecal mass
4. ___ Draw water into the intestinal lumen, causing the fecal mass to soften and swell, thereby stretching the intestinal wall, which stimulates peristalsis

   a. Bulk forming
   b. Osmotic
   c. Stimulant
   d. Surfactant

CRITICAL THINKING, PRIORITIZATION, AND DELEGATION QUESTIONS

5. Which is a reason to use castor oil?
   a. Avoid straining with defecation.
   b. Compensate for lack of dietary fiber.
   c. Prevent opioid-related constipation.
   d. Prepare for a diagnostic colonoscopy.

✳ 6. When clarifying a patient's report of constipation, which is the priority information to obtain?
   a. Amount of stool.
   b. Color of stool.
   c. Consistency of stool.
   d. Frequency of stool.

7. The nurse is teaching a patient about measures to prevent and treat constipation. Which statement made by the patient indicates a need for additional instruction?
   a. "Eight glasses of water each day will keep my bowels regular."
   b. "Eating vegetables every day will help prevent constipation."
   c. "I should eat more whole grains if my stool is hard."
   d. "Laxatives do not normally work overnight."

8. Which is the best source of fiber to promote proper colon function?
   a. Dietary bran
   b. Methylcellulose
   c. Psyllium
   d. Vegetable fiber

9. A nursing student is sharing research on laxatives. Which statement by the student would indicate a need for further study?
   a. "Without enough fluid, bulk-forming agents can form a mass in the esophagus."
   b. "Cathartics are useful as bowel preparations for gastrointestinal procedures."
   c. "Patients should be taught stimulant laxatives can cause electrolyte imbalances."
   d. "Stimulant laxatives are used to prevent constipation associated with pregnancy."

▶ 10. Which is the most important teaching the nurse should provide regarding bulk-forming laxatives?
   a. They should never be taken more than once a day.
   b. Take the drug with at least 8 oz of water or juice.
   c. Fiber increases bulk but has no effect on peristalsis.
   d. They are contraindicated in irritable bowel syndrome.

11. Which directive should be included in the instructions for administration of bisacodyl tablets?
   a. "The drug will work best if you take it with a meal."
   b. "Chew the bisacodyl tablets to achieve the maximum effect."
   c. "Do not take antacids within 1 hour of taking the laxative."
   d. "You should take the laxative with a full glass of milk."

12. Which is a sign of magnesium toxicity?
   a. Hypertension
   b. Paresthesia
   c. Twitching
   d. Weakness

✳ 13. The nurse is administering lactulose 30 mL to a patient with hepatic encephalopathy. Which is a priority outcome for this patient?
   a. Ammonia 110 mcg/dL
   b. Total bilirubin 0.8 mg/dL
   c. A formed stool within 24 hours
   d. Relief of constipation

▶14. Which result would be a reason withhold milk of magnesia as needed and consult the provider?
   a. Potassium 4.2 mEq/L
   b. Creatinine 2.3 mg/dL
   c. Magnesium 1.4 mEq/L
   d. Sodium 146 mEq/L

15. A patient has a history of type 2 diabetes mellitus (T2DM) and hypertension and takes insulin, hydrochlorothiazide, and valsartan. The patient is having bowel preparation for a colonoscopy. The patient asks why the provider has ordered polyethylene glycol-electrolyte solution instead of the sodium phosphate that they took in the past. Which is the appropriate nursing response?
   a. "Polyethylene glycol-electrolyte solution causes electrolyte imbalances."
   b. "Sodium phosphate harms the liver, but it won't hurt the kidneys."
   c. "You are at risk for kidney damage due to your medical history."
   d. "Sodium phosphate can cause electrolyte disturbances."

✳16. A healthy pregnant patient reports chronic constipation. Which would be the best initial intervention?
   a. Bulk-forming laxative daily
   b. Increase fiber and fluid in the diet
   c. Stool softener each day at bedtime
   d. Moderate exercise before meals

17. Which would be a reason to withhold administration of lubiprostone and consult the provider?
   a. P450 enzyme drug interaction
   b. Mild nausea after taking the drug
   c. The patient is older than 60 years
   d. Opioid-induced constipation in a cancer patient

✳18. A patient has been using mineral oil daily as a laxative. Which is a priority to report to the provider?
   a. Bruising
   b. Fatigue
   c. Pallor
   d. Sore tongue

19. Which laxative is best for reestablishing normal bowel functioning when discontinuing chronic stimulant laxative use?
   a. Castor oil
   b. Glycerin suppository
   c. Lactulose
   d. Mineral oil

DOSE CALCULATION QUESTIONS

20. Milk of magnesia, 1 oz, is prescribed. How many milliliters will the nurse administer?

21. Lubiprostone, 0.008 mg twice a day, is prescribed for irritable bowel syndrome with constipation. Available are 8-mcg soft gelatin capsules. How many capsules should the nurse administer at each dose?

CASE STUDY

During a routine physical examination, the nurse discovers that an older adult who lives alone uses several over-the-counter (OTC) laxatives each day in order to have a bowel movement. They have a history of hypertension and heart failure.

1. What additional information does the nurse need to know about this patient before addressing the problem of laxative overuse?

Further data collection reveals that this patient describes their daily bowel movement as light brown, mushy, and with some watery discharge.

2. What lifestyle changes are appropriate to help establish an acceptable bowel pattern for this patient?

3. What problems does this patient's medical history present when trying to address normalizing bowel patterns and laxative use for this patient?

4. What laxatives are contraindicated for this patient?

84 Other Gastrointestinal Drugs

STUDY QUESTIONS

Completion

1. The vomiting center is a group of neurons located in the ________________ ________________.
2. Vomiting is a(n) ________________ action.
3. Chemotherapy drugs cause vomiting by directly stimulating the ________________ ________________ ________________.
4. Signals that stimulate nausea and vomiting travel via the ________________ nerve.
5. Drugs for chemotherapy-induced nausea and vomiting (CINV) are most effective if administered ________________ ________________.
6. Ondansetron exerts its antiemetic action by blocking ________________ receptors.
7. The effectiveness of ondansetron is increased by also administering ________________.
8. First-line therapy for nausea and vomiting of pregnancy is ________________ plus ________________.
9. Slowing down intestinal motility with drugs in uncomplicated diarrhea can ________________ traveler's diarrhea.
10. ____________ ______________ ____________ is the most common disorder of the GI tract.

CRITICAL THINKING, PRIORITIZATION, AND DELEGATION QUESTIONS

✳11. The nurse is caring for a patient who is prescribed aprepitant plus ondansetron and dexamethasone for CINV. The patient reports diarrhea. Which is the priority laboratory result for the nurse to monitor?
   a. Alanine aminotransferase
   b. Blood urea nitrogen (BUN)
   c. Complete blood count (CBC)
   d. Prothrombin time (PT)

12. Which is the primary reason why aprepitant is often used with other antiemetics for CINV?
   a. It is only moderately effective when given alone.
   b. When given with other drugs, it has few side effects.
   c. It is more effective than serotonin receptor blockers.
   d. The drug is effective only for acute nausea and vomiting.

►13. A postoperative patient is prescribed intravenous (IV) prochlorperazine as needed for nausea and vomiting. After being transferred from the bed to a chair with the assistance of three people, the patient vomits and requests the medication. Which is the appropriate nursing action? (**Select all that apply.**)
   a. Administer while the patient is sitting in the chair.
   b. Assess vital signs before and after administration.
   c. Hold the medication if the patient is hypertensive.
   d. Incorporate safety precautions after administration.
   e. Transfer patient back to the bed before administration.

✳14. Which action would be priority if a patient with postoperative vomiting reports burning at the IV promethazine infusion site?
   a. Apply ice to the site.
   b. Contact the provider.
   c. Page the IV team.
   d. Stop the IV infusion.

15. Which is an appropriate nursing focus when a patient is prescribed haloperidol for nausea and vomiting after knee replacement surgery?
   a. Anxiety
   b. Body image
   c. Safety
   d. Swallowing

✳16. It would be priority to report to the provider which new finding when a patient is prescribed dronabinol for CINV?
   a. Need to take two naps per day
   b. Blood pressure of 110/72 mm Hg
   c. Pulse increase from 82 to 122 beats/min
   d. Two-pound weight gain in the past month

17. It is recommended that a patient with nausea and vomiting of pregnancy take doxylamine at which time?
   a. Two hours after breakfast.
   b. At bedtime.
   c. With dinner.
   d. Upon waking.

18. Which planned activity would be of most concern if a patient has a new prescription for scopolamine for motion sickness?
   a. Taking a charter fishing trip
   b. Going on a cross-country rail trip
   c. Driving a delivery truck for work
   d. Flying on a 2-week trip to Europe

19. Which symptoms would be of concern when a patient is experiencing prolonged diarrhea?
    a. BUN 22 mg/dL
    b. Hematocrit 35%
    c. K 3.3 mEq/L
    d. Na 135 mEq/L

20. Which is the primary reason why diphenoxylate contains atropine in addition to diphenoxylate?
    a. It limits abuse of the drug.
    b. Opiate effects are antagonized.
    c. Inhibits gastric acid secretion.
    d. Relieves pylorospasm.

21. Which is the best intervention for a healthy child who has had two loose stools in the past 12 hours?
    a. Difenoxin
    b. Loperamide
    c. Paregoric
    d. Watchful waiting

►22. Persons taking bismuth subsalicylate should be warned about which effect of the drug?
    a. GI irritation
    b. Black tongue
    c. Poor appetite
    d. Confusion

23. A patient is prescribed alosetron 1 mg once a day. The patient should be told to call the provider if which occurs?
    a. Abdominal pain
    b. Two loose stools a day
    c. Decreased fecal urgency
    d. Constipation

24. It is important for the nurse to teach a patient who is taking alosetron to stop taking the medication and call their provider immediately if they experience which symptom?
    a. Dyspepsia
    b. Back pain
    c. Constipation
    d. Headache

25. A patient is prescribed sulfasalazine for moderate ulcerative colitis. The nurse would consult the provider if which allergy was listed on the patient's chart? (**Select all that apply.**)
    a. Cefazolin
    b. Glipizide
    c. Meperidine
    d. Nafcillin
    e. Quinapril
    f. Sulfamethoxazole

►26. Which laboratory result suggests possible adverse effects of sulfasalazine?
    a. Hemoglobin 14 g/dL
    b. Platelet count 250,000/μL
    c. Mean corpuscular volume 105 fL
    d. White blood cell (WBC) 10,500/mm^3

27. A patient has relief with dexamethasone for an exacerbation of Crohn disease of the ascending colon. They are concerned because the provider is discontinuing this drug and prescribing budesonide. Which is the appropriate nurse response? (**Select all that apply.**)
    a. "Systemic effects are lower than with dexamethasone."
    b. "Budesonide is released in the colon where it needs to work."
    c. "The drugs are the same, but budesonide is less expensive."
    d. "Tolerance develops to long-term use of dexamethasone."
    e. "Long-term use of dexamethasone may lead to Addison disease."

►28. Which laboratory test result would be of most concern to the nurse when caring for a patient who is receiving cyclosporine for severe Crohn disease?
    a. BUN 22 mg/dL
    b. Creatinine 3.6 mg/dL
    c. Platelet count 250,000/μL
    d. Blood glucose 122 mg/dL

✳29. It would be priority for a patient who is prescribed infliximab to report which symptom if it persists for over 6 weeks?
    a. Abdominal pain
    b. Dyspepsia
    c. Fatigue
    d. Productive cough

30. The nurse would consult the provider if a patient with Crohn disease reported new paresthesias after prolonged use of which drug?
    a. Budesonide
    b. Ciprofloxacin
    c. Infliximab
    d. Cyclosporine

31. A patient with diabetes has been experiencing episodes of abdominal pain, nausea, and vomiting of undigested food, especially at night. They are prescribed metoclopramide for gastroparesis. Which should be included in patient teaching?
    a. You may develop a rash while taking this drug
    b. Call the provider if you experience involuntary movements
    c. This drug is known to cause discoloration of the tongue
    d. You may become sensitive to light while taking this drug

►32. Which outcome would be expected for a patient who is taking palifermin?
    a. Absence of vomiting after chemotherapy
    b. Soft stool at least every other day
    c. Consumption of 70% of meals each day
    d. Weight gain of 1 lb each week

33. The school nurse cares for a student with cystic fibrosis, who takes pancrelipase. The nurse understands the drug is made from lipases, amylases and proteases that come from which animal?
    a. Hog
    b. Rabbit
    c. Horse
    d. Cow

DOSE CALCULATION QUESTIONS

34. Dronabinol 5 mg is prescribed 2 hours before the start of chemotherapy for a patient who is 4′2″ and weighs 70 lb. Based on body surface area (BSA), is the dose safe and effective?

35. What is a safe and effective maintenance dose of infliximab for a 166-lb male with ulcerative colitis?

CASE STUDIES

Case Study 1

A patient who has a history of motion sickness receives a prescription for a scopolamine patch for use when flying cross-country and embarking on a 7-day cruise. The patient has many questions, so the provider asks the office nurse to explain the use of this medication.

1. How should the nurse describe the medication's action and administration?

2. Research the drug in a drug handbook and list precautions that the nurse should teach the patient to take.

3. What interventions can the nurse suggest to prevent adverse effects?

Case Study 2

A patient diagnosed with diarrhea-predominant irritable bowel syndrome (IBS) comes to the office reporting that previously prescribed drugs have not provided any relief. When questioned by the nurse, the patient reports they have tried hyoscyamine, psyllium, and amitriptyline over the last year, but symptoms persist, including abdominal pain and bloating and mucous loose stools.

4. What nonpharmacologic measures can the nurse teach to assist this patient with controlling their IBS?

5. Alosetron is prescribed. The patient should stop taking the medication and return to the office if they experience what symptoms?

85 Vitamins

STUDY QUESTIONS

Matching

Match the term with its definition

1. ___ Average daily dietary intake sufficient to meet the nutrient requirements of nearly all healthy individuals
2. ___ An estimate of the average daily intake required to meet nutritional needs
3. ___ Five reference values on dietary intake
4. ___ The highest average daily intake that can be consumed by nearly everyone without a significant risk of adverse effects
5. ___ The level of intake that will meet nutrition requirements for 50% of the healthy individuals in any life stage or gender group

a. Adequate intake (AI)
b. Dietary reference intakes (DRIs)
c. Estimated average requirement (EAR)
d. Recommended dietary allowance (RDA)
e. Tolerable upper intake (UI)

CRITICAL THINKING, PRIORITIZATION, AND DELEGATION QUESTIONS

6. The nurse knows which statement is true about vitamins?
   a. They are inorganic compounds.
   b. They are needed for energy transformation.
   c. They are required in megadoses for growth.
   d. They are sources of energy.

7. The nurse knows which statement is true about published RDAs?
   a. Do not consider increased needs during illness.
   b. Include values for health maintenance of older adults.
   c. May be excessive for a chronically ill person.
   d. Need to be ingested at the same time each day.

8. Routine vitamin supplementation is recommended with which vitamin? **(Select all that apply.)**
   a. Vitamin E
   b. Vitamin C
   c. β-Carotene
   d. Vitamin B_{12}
   e. Folic acid

✳9. It would be a priority for the nurse to report which laboratory results when a patient takes high doses of vitamin A?
   a. Alanine aminotransferase (ALT) 250 IU/L
   b. Blood urea nitrogen (BUN) 20 mg/dL
   c. Human chorionic gonadotropin (hCG) 0.6 mIU/mL
   d. International normalized ratio (INR) 1

10. The nurse teaches a group of young adults in a childbirth education class about which food that is high in niacin? (**Select all that apply**.)
   a. Pork
   b. Chicken
   c. Dairy products
   d. Peanuts
   e. Bran cereal

►11. The preoperative patient's medication history includes hydrochlorothiazide 25 mg once a day, calcium 400 mg four times a day, a senior multivitamin once a day, cholestyramine 4 g four times a day, and vitamin E 1000 mg twice a day. The nurse should document the findings and notify the surgeon of the medication history because the patient is at risk for which issue?
   a. Bleeding
   b. Hypotension
   c. Hyponatremia
   d. Vomiting

12. The nurse would teach a patient who follows a vegan diet the importance of supplementation with which vitamin?
   a. α-Tocopherol
   b. Ascorbic acid
   c. Cyanocobalamin
   d. Folic acid

✳13. It would be a priority to educate which patient about the possible adverse effects of self-prescribing megadoses of vitamin A for healthy skin?
   a. Adolescent female
   b. Young adult male
   c. Older adult female
   d. Middle-aged male

14. The nurse should be aware that which disorder puts the patient at greatest risk for bleeding and bruising because of vitamin K deficiency?
    a. Addison disease
    b. Celiac disease
    c. Acid reflux
    d. Peptic ulcer disease

*15. Persons who take high doses of vitamin E increase their risk for which conditions?
    a. Heart failure
    b. Hypertension
    c. Kidney dysfunction
    d. Macular degeneration

16. The nurse includes in her health promotion teaching that vitamin C supplementation has been approved for which use?
    a. Exercise-induced asthma
    b. Prevention of colds
    c. Wound healing
    d. Treatment of scurvy

17. An oncology nurse is providing health teaching to a patient who is starting chemotherapy. The patient has heard that chemotherapy can cause painful mouth ulcers. The patient would like to know if there is anything that they can do to help prevent these ulcers. The nurse could teach about adequate consumption of which foods? (**Select all that apply**.)
    a. Strawberries
    b. Carrots
    c. Fish oil
    d. Rye breads
    e. Tomatoes

*18. The nurse is providing nutritional teaching to a patient with advanced esophageal cancer. It is important for the nurse to assess if the patient is self-medicating with which vitamin?
    a. Vitamin A
    b. Vitamin B
    c. Vitamin C
    d. Vitamin E

DOSE CALCULATION QUESTIONS

19. Niacinamide is available in 100-mg tablets. The medication administration record indicates the dose is 150 mg. How many tablets should the nurse administer?

20. Vitamin K_1 0.5 mg intramuscular (IM) is ordered for a neonate. Available is vitamin K_1 2 mg/mL. Calculate the dose.

CASE STUDY

A middle-aged patient has been admitted to a medical unit after 4 days in an alcohol detoxification center. They were admitted due to reports of extreme weakness and an unsteady gait. The patient's partner provided a history that the patient's alcohol intake has steadily increased since losing their job 3 years ago. During the past 6 months, the patient has been living on the street and drinking one to two bottles of wine daily. They are a poor historian and do not recall being admitted to the hospital. When asked about their diet, the patient responds, "Whatever I can get." Physical assessment reveals ataxia, edema of the lower extremities, nystagmus, dry skin with cracks in the corners of the mouth, bleeding gums, and multiple bruises. The patient states that the bruises are caused by any slight pressure. They are anorexic, taking sips of fluid and eating only a few bites of lunch. The patient reports that their mouth is "too sore" to eat many foods. Endoscopy reveals severe gastritis with no obvious bleeding. The patient is diagnosed with Wernicke-Korsakoff syndrome and started on an IV infusion with one 10-mL vial of multivitamin and 100 mg thiamine hydrochloride.

1. Describe the symptoms exhibited that suggest deficiency of the following vitamins.

    a. Thiamine

    b. Niacin

    c. Riboflavin

    d. Ascorbic acid

    e. Cyanocobalamin and folic acid

2. Why is the patient less likely to be showing symptoms of fat-soluble vitamin deficiencies?

3. Blood studies include hemoglobin 8.4 g and hematocrit 25%. Which vitamins are essential in red blood cell production?

4. The patient's partner has agreed that the patient may come home with them after discharge from the hospital as long as they continue to stay in an outpatient rehabilitation program and do not drink. The partner asks the nurse to tell them some of the foods that should be prepared to be certain that the necessary vitamins are provided. What foods or food groups would you suggest to ensure intake of vitamin A, vitamin C, niacin, pyridoxine, riboflavin, thiamine, and folate?

5. The patient's partner asks the nurse whether it would be a good idea to go to the health food store and buy some high-dose vitamin pills that include all vitamins. What is the best response?

86 Drugs for Weight Loss

STUDY QUESTIONS

Matching

Match the drug with its mechanism of action.

1. ___ Suppresses appetite and induces a sense of satiety, possibly by antagonism of glutamate.
2. ___ Acts in the GI tract to reduce absorption of fat.
3. ___ Hypothesized to promote weight loss by acting on the regulation of appetite in the hypothalamus and on the mesolimbic dopamine system.
4. ___ Acts by slowing gastric emptying, which increases the feeling of fullness and decreases food intake.

a. Orlistat
b. Phentermine/topiramate
c. Liraglutide
d. Naltrexone/bupropion

True or False

For each of the following statements, enter T for true or F for false.

5. ____ Research on drugs for weight loss suggests that some patients will lose weight even when receiving a placebo.
6. ____ Childhood obesity increases the risk for asthma.
7. ____ Obesity can be cured.
8. ____ Health risk is determined by body mass index (BMI), waist circumference, and cardiovascular risk factors.
9. ____ A BMI exceeding 30 is considered severe obesity.
10. ____ Waist circumference is an independent risk factor for obesity-related diseases.
11. ____ Research has determined that weight is controlled by a complex hormonal system in combination with genetic contributions.

CRITICAL THINKING, PRIORITIZATION, AND DELEGATION QUESTIONS

12. The school nurse is teaching health promotion to a group of adolescent girls. Developmentally, which health risk would most likely be a motivator for change to healthier eating and exercise habits?
    a. Cardiovascular disease
    b. Increases risk of fetal death
    c. Diabetes mellitus
    d. Hypertension

13. Which is the most important factor when the nurse devises a patient's weight management plan?
    a. Developing strategies to help the patient minimize stress
    b. Including aerobic exercise, as possible, in the patient's plan
    c. Advising the patient to limit overly processed foods in the diet
    d. Self-monitoring of eating and exercise habits

14. Which statement, if made by a patient who has been prescribed a drug for weight loss, suggests that the patient needs additional teaching?
    a. "If I exercise, I should be able to lose 4 pounds the first month."
    b. "I may need to take the drug long term to maintain weight loss."
    c. "Drug therapy was started because I lost very little weight with lifestyle changes."
    d. "My doctor is starting drug therapy for me because I am too heavy to exercise."

*15. Which laboratory result would be a priority to report to the provider if a patient has self-prescribed orlistat while taking warfarin?
    a. Alanine aminotransferase (ALT) 30 IU/L
    b. Blood urea nitrogen (BUN) 22 mg/dL
    c. International normalized ratio (INR) 5.2
    d. Potassium 5.2 mEq/L

16. Which result would be priority if a patient is prescribed phentermine/topiramate?
    a. Blood pressure (BP) 180/98 mm Hg
    b. Pulse 52 beats/min
    c. Respiration 24/minute
    d. Temperature 102.2°F (39°C)

17. A patient who is prescribed levothyroxine for hypothyroidism has self-prescribed over-the-counter (OTC) orlistat for weight loss. Which teachings would be important for this patient? (**Select all that apply.**)
    a. It is important to take a daily multivitamin supplement.
    b. It is important to take supplements of vitamins B and C.
    c. Omit the orlistat dose if the meal does not contain fat.
    d. Levothyroxine and orlistat should be taken 4 hours apart.
    e. Taking fiber supplements can reduce gastrointestinal (GI) effects.

DOSE CALCULATION QUESTIONS

18. A prescription orlistat dose is equal to how many capsules of OTC orlistat?

19. Phentermine 18.75 mg is prescribed twice a day. Available are 37.5-mg tablets. How many tablets should be administered at each dose?

CASE STUDY

A middle-aged patient with a history of sleep apnea, hypertension, and type 2 diabetes weighs 285 lb and is 5′ 8″ tall. Their waist circumference is 44″, and total cholesterol is 330 mg.

1. What is this patient's BMI?

2. The patient asks the nurse what is considered a realistic goal for weight loss and how much they need to cut back on eating. How should the nurse respond?

3. The patient is prescribed orlistat 120 mg three times a day with meals. What strategies can the nurse suggest to minimize adverse effects, which can be serious?

    a. GI effects

    b. Liver damage

    c. Reduced absorption of vitamins A, D, E, and K

4. The patient is concerned about the adverse effects of orlistat and asks if there are ways to improve their health without taking diet drugs. How should the nurse respond?

87 Complementary and Alternative Therapy

STUDY QUESTIONS

Matching Group 1

Match the dietary supplement to its primary use or side effect.

1. ___ Taken orally may prevent common colds
2. ___ May decrease the rate of atherosclerosis development
3. ___ Used to treat symptoms of menopause
4. ___ Has been promoted as a natural alternative to benzodiazepines
5. ___ Can cause hepatic veno-occlusive disease when taken orally
6. ___ Prevention and treatment of morning sickness
7. ___ Beneficial in the management of irritable bowel syndrome
8. ___ May reduce the frequency of migraine headaches

a. Black cohosh
b. Peppermint
c. Echinacea
d. Comfrey
e. Kava
f. Feverfew
g. Garlic
h. Ginger root

Matching Group 2

Match the dietary supplement to its primary use or side effect.

9. ____ Used primarily to improve memory
10. ____ Taken to relieve urinary symptoms associated with BPH
11. ____ Appears to relieve nasal allergy symptoms
12. ____ May have mild sedative effects
13. ____ Important food source of phytoestrogens
14. ____ Appears equal to tricyclic antidepressants in treating mild depression
15. ____ Antioxidant promoted for antiaging effects
16. ____ Contains a compound that can elevate blood pressure

a. Butterbur
b. Resveratrol
c. Ginkgo biloba
d. Flaxseed
e. Ma Huang
f. St. John wort
g. Saw palmetto
h. Valerian

True or False

For each of the following statements, enter T for true or F for false.

17. ___ Natural products are always better and safer than synthetic products.
18. ___ Products marketed as dietary supplements do not require rigorous evaluation before marketing.
19. ___ The FDA cannot remove a dietary supplement from the market even if there is evidence that it causes harm.
20. ___ Dietary supplement labels can insinuate they provide specific benefits.
21. ___ Dietary supplements have been found to contain harmful ingredients such as arsenic, mercury, and lead.
22. ___ Dietary supplements have been found to not contain the stated ingredients in the amount listed on the label.
23. ___ Dietary supplement labels may claim to treat a specific disease without adequate research supporting the claim.
24. ___ There is conflicting evidence that dietary supplements are effective or safe.

CRITICAL THINKING, PRIORITIZATION, AND DELEGATION QUESTIONS

25. Which is the purpose of the Current Good Manufacturing Practices (CGMPs) rule?
    a. Supplements must list their active and inert ingredients.
    b. All socioeconomic groups must have access to supplements.
    c. Generic names must be used with supplements.
    d. Designates health promotion as the use for supplements.

*26. Which is the priority teaching when a patient chooses to use a dietary supplement?
  a. Do not focus on the cost of the supplements.
  b. Take the supplement with at least 8 oz of water.
  c. Use products that have the US Pharmacopeia seal.
  d. Take the lowest dose of the supplement possible.

*27. Which is the priority nursing action when a nurse discovers that a patient self-prescribes supplements?
  a. Assess for adverse effects of the product.
  b. Ensure the patient is making an informed choice.
  c. Discuss alternatives to taking the supplement.
  d. Inform the provider about the supplements.

28. A patient who is taking warfarin is at risk for bleeding if also taking which of the following? (**Select all that apply.**)
  a. Feverfew
  b. Garlic
  c. St. John wort
  d. Ma Huang
  e. Ginkgo

29. The patient asks how peppermint oil is effective in managing irritable bowel syndrome. Which is the appropriate nursing response?
  a. "Its effects are probably due to caffeine."
  b. "It inhibits smooth muscle activity."
  c. "It blocks serotonin 5 HT_3 receptors."
  d. "It suppresses inflammation."

30. Research suggests which is the possible effect of cranberry juice?
  a. It increases excretion of bacteria.
  b. It acidifies urine to kill the bacteria.
  c. Bacteria cannot adhere to the bladder wall.
  d. It prevents the development of kidney stones.

31. Which is true about echinacea? (**Select all that apply.**)
  a. Should be avoided in those with autoimmune disorders
  b. Can produce allergic reactions in patients allergic to ragweed
  c. May suppress the immune system with long-term use
  d. Decreases symptom severity of colds and influenza
  e. Prevents development of common cold symptoms

*32. The nurse is assessing a new admission. The patient lists echinacea, garlic, and kava among the products that they use regularly. On first observation, the nurse notes that the patient's skin has a yellowish color. Which is the priority nursing action?
  a. Continue to assess the patient.
  b. Document findings in the electronic health record (EHR).
  c. Notify the health care provider.
  d. Have patient stop taking supplements.

33. A patient who regularly took feverfew to prevent migraine headaches stopped taking the supplement before elective surgery. The nurse should assess the patient for which possible symptom?
  a. Bleeding
  b. Flatulence
  c. Insomnia
  d. Nausea

*34. A patient who is prescribed glipizide for type 2 diabetes mellitus and celecoxib for inflamed joints informs the nurse that they have started taking ginger because they read in a magazine that it helps arthritis. Which information should be included in patient teaching?
  a. Dry, itchy skin may be a drug side effect.
  b. The drug combination may cause headaches.
  c. Taking ginger may cause loss of appetite.
  d. Be aware of developing shaking and sweating.

*35. It is a priority to inform patients with which disorder that ginkgo biloba can aggravate their condition?
  a. Diabetes mellitus
  b. Hay fever
  c. Hypertension
  d. Seizures

*36. Which is an expected outcome for a 12-year-old child taking probiotics prescribed during a rotavirus infection?
  a. Soft, formed stool
  b. No bacterial growth in urine
  c. Temperature 98–99°F
  d. No adventitious lung sounds

37. Which is a priority nursing concern when a patient self-prescribes St. John wort?
  a. Drug-drug interactions
  b. Constipation
  c. Photosensitivity
  d. Potency of the preparation

38. The nurse is aware that which herbal supplement has been associated with liver failure?
  a. Black cohosh
  b. Ginger
  c. Kava
  d. Valerian

*39. The nurse is caring for a patient who admits to using mail-order Ma Huang for weight loss. Which is the priority nursing intervention?
  a. Assess mental status.
  b. Monitor vital signs.
  c. Avoid sedatives.
  d. Assess daily weights.

CASE STUDIES

Case Study 1

A middle-aged adult is admitted with chest pain. Assessment findings include height 5′8″, weight 220 lb, waist circumference 42″, BP 145/86 mm Hg, and pulse 78 beats/min. Lab results include triglycerides 380 mg/dL, low-density lipoprotein (LDL) 240 mg/dL, and HDL 34 mg/dL. The patient is diagnosed with gastroesophageal reflux disease and metabolic syndrome. They inform their health care provider that they want to try natural therapy and have heard that garlic can help with many things. The health care provider asks the nurse to discuss garlic therapy with this patient.

1. What are possible positive effects of garlic supplementation for this patient?

2. The health care provider recommends enteric-coated garlic supplements. What can the nurse teach the patient to ensure that the product that the patient purchases contains effective amounts of allicin?

3. Why is it important for the patient to inform all health care providers and their pharmacist that they are using garlic therapy?

Case Study 2

An older adult with atrial fibrillation is being treated with digoxin and warfarin. At times, the patient is fatigued and forgetful. Their friend suggests taking ginkgo biloba to boost their energy.

4. What possible complications can occur with this combination of drugs and supplement?

5. What teaching should the nurse provide this patient regarding the use of supplements?

6. The patient informs the nurse that they are not going to get their annual flu shot because they have purchased a bottle of echinacea. How should the nurse respond?

88 Basic Principles of Antimicrobial Therapy

STUDY QUESTIONS

True or False

For each of the following statements, enter T for true or F for false.

1. ___ Mammalian cells do not have a rigid cell wall.
2. ___ Patients should not take folic acid supplements when prescribed sulfonamide drugs.
3. ___ Cephalosporins kill bacteria by weakening the cell wall and promoting bacterial lysis.
4. ___ Aminoglycosides inhibit folic acid production by the microbe.
5. ___ Metronidazole inhibits DNA synthesis in certain microbes.
6. ___ Many drugs that are prescribed for HIV infection inhibit enzymes needed for viral reproduction.
7. ___ Methicillin-resistant *Staphylococcus aureus* (MRSA), vancomycin-resistant enterococci (VRE), and *Clostridioides difficile* are a problem because infection with these microbes is usually fatal.
8. ___ When patients take antibiotics as prescribed, resistance to antibiotics does not occur.
9. ___ Bacteria can become resistant to antibiotics by producing enzymes that inactivate the antibiotic.
10. ___ If a bacterium changes its receptors, an antibiotic may not be able to bind to the microbe and exert effects.
11. ___ The human body can make compounds that prevent an antibiotic from exerting the desired effect.
12. ___ Some microbes can change so that they stop taking antibiotics into the cell.
13. ___ The New Delhi metallo-β-lactamase 1 (NDM-1) gene is common in people of Indian or Pakistani descent.
14. ___ Broad-spectrum antibiotics kill more competing organisms than do narrow-spectrum drugs and do the most to facilitate emergence of resistance.
15. ___ Narrow-spectrum antibiotics tend to promote overgrowth of normal flora that possess mechanisms for resistance.
16. ___ Antibiotics have difficulty penetrating an abscess.
17. ___ The American Heart Association has recently stressed that prophylactic use of antibiotics is more important than previously thought.
18. ___ The use of antibiotics in the livestock and poultry industries has created a large reservoir of drug-resistant bacteria, some of which now infect humans.

CRITICAL THINKING, PRIORITIZATION, AND DELEGATION QUESTIONS

*19. A patient is admitted to a medical unit and prescribed intravenous (IV) ampicillin/sulbactam after a specimen was sent for culture and sensitivity (C&S). Which is the priority reason for notifying the provider of culture results as soon as they are available?
   a. Ampicillin/sulbactam has more adverse effects than other antibiotics.
   b. There may be an effective narrow-spectrum antibiotic alternative.
   c. A less expensive alternative antibiotic may be effective.
   d. The drug may not be sensitive to the cultured organism.

20. Which patient would most likely have an infection that is resistant to antibiotic therapy?
   a. Child with asthma who develops pneumonia
   b. Construction worker who developed giardiasis
   c. Patient who developed a wound infection after surgery
   d. Older adult who developed infection from a paper cut

21. Which infection would be classified as a superinfection?
   a. Monilial vaginal infection that develops during antibiotic therapy
   b. Peritonitis that develops after surgery for a ruptured appendix
   c. Pneumonia in a patient with chronic bronchitis
   d. Varicella outbreak after injection with varicella vaccine

22. Microscopic examination of Gram-stained preparations has which advantage? (**Select all that apply.**)
    a. It detects microbes when minute amounts are present.
    b. It is the simplest test to identify microorganisms.
    c. It provides quickest microorganism identification.
    d. It is the most versatile technique to identify organisms.
    e. It can be done on a variety of body fluids.

✳23. The nurse has consulted the provider because a patient reports an allergy to the prescribed penicillin antibiotic. The provider is aware of the allergy, but the patient is experiencing a life-threatening infection and no other suitable antibiotic is available. Which is the priority nursing action?
    a. Obtain consent for administering the antibiotic.
    b. Ask the patient if they are willing to take the antibiotic.
    c. Obtain orders for treatment of a possible allergic reaction.
    d. Consult with the charge nurse about administering the drug.

✳24. It would be a priority to report which test result if a patient is prescribed tetracycline?
    a. Creatinine 1.5 mg/dL
    b. hCG 5325 mIU/mL
    c. Glucose 125 mg/dL
    d. Sodium 132 mEq/L

25. Which test results should the nurse monitor when caring for a patient who has red blood cells that are deficient in glucose-6-phosphate dehydrogenase and is prescribed a sulfonamide antibiotic?
    a. Total bilirubin
    b. Blood urea nitrogen
    c. Hemoglobin A1c
    d. Hematocrit

26. To be effective, which relationship to the minimum inhibitory concentration (MIC) must be achieved by the antibiotic concentration at the site of infection?
    a. Equal to MIC
    b. 2–4 times the MIC
    c. 4–8 times the MIC
    d. 10 times the MIC

27. Which are valid reasons for prescribing two different antibiotics? (**Select all that apply.**)
    a. Cases of infection with *Mycobacterium tuberculosis*
    b. Sensitivity results indicate multiple drugs are effective
    c. Mixed infection with differing drug susceptibilities
    d. Enhance the antibacterial action
    e. Decrease the development of toxicity

28. Which is an acceptable reason for giving antibiotic prophylaxis?
    a. Before cardiac surgery
    b. With ophthalmic dilation
    c. Yellow-green nasal discharge
    d. Whenever a patient has a fever

CASE STUDIES

Case Study 1

An older adult nursing home resident with a history of hypertension, type 2 diabetes mellitus, and chronic obstructive pulmonary disease is brought into the emergency department (ED) with a history of fever for 72 hours and moist cough. The nursing report states that the patient was very irritable last night and then was difficult to awaken this morning. Assessment findings include temperature 103°F (39.4°C), pulse 112 beats/min, BP 100/56 mm Hg, respirations 26 and labored, and rales throughout the lung fields. Chest X-ray demonstrates lung consolidation. IV fluids are infusing. Other orders include sputum C&S.

1. What are nursing responsibilities regarding these orders?
2. What type of antibiotic would the nurse expect to be ordered and why?
3. Cefotetan 1 g every 12 hours is ordered. The unit nurse reviews the following C&S results. What action should the nurse take?

Organism: *Moraxella Catarrhalis*

Antibiotic	**Sensitivity**
Amikacin	R
Amoxicillin	R
Azithromycin	S
Cefepime	R
Cefotetan	R
Clarithromycin	R
Gatifloxacin	S
Levofloxacin	S
Piperacillin	R
Tobramycin	R

R, Resistant; *S*, sensitive.

4. The cultured organism is sensitive to more than one drug. In this case, what other factors are considered when choosing among the effective antibiotics?

5. What assessment should be monitored by the nurse to determine clinical response to the antibiotic?

Case Study 2

A neighbor asks a student nurse why their provider will not phone in prescriptions when they have a "sinus infection" anymore.

6. How can the nurse explain these changes in antibiotic prescription practices?

7. The neighbor states that they have antibiotics left over from the last infection. "I always save some in case I need them," they say. The neighbor asks the nurse if it is okay to take the leftover drug, since it was prescribed for them. How should the student nurse respond?

8. The neighbor asks what they can do to prevent resistance to antibiotics. What suggestions should the student nurse make?

9. Where can the student nurse direct people for more information on preventing antibiotic resistance?

89 Drugs That Weaken the Bacterial Cell Wall I: Penicillins

STUDY QUESTIONS

True or False

For each of the following statements, enter T for true or F for false.

1. ___ All penicillins are able to penetrate the Gram-negative cell membrane.
2. ___ Penicillins are able to destroy many bacteria when taken as prescribed.
3. ___ Penicillins are in the same antibiotic family as macrolide antibiotics.
4. ___ Penicillins are only active against bacteria that are undergoing growth and division.
5. ___ Penicillins are more effective against Gram-negative than Gram-positive bacteria.
6. ___ Penicillins are toxic to human tissue when prescribed in high doses.
7. ___ In patients with a history of penicillin allergy, a skin test may be performed to determine current allergic status.
8. ___ Penicillins must bind to special proteins on the outer surface of the cytoplasmic membrane to be effective.
9. ___ People can drastically reduce their chance of catching methicillin-resistant *Staphylococcus aureus* (MRSA) by simple hygiene measures.
10. ___ MRSA can be treated by penicillinase-resistant penicillin such as nafcillin.
11. ___ Many people have MRSA in their nose and do not know it.
12. ___ Most infections with MRSA come from sports equipment.
13. ___ The germ that causes MRSA is commonly found on the skin.

CRITICAL THINKING, PRIORITIZATION, AND DELEGATION QUESTIONS

*14. Which assessment is priority for the nurse to complete before administering a penicillin antibiotic?
   a. Allergy history
   b. Blood urea nitrogen
   c. Temperature
   d. Wound drainage

15. Parents ask why their child has been prescribed amoxicillin and clavulanate if amoxicillin has been ineffective in the past. Which is the best response based on the addition of clavulanate?
   a. Aids the penicillin in attaching to microbial proteins
   b. Affects a wider spectrum of infecting organisms
   c. Prevents penicillinase from inactivating the amoxicillin
   d. Provides additional activity to disrupt the bacterial cell wall

16. Oxacillin is clinically useful for which microorganism?
   a. *Clostridium perfringens*
   b. *Neisseria gonorrhoeae*
   c. *Streptococcus pneumoniae*
   d. *Treponema pallidum*

17. A child is prescribed amoxicillin. When asked if their child is allergic to penicillin, the child's parents state that the child has never received any medication except immunizations. Which is the reason to assess for an allergic response despite this history?
   a. The first allergic response occurs in childhood.
   b. Penicillin allergies are poorly understood.
   c. Parents are poor historians concerning allergies.
   d. Initial exposure may occur from antibiotics in foods.

*18. Which assessment finding would be priority to report to the provider if it occurred after administration of a large intravenous (IV) dose of penicillin?
   a. IV site pain
   b. Fever
   c. Wheezing
   d. Nausea

▶19. The nurse is preparing to administer 8 a.m. medications to a patient prescribed nafcillin 2 g via a secondary IV infusion. The drug is dissolved in 100 mL of normal saline solution. The drug handbook states that the drug should be infused over 30–90 minutes. Just before the nurse hangs the nafcillin, the nurse is informed the patient is to go off the unit for a diagnostic test in 30–45 minutes. The patient is expected to be off the unit for 30 minutes. Which is the appropriate nursing intervention?
   a. Hold the drug infusion until the patient returns from the test.
   b. Administer over 30 minutes before the patient leaves the unit.
   c. Run the drug over 45 minutes while waiting for patient transport.
   d. Infuse over 90 minutes, as the technician can monitor the IV.

20. Which is the appropriate nursing action when assisting with skin testing for penicillin allergy with the minor determinant mixture (MDM)?
   a. Instruct the patient to monitor for local reaction.
   b. Tell the patient MDM carries little risk of systemic reaction.
   c. Ensure respiratory support and epinephrine are available.
   d. Teach the patient what will happen during skin testing.

21. The nurse would be concerned about the increased possibility of an allergic reaction when administering which antibiotic if the patient's record includes penicillin allergy? **(Select all that apply.)**
   a. Ampicillin/sulbactam
   b. Azithromycin
   c. Clindamycin
   d. Gatifloxacin
   e. Piperacillin/tazobactam
   f. Vancomycin

*22. If blood levels of penicillin G become too high, which may occur?
   a. Sensory dysfunction
   b. Gangrene
   c. Hallucinations
   d. Motor dysfunction

23. The nurse would be concerned about toxicity if a patient receiving penicillin G had which laboratory result?
   a. Glucose 124 mg/dL
   b. BUN 20 mg/dL
   c. Creatinine 2.6 mg/dL
   d. Potassium 3.3 mEq/L

DOSE CALCULATION QUESTIONS

24. Amoxicillin 125 mg every 6 hours for 10 days is prescribed for a child with acute otitis media who weighs 16.5 lb. The recommended dose is 20–40 mg/kg per day. Is the prescribed dose safe?

25. Ampicillin 1 g/sulbactam 0.5 g is supplied in 50 mL of solution to be infused over 15 minutes. The nurse should program the IV pump to deliver how many milliliters per hour?

CASE STUDIES

Case Study 1

A child is diagnosed with streptococcal pharyngitis. They are prescribed amoxicillin 500 mg twice daily for 10 days.

1. What important information should the nurse obtain before the penicillin is administered?

2. What information about the possible side effects and adverse reactions of penicillin does the nurse need to provide to the child's parents?

3. Describe the types of allergic reactions that might develop with the administration of penicillin and the interventions that should be included in nursing care to prevent complications from an allergic reaction.

4. The patient's parents ask how and when amoxicillin should be given. How should the nurse respond?

5. Why is it critical that the nurse teach the patient's parents not to stop the medication even if the child's throat stops hurting in 4–5 days?

6. What outcome would indicate that the antimicrobial effects were successful?

Case Study 2

The nurse is working in a public health clinic. A young adult with no known allergies is diagnosed with syphilis and prescribed one dose of 2.4 million units of benzathine penicillin G intramuscularly (IM).

7. Why is this drug a good choice for this patient?

8. The patient asks why they cannot get this medication in a pill. How should the nurse respond?

9. The patient has denied an allergy to penicillin. Why does the nurse need to be cautious about possible allergy?

10. What actions/policies should the clinic have in place to prevent death from an anaphylactic reaction?

90 Drugs That Weaken the Bacterial Cell Wall II: Other Drugs

STUDY QUESTIONS

Completion

1. Cephalosporins are often resistant to ____________.
2. First-generation cephalosporins are highly active against Gram-_________________ bacteria.
3. First-generation cephalosporins are not effective against _________________.
4. Second-generation cephalosporins have _____ ____ _____ resistance to β-lactamases produced by Gram-negative organisms.
5. Third-generation cephalosporins are considerably more active against Gram-____________ aerobes.
6. _________________ is the only cephalosporin with activity against methicillin-resistant *Staphylococcus aureus* (MRSA).
7. Penetration of cerebrospinal fluid (CSF) by fourth-generation cephalosporins is ___________.

CRITICAL THINKING, PRIORITIZATION, AND DELEGATION QUESTIONS

∗8. A patient is prescribed cefotaxime. Which result would be priority to report to the provider?
   a. Albumin 3.4 g/dL
   b. Total bilirubin 0.8 mg/dL
   c. Creatinine 2.0 mg/dL
   d. Platelets 150×10^9/L

∗9. A patient is prescribed ceftriaxone. Which result would be priority to report to the provider?
   a. Albumin 3.4 g/dL
   b. Creatinine 1.2 mg/dL
   c. Hemoglobin 9.2 g/dL
   d. Glucose 100 mg/dL

∗10. When performing their shift assessment, the nurse notes a maculopapular rash over the trunk of a patient who has been taking ceftriaxone for 4 days. Which is the priority nursing action?
   a. Administer epinephrine.
   b. Complete the assessment.
   c. Consult the provider.
   d. Withhold the ceftriaxone.

11. A patient who is receiving ceftazidime has three loose brown bowel movements in 24 hours. Which is the appropriate nursing intervention?
   a. Document the finding.
   b. Notify the provider.
   c. Withhold the drug.
   d. Notify the pharmacy.

12. A patient with hospital-acquired pneumonia has been prescribed cefotaxime and probenecid. The patient has no history or evidence of gout. Which is the appropriate nursing intervention?
   a. Administer both drugs.
   b. Give cefotaxime only.
   c. Call the pharmacy.
   d. Verify with the charge nurse.

∗13. An alert and oriented patient with a history of penicillin allergy is prescribed cephalexin. Which is the priority nursing intervention?
   a. Administer the cephalexin as ordered.
   b. Assess for reaction after drug administration.
   c. Determine the type of reaction to penicillin.
   d. Notify the provider of the drug allergy.

14. The nurse is reviewing new laboratory results, including estimated glomerular filtration rate (eGFR) of 82 mL/min for a patient receiving cefotetan 2 g every 12 hours. Which is the appropriate nursing intervention?
   a. Administer the medication.
   b. Withhold the medication.
   c. Call the provider about results.
   d. Call pharmacist to reduce dose.

15. Cefazolin has been prescribed at discharge for a patient with pelvic inflammatory disease. Due to the possibility of a disulfiram-like reaction, during discharge teaching, which is important for the nurse to teach the patient to avoid consuming?
   a. Alcohol
   b. Antacids
   c. Aspirin
   d. Ibuprofen

16. The nurse is preparing to administer an IV minibag of ceftriaxone in 50 mL of 5% dextrose to an infant. The infant has an IV of lactated Ringer solution infusing at 35 mL/h. Which is the appropriate nursing intervention?
   a. Start a second IV.
   b. Infuse as a piggyback.
   c. Consult with the provider.
   d. Interrupt the IV to infuse the drug.

▶17. Which laboratory result would cause the nurse to hold cefotetan and notify the provider?
   a. Alanine aminotransferase (ALT) 254 IU/L
   b. Alkaline phosphatase (Alk Phos) 147 IU/L
   c. Brain natriuretic peptide (BNP) 150 pg/mL
   d. International normalized ratio (INR) 1.2

✳18. When imipenem and valproate are prescribed for a patient, which is the priority nursing concern?
   a. Hydration
   b. Nutrition
   c. Safety
   d. Skin integrity

19. Which is the purpose of adding cilastatin to imipenem?
   a. Decrease adverse effects of nausea and vomiting
   b. Improve absorption in the gastrointestinal (GI) tract
   c. Prevent destruction of the antibiotic by β-lactamase
   d. Avoid inactivation by an enzyme present in the kidney

20. Vancomycin is being administered by mouth for pseudomembranous colitis caused by *Clostridioides difficile.* The nurse receives laboratory results on the patient that include creatinine 2.2 mg/dL. Which is the priority nursing intervention?
   a. Administer the medication.
   b. Hold the medication.
   c. Decrease dose by half.
   d. Notify the provider.

21. Which predrug administration assessment finding would be of most concern when a patient is prescribed telavancin?
   a. Facial flushing
   b. Foamy urine
   c. Maculopapular rash
   d. Bibasilar crackles

DOSE CALCULATION QUESTIONS

22. Telavancin 0.75 g is prescribed for a patient who weighs 72 kg and whose eGFR is 34 mL/min. Is the dose safe?

23. Meropenem 250 mg is prescribed every 8 hours for a 14-lb child. The recommended safe pediatric dose of meropenem for meningitis is 120 mg/kg per day divided every 8 hours. Is this a safe dose?

CASE STUDIES

Case Study 1

A middle-aged adult is admitted to the nursing unit with the diagnosis of acute diverticulitis. They report abdominal pain, nausea, and vomiting. The patient has a temperature of 101°F and a white blood cell count of 18,000/mm^3. A nasogastric tube is placed, an IV is started, and 1 g of ceftriaxone is ordered every 12 hours. Pain management is provided by IV morphine.

1. The nurse should assess the patient for which possible adverse reactions to the antibiotic?

2. Why would a broad-spectrum antibiotic not be prescribed for this patient?

3. What should the nurse do if they discover the patient has had an anaphylactic reaction to penicillin?

Case Study 2

A patient is prescribed vancomycin 1 g every 12 hours scheduled at 0900 and 2100. The pharmacy provides a solution of 1 g in 200 mL.

4. Why is it critical to use an IV pump when administering this drug rather than hanging this drug by gravity?

5. If the drug is administered at 0900, at what time should blood be drawn to assess trough levels of the drug?

6. The drug will reach its therapeutic level after how many doses of the drug?

7. Describe red man syndrome and the nursing measures that can be taken to prevent this reaction.

8. Does experiencing a red man syndrome create a contraindication for further administration of vancomycin?

9. Describe how the nurse will assess for the possible adverse effects of

   a. Ototoxicity.

   b. Immune-mediated thrombocytopenia.

91 Bacteriostatic Inhibitors of Protein Synthesis: Tetracyclines, Macrolides, and Others

STUDY QUESTIONS

True or False

For each of the following statements, enter T for true or F for false.

1. ___ Most oral tetracyclines should be taken on an empty stomach.
2. ___ Low doses of doxycycline can be used to prevent destruction of gingival connective tissue.
3. ___ Resistance to tetracycline is increasing.
4. ___ Tetracyclines are the drugs of choice for most infections.
5. ___ Tetracycline easily crosses mammalian cell membranes.
6. ___ Tetracycline is active against the bacilli that cause anthrax.
7. ___ Tetracycline is a narrow-spectrum antibiotic.
8. ___ Tetracyclines are bactericidal.
9. ___ Minocycline is used topically to treat periodontal disease.
10. ___ Tetracycline should be used for mild acne.

CRITICAL THINKING, PRIORITIZATION, AND DELEGATION QUESTIONS

11. The nurse teaches a patient who has been prescribed oral tetracycline that the medication should not be taken with which over-the-counter medication? **(Select all that apply.)**
    a. Ascorbic acid
    b. Centrum Silver
    c. Ferrous sulfate
    d. Folic acid
    e. Calcium

►12. A patient who was admitted with severe abdominal pain has been diagnosed with *Helicobacter pylori*–associated peptic ulcer. Tetracycline 500 mg, metronidazole 250 mg, and bismuth subsalicylate 524 mg have been prescribed to be taken four times a day. The nurse notes that the patient's 24-hour fluid intake has been approximately 2500 mL and urine output has been 600–800 mL for each of the past 2 days. Which is the appropriate nursing action?
    a. Administer the medications.
    b. Document the assessment.
    c. Withhold the medication.
    d. Notify the provider.

13. A patient is prescribed tetracycline. Which information should the nurse provide the patient to minimize the risk of esophageal ulceration?
    a. Take two hours before a meal.
    b. Avoid taking the drug at bedtime.
    c. Take the medication with an antacid.
    d. Take the medication with milk.

14. A patient is prescribed a tetracycline antibiotic. Which patient information is a reason for the medication to be withheld and the provider consulted?
    a. Allergy to penicillin
    b. Creatinine 1.4 mg/dL
    c. Unknown pregnancy status
    d. Prescribed theophylline

15. Patient education concerning which drug would include that the drug can be taken with or without food, as absorption is not affected by food?
    a. Demeclocycline
    b. Doxycycline
    c. Minocycline
    d. Tetracycline

✳16. A patient is prescribed tetracycline for *Chlamydia trachomatis.* Which change in assessment findings would be a priority to report to the provider?
    a. Burning on urination
    b. Perineal itching
    c. Vaginal discharge
    d. Watery stool

17. A patient with a penicillin allergy is prescribed erythromycin ethylsuccinate 250 mg every 6 hours for pneumonia caused by *Haemophilus influenzae.* The medication administration record (MAR) has the medication scheduled at 0600, 1200, 1800, and 2400. On the second day of therapy, the patient states they do not like taking the drug because it causes heartburn. Which is an appropriate nursing intervention?
    a. Administer the drug with food.
    b. Change dosing to twice daily.
    c. Explain how food alters drug absorption.
    d. Withhold the drug and notify the provider.

18. Which is the appropriate way to administer enteric-coated erythromycin base? **(Select all that apply.)**
    a. On empty stomach
    b. Once a day
    c. Whole, not chewed
    d. With full glass of water
    e. With food

19. Because of the risk of prolonged QT interval and torsades de pointes, the nurse would consult the provider before administering erythromycin to which patient?
    a. Chronic migraine headaches
    b. Reports a fear of needles
    c. History of fainting
    d. Poorly controlled asthma

20. Erythromycin can increase the plasma levels of which drugs? **(Select all that apply.)**
    a. Theophylline
    b. Digoxin
    c. Warfarin
    d. Selegilene
    e. Lexapro

21. Which patient teaching helps decrease the development of antibiotic resistance?
    a. Avoid people with symptoms of communicable disease.
    b. Only take antibiotics when symptoms are present.
    c. Ask the provider for antibiotics for all infections.
    d. Take the full antibiotic course even if symptoms are gone.

22. It is important for the nurse to monitor which laboratory results when a patient is prescribed azithromycin or erythromycin and they also take warfarin?
    a. Blood urea nitrogen (BUN)
    b. Creatine kinase-skeletal muscle (CK-MM)
    c. International normalized ratio (INR)
    d. Red blood cell (RBC)

23. The nurse is caring for a patient who, following treatment with clindamycin, develops profuse, watery diarrhea. The nurse anticipates which drug will be started?
    a. Trimethoprim-sulfamethoxazol orally.
    b. Daptomycin orally
    c. Vancomycin orally
    d. Ceftriaxone orally

►24. A patient with diabetes is receiving clindamycin for gas gangrene. Which drug concurrently administered drug could decrease bowel motility and worsen symptoms of *Clostridioides difficile*?
    a. Bethanechol
    b. Digoxin
    c. Meperidine
    d. Warfarin

25. The nurse would consult the provider regarding administration of linezolid oral suspension if the nurse discovered the patient has a history of which disorder?
    a. Asthma
    b. Celiac disease
    c. Gout
    d. Phenylketonuria

✳26. It would be a priority to monitor which laboratory test when a patient is prescribed linezolid?
    a. Aspartate aminotransferase (AST)
    b. Blood urea nitrogen (BUN)
    c. Complete blood count (CBC)
    d. Fasting blood glucose (FBG)

27. A patient with a history of hypertension controlled by lisinopril is prescribed linezolid for a vancomycin-resistant enterococcal (VRE) infection. The patient should be instructed to avoid consuming which substance while on this antibiotic?
    a. Aged cheese
    b. Milk
    c. Red meat
    d. Seafood

28. The nurse should teach a patient who's been prescribed linezolid to call the provider if which symptoms occur?
    a. Dizziness
    b. Headache
    c. Numbness
    d. Vomiting

29. When used to treat colonized Methicillin-resistant *Staphylococcus aureus* (MRSA), mupirocin is administered in which way?
    a. Intranasally
    b. Intravenously
    c. Orally
    d. Topically

DOSE CALCULATION QUESTIONS

30. Erythromycin oral suspension, 200 mg four times a day, has been prescribed for a child. The pharmacy provided erythromycin 250 mg/5 mL. How much erythromycin should the nurse teach the parent to administer per dose?

31. Eravacycline 1 mg/kg/dose is prescribed intravenous (IV) every 12 hours for a 275-pound patient. How many milligrams will the patient receive IV every 12 hours?

CASE STUDIES

Case Study 1

An attorney reports to the health care facility with a fever of 101°F and a nonproductive cough that has lasted 10 days. Their medical history reveals that they have asthma, take theophylline, and are allergic to penicillin. On physical examination, respiratory rate is 24/min and nonlabored, and bibasilar rhonchi are heard on auscultation. The patient is given a prescription for erythromycin 250 mg four times a day for 10 days to treat what is suspected to be mycoplasma pneumonia. They are advised to take acetaminophen 325 mg every 4 hours for fever, increase fluids to 6–8 glasses of water per day, and stay home from work for 2–3 days.

1. What serious adverse effect is this patient at risk for based on drug interactions, and what symptoms would suggest this syndrome?

2. What should the nurse do regarding the possibility of this syndrome?

Case Study 2

A pediatric patient is readmitted following an appendectomy with shaking chills, fever of 103°F, and purulent drainage from the incision site. Culture and sensitivity results of the wound drainage reveal vancomycin-resistant *Enterococcus faecium*. Linezolid 20-mg oral suspension every 12 hours is prescribed.

3. Which laboratory test should the nurse monitor to assess for myelosuppression? How often should the laboratory test be ordered?

4. Explain why linezolid poses a risk of hypertensive crisis? Which foods should the patient avoid?

5. Patients with which disorder should not use linezolid oral suspension, and why?

92 Aminoglycosides: Bactericidal Inhibitors of Protein Synthesis

STUDY QUESTIONS

Completion

1. Aminoglycosides kill bacteria, so their action is ______________________.
2. Aminoglycosides are highly polar polycations and therefore do not enter the __________________ __________________.
3. Aminoglycosides are rapidly excreted by the ______________________.
4. Aminoglycosides are ________________-spectrum antibiotics.
5. Aminoglycosides are primarily used to treat serious infections with aerobic Gram-______________________ bacilli.
6. Aminoglycosides can kill bacteria for several ______________________ after serum levels drop below the minimal bactericidal concentration.
7. Cell kill by aminoglycosides is __________________ ________ ___________________________.
8. The principal cause of bacterial resistance is production of ______________________ that can inactivate aminoglycosides.
9. Aminoglycosides cannot kill __________________ __________________.

CRITICAL THINKING, PRIORITIZATION, AND DELEGATION QUESTIONS

10. Major adverse effects of aminoglycoside antibiotics include damage to which structures? **(Select all that apply.)**
    a. Cochlea
    b. Heart
    c. Kidneys
    d. Lungs
    e. Stomach
    f. Vestibular apparatus
11. Aminoglycosides are inactive against facultative bacteria living in which condition?
    a. Anaerobic
    b. Extreme heat
    c. Aerobic
    d. Severe cold

*12. A patient who is prescribed tobramycin reports a headache. Which is the priority nursing intervention?
    a. Assess headache characteristics.
    b. Administer acetaminophen.
    c. Withhold the tobramycin.
    d. Notify the provider.

*13. The nurse is obtaining history from a patient's partner, who was admitted with sepsis and prescribed an aminoglycoside antibiotic. Which is the most important question to ask the patient's partner?
    a. "Has your partner ever had surgery?"
    b. "Which diet does your partner follow?"
    c. "Did your partner have the flu vaccine this year?"
    d. "What medications is your partner currently taking?"

*14. The nurse is assessing for adverse effects of intravenous (IV) tobramycin. Which change would be a priority to report to the provider?
    a. Dilute urine
    b. Headache
    c. Very weak muscles
    d. Ringing in the ears

15. The nurse is aware that the risk of ototoxicity is significantly increased if a hypertensive patient is also receiving which medication?
    a. Bumetanide
    b. Ethacrynic acid
    c. Furosemide
    d. Hydrochlorothiazide

*16. Which is the priority nursing action before administering an aminoglycoside to a patient with an estimated glomerular filtration rate (eGFR) of 50 mL/min?
    a. Ask the patient if they have a headache.
    b. Assess peak levels of the drug.
    c. Determine intake and output.
    d. Compare prescribed to recommended dose.

17. When an aminoglycoside is prescribed IV as a once-daily dose, which is the appropriate time for trough levels to be drawn?
    a. 30 minutes before the next dose
    b. 1 hour after completing the infusion
    c. 1 hour before the next dose
    d. 30 minutes after completing the infusion

▶18. The nurse is caring for a patient who is receiving gentamicin twice a day. Peak and trough levels were drawn around the fourth dose. Results were peak 3 mcg/mL and trough 0.6 mcg/mL. Which is the appropriate nursing action?
   a. Administer an additional dose.
   b. Continue nursing care.
   c. Consult with the provider.
   d. Withhold the gentamicin.

✳19. Which laboratory results would be a priority for the nurse to evaluate when a patient is prescribed an aminoglycoside?
   a. Creatinine
   b. Glucose
   c. Sodium
   d. Potassium

▶20. A patient received a neuromuscular blocking agent during surgery. In the postanesthesia care unit, the provider orders gentamicin 40 mg IV STAT. Which is the appropriate nursing action?
   a. Administer the drug.
   b. Assess vital signs.
   c. Clarify the order.
   d. Call the pharmacist.

DOSE CALCULATION QUESTIONS

21. Based on the recommended dose of gentamicin, what is the dose range for a patient with a Gram-negative infection, who weighs 220 lb, if the gentamicin is to be administered every 8 hours?

22. A patient weighs 65 kg and has been prescribed amikacin 175 mg every 8 hours. Is the prescribed dose appropriate for this patient?

CASE STUDIES

Case Study 1

An older adult with a history of type 2 diabetes mellitus (T2DM) and rheumatoid arthritis is readmitted to the hospital with sepsis following resection of the prostate. Home medications include metformin and naproxen. Assessment findings include BP 100/70 mm Hg, pulse 98 beats/min, respirations 24/min, and temperature 104°F (40°C). The patient is difficult to arouse, and skin is hot and dry. *Escherichia coli* cultured from the wound drainage is sensitive to amikacin. The dose of amikacin is less than the normal recommended dose.

1. What are possible reasons for the prescribed dose not being equivalent to the recommended dose?

2. The drug is to be administered at 0600, 1400, and 2200. Peak and trough levels of the amikacin are ordered. When will the nurse schedule the collection of the blood sample for this testing?

3. Why are serum trough levels more significant than serum peak levels?

4. The trough level of the amikacin is 15 mcg/mL. What should the nurse do?

Case Study 2

A middle-aged patient is recovering in the trauma unit from a major accident. They are on a ventilator and have a central line for IVs and antibiotics, a Swan-Ganz catheter to measure cardiac status, an arterial line to measure continuous BP, a small-bore feeding tube, two chest tubes, and a Foley catheter. After 3 days, the patient develops Gram-negative septicemia and pneumonia and is started on gentamicin sulfate and ampicillin IV.

5. Describe the assessments the nurse should perform to detect nephrotoxicity and neurotoxicity.

6. How does nephrotoxicity increase the risk of developing ototoxicity?

7. Which toxicity is most likely to be permanent?

8. How can the nurse prevent drug interactions?

9. What type of urine collection bag should the nurse use with this patient?

10. What changes in the dosages of medications would be necessary if the patient were an older adult, rather than middle-aged?

93 Sulfonamide Antibiotics and Trimethoprim

STUDY QUESTIONS

True or False

For each of the following statements, enter T for true or F for false.

1. ___ Sulfonamides are narrow-spectrum antibiotics.
2. ___ Sulfonamides are no longer active against many microbes for which they initially were effective.
3. ___ Sulfonamides are often used to treat urinary tract infections.
4. ___ Sulfonamides are usually administered intramuscularly or intravenously.
5. ___ Sulfonamides are widely used because of low toxicity.
6. ___ Sulfonamides are effective in treating a fungus infection that occurs in immunocompromised patients.
7. ___ Sulfonamides cause folic acid deficiency in the patient.
8. ___ Sulfonamides cross the placenta.
9. ___ Sulfssonamides do not cause toxicity when applied topically.
10. ___ Sulfonamides inhibit microbial synthesis of folic acid.
11. ___ Sulfonamides were the first systemic antibiotics developed.

CRITICAL THINKING, PRIORITIZATION, AND DELEGATION QUESTIONS

*12. Which signs would most likely indicate the start of Stevens-Johnson syndrome when a patient is receiving sulfonamides?
   a. Crusty rash on the cheeks
   b. Papular rash on the shoulders
   c. Pruritic rash on lower arms
   d. Blisters in the mouth

*13. Which is the priority reason why the nurse teaches a patient who is prescribed sulfamethoxazole to take this medication with a full glass of water?
   a. Decrease risk of esophageal irritation
   b. Minimize crystal formation in the urine
   c. Prevent nausea and vomiting
   d. Stimulate frequent voiding

*14. Which laboratory test result would be a priority to report to the provider of a patient prescribed a sulfonamide?
   a. Mean corpuscular volume 90 fL
   b. Lactate dehydrogenase 200 U/L
   c. Hemoglobin 10.0 g/dL
   d. Reticulocyte count 1%

15. Which is the presentation of sulfonamide-induced kernicterus?
   a. Whole-body limpness
   b. Ureteral obstruction
   c. Shortness of breath
   d. Sensitivity to sunlight

16. A patient who takes glyburide for type 2 diabetes mellitus (T2DM) is prescribed trimethoprim-sulfamethoxazole (TMP/SMZ) for a urinary tract infection (UTI). Which is a priority assessment?
   a. Oral intake
   b. Blood glucose
   c. Temperature
   d. Neurologic status

17. The patient has been receiving mafenide application to a second-degree burn for over 2 weeks. Which symptoms suggest the drug might be causing acidosis?
   a. Tachypnea
   b. Hypervigilance
   c. Bradycardia
   d. Constipation

*18. The nurse is preparing to apply topical mafenide to second-degree burns on the anterior arms, upper legs, and trunk of a patient. Which is the priority nursing intervention?
   a. Aseptic technique
   b. Patient teaching
   c. Pain management
   d. Cleansing skin

19. The nurse is administering trimethoprim to a patient who has a history of alcohol use disorder. Because folate deficiency is associated with alcohol use disorder, the nurse should assess for which possible adverse effects of trimethoprim?
   a. Vomiting
   b. Flushing
   c. Oral ulcers
   d. Constipation

*20. Due to the risk of hyperkalemia when trimethoprim is prescribed, it is a priority for the nurse to teach the patient to report which symptom?
   a. Bruising
   b. Weakness
   c. Pallor
   d. Sore throat

21. The nurse is preparing to administer trimethoprim 50 mg orally every 12 hours. Laboratory results include estimated glomerular filtration rate (eGFR) 30 mL/min. Which is the appropriate nursing action?
   a. Administer the drug.
   b. Check intake and output.
   c. Consult the provider.
   d. Withhold the drug.

22. Which is a benefit of TMP/SMZ over each component used alone?
   a. Decreased hematologic effects.
   b. Lower dose of both drugs.
   c. Antibiotic resistance is reduced.
   d. Lower incidence of toxicity.

23. A provider gives a verbal order for TMP/SMZ. The nurse would discuss the orders with the provider if the patient has a history of which condition?
   a. Megaloblastic anemia
   b. Congestive heart failure
   c. Diabetes mellitus
   d. Tobacco use disorder

24. A patient on long-term warfarin therapy for atrial fibrillation is prescribed a sulfonamide. The nurse would contact the provider about which international normalized ratio (INR)?
   a. INR 2
   b. INR 2.5
   c. INR 3
   d. INR 3.5

DOSE CALCULATION QUESTION

25. An 88-lb child is prescribed TMP/SMZ at 8 mg/kg per day in two divided doses. Available is an oral suspension of TMP 40 mg/SMZ 200 mg per 5 mL. How many milliliters should the nurse administer in each dose?

CASE STUDIES

Case Study 1

An HIV-positive patient has been treated with zidovudine for more than a year. They present to the clinic with a low-grade fever, nonproductive cough, and shortness of breath. A chest X-ray shows diffuse infiltrates. A diagnosis of pneumocystis pneumonia (PCP) caused by *Pneumocystis jiroveci* is made.

1. The patient states that they know about getting pneumonia from *Pneumocystis carinii.* Now they have something new and are afraid of dying. How should the nurse respond?

2. The patient is started on TMP/SMZ. Why is TMP/SMZ a good choice for this patient?

3. Why is it important to wait for the results of human chorionic gonadotropin (hCG) levels before this patient starts taking TMP/SMZ?

4. What adverse effects should the nurse teach the patient to report, should they occur?

5. What can the nurse teach to decrease the incidence and severity of these possible adverse effects of TMP/SMZ?

   a. Photosensitivity

   b. Stevens-Johnson syndrome

   c. Renal damage

6. What forms of sulfonamide drugs have less risk of Stevens-Johnson syndrome?

94 Drug Therapy for Urinary Tract Infections

STUDY QUESTIONS

Matching

Match the term with its definition.

1. ___ Inflammation of the kidney and its pelvis
2. ___ Inflammation of the urethra
3. ___ Inflammation of the prostate
4. ___ Inflammation of the urinary bladder
5. ___ Recolonization with the same organism
6. ___ Colonization with a new organism
   a. Cystitis
   b. Prostatitis
   c. Pyelonephritis
   d. Reinfection
   e. Relapse
   f. Urethritis

CRITICAL THINKING, PRIORITIZATION, AND DELEGATION QUESTIONS

7. Which is an example of a complicated urinary tract infection (UTI)?
   a. Acquired in the hospital
   b. Caused by prostatic hypertrophy
   c. Multiple organisms are present
   d. In a pregnant female

✳ 8. The nurse is caring for a patient who has frequent UTIs caused by *Escherichia coli*, which have been treated with trimethoprim-sulfamethoxazole (TMP/SMZ). The patient states they use proper perineal hygiene and void after intercourse. Which is the priority action to prevent the recurrence of infection?
   a. Assessing vital signs every 4 hours.
   b. Prophylaxis with nitrofurantoin for 6 months
   c. Encouraging intake of 2000 mL of fluids daily.
   d. Offering cranberry juice with each meal.

9. A patient has been prescribed an antibiotic for 3 days. Which is an advantage of shorter courses of therapy? **(Select all that apply.)**
   a. Fewer adverse effects
   b. Decreased antibiotic resistance
   c. Lower cost to the patient
   d. Greater likelihood of adherence
   e. Treats upper and lower urinary tract

✳10. A provider's orders for a new admission include urine culture and sensitivity and ciprofloxacin 400 mg intravenously (IV) every 12 hours. Which is the priority nursing intervention?
   a. Calculate the drip rate for the IV infusion.
   b. Teach the patient about possible side effects.
   c. Mix the antibiotic in the correct IV solution.
   d. Obtain urine specimen before starting the drug.

11. Which is true about nitrofurantoin and methenamine?
   a. They are first-line agents for prostatitis.
   b. There is no gastrointestinal (GI) tract absorption.
   c. Therapeutic levels are achieved only in urine.
   d. There are few adverse drug effects.

✳12. The nurse is caring for a patient prescribed nitrofurantoin for a UTI. Which of these assessment findings should the nurse report to the provider immediately?
   a. Discolored urine
   b. Dyspnea
   c. Nausea
   d. Headache

13. Which is the appropriate dosing of nitrofurantoin for prophylaxis of frequent reinfection?
   a. 50 mg orally (PO) daily for 6 months
   b. 50 mg PO twice daily for life
   c. 100 mg PO twice daily for 5 days
   d. 100 mg PO daily for 7 days

14. A patient has been prescribed nitrofurantoin for recurrent UTIs. Which should be included in patient teaching? **(Select all that apply.)**
   a. Do not take the drug if you become pregnant.
   b. Report shortness of breath.
   c. Call for new-onset numbness.
   d. Take on an empty stomach.
   e. May take with milk or a meal.

✳15. Which laboratory result is priority to review before the nurse administers nitrofurantoin?
   a. Potassium
   b. Alanine transaminase
   c. Creatinine
   d. Sodium

16. The nurse is reviewing the drugs taken by a patient who has been prescribed methenamine. Which of these drugs, taken to self-medicate, can reduce the urinary antiseptic action of methenamine?
    a. Alka-Seltzer
    b. Pepto Bismol
    c. Tylenol PM
    d. Ibuprofen

DOSE CALCULATION QUESTIONS

17. Nitrofurantoin macrocrystals 50 mg twice a day is prescribed. Available are 25-mg capsules. How many should be administered per dose?

18. Methenamine hippurate 500 mg twice a day is prescribed for a 10-year-old child. The pharmacy dispenses methenamine Hippurate 1-g tablets. How many tablets should be administered at each dose?

CLINICAL JUDGMENT CASE STUDY

HEALTH HISTORY	NURSE'S NOTES	PHYSICIAN'S ORDERS	LABORATORY PROFILE
1000 hrs:			

Student comes to the university health center reporting burning, urgency, and frequency. These symptoms are accompanied by nausea, chills, and malaise. Vital signs are blood pressure 124/84 mm Hg, pulse 110 bpm, respirations 16 bpm, and temperature 101.8°F. The student states that they took Bactrim DS for a prior UTI, and they are allergic to it. The student lives in the dorms on campus, carries a full load of coursework, and works part time at a nearby fast-food restaurant. The student admits they do not drink much water, snack on convenience food most of the day rather than eating set meals, and drink sodas and energy drinks.

Notified the provider concerning results of urinalysis:

- Urine is cloudy, pH 5.0, nitrite negative and leukocyte esterase 2+, RBC 5/high power field (hpf), WBC >50/hpf, and bacteria 100,000 CFU/mL.

Received verbal orders for nitrofurantoin 100 mg ER PO every 12 hours for 5 days.

For each of the following nursing interventions, place an X in the appropriate column to indicate whether the action should be implemented or not implemented.

NURSING ACTION	IMPLEMENT	DO NOT IMPLEMENT
Obtain urine culture within 24 hours of beginning nitrofurantoin.		
Teach patient to report symptoms of numbness and tingling.		
Instruct patient to avoid taking the drug with milk.		
Obtain serum pregnancy test.		
Teach patient to report yellow discoloration of skin and eyes.		

95 Antimycobacterial Agents: Drugs for Tuberculosis

STUDY QUESTIONS

True or False

For each of the following statements, enter T for true or F for false.

1. ___ The principal cause underlying the emergence of resistance is inadequate drug therapy.
2. ___ Microscopic examination of sputum is the best way to diagnose tuberculosis (TB).
3. ___ Culture and sensitivity for *Mycobacterium tuberculosis* takes 24–48 hours.
4. ___ Individuals infected with TB but who are symptom free cannot infect other people.
5. ___ Individuals infected with TB have a risk of developing active TB without additional exposure to the bacteria even if the infection has been dormant for many years.
6. ___ Infection with TB is best treated in the hospital.
7. ___ TB is an infection limited to the lungs.
8. ___ TB is more prevalent in jails and homeless populations than the general population.
9. ___ Primary infection with TB usually is evident on chest X-ray.
10. ___ Infection with multidrug-resistant organisms greatly increases the risk of death.
11. ___ Anti-TB regimens must always include two or more drugs.

CRITICAL THINKING, PRIORITIZATION, AND DELEGATION QUESTIONS

12. A patient who has been diagnosed with active TB has been prescribed isoniazid, rifampin, ethambutol, and pyrazinamide. The patient asks the nurse why they must take so many drugs. The basis of the nurse's response should include that this multidrug therapy has which effect? **(Select all that apply.)**
    a. Decreases adverse effects of any single drug
    b. Less risk of relapse by killing all bacilli present
    c. Superinfection is less likely to develop
    d. Active against active and dormant organisms
    e. Eliminates the development of drug resistance

13. An HIV-infected patient who is receiving drug therapy, including delavirdine and saquinavir, is diagnosed with an active TB infection. This patient should not be prescribed which drug?
    a. Ethambutol
    b. Isoniazid
    c. Pyrazinamide
    d. Rifampin

14. A nursing student with no history of medical conditions, no symptoms of disease, and no risk factors for contracting TB is being screened for TB prior to starting a clinical nursing course. They develop a 20-mm area of erythema surrounding an 11-mm area of induration 48 hours after receiving a purified protein derivative (PPD) tuberculin test. Chest X-ray and sputum culture are negative. The nurse would expect prophylactic treatment to involve:
    a. multidrug therapy.
    b. watchful waiting.
    c. isoniazid.
    d. rifampin.

*15. A nurse is receiving isoniazid therapy for latent TB. It would be priority to contact the provider if the nurse experiences which symptom?
    a. Headache
    b. Dry mouth
    c. Dyspepsia
    d. Anorexia

16. The public health nurse would withhold administration of drug therapy with rifampin and pyrazinamide and contact the provider for which laboratory result?
    a. Albumin 4.5 g/dL
    b. Total bilirubin 3 mg/dL.
    c. Total protein 75 g/L.
    d. Alkaline phosphatase 100 IU/L.

17. Intake and output and serum creatinine should be carefully monitored when a patient is receiving which antitubercular drug? **(Select all that apply.)**
    a. Amikacin
    b. Pyrazinamide
    c. Kanamycin
    d. Isoniazid
    e. Streptomycin

18. A patient with a history of peripheral vascular disease, type 2 diabetes mellitus, and latent TB is prescribed isoniazid and pyridoxine. Which is the purpose of prescribing pyridoxine?
    a. Improve arterial blood flow
    b. Avoid the development of seizures
    c. Prevent peripheral neuropathy
    d. Treat intracellular mycobacteria

19. The interaction between isoniazid and phenytoin may result in which outcome?
    a. Isoniazid blood levels become subtherapeutic.
    b. Blood levels of phenytoin become toxic.
    c. Phenytoin levels become subtherapeutic.
    d. Risk of developing hepatotoxicity is increased.

20. A patient with paranoid schizophrenia, involuntarily committed to a psychiatric institution, has been diagnosed with latent TB and is refusing oral drug therapy with isoniazid. Which is an appropriate nursing action?
    a. Request intramuscular drug administration.
    b. Rationalize the importance of drug therapy.
    c. Isolate the patient until they agree to take the drug.
    d. Withhold the drug; the patient cannot infect others.

21. A patient on long-term warfarin therapy for atrial fibrillation is diagnosed with TB. They are prescribed antitubercular drugs, including rifampin. Due to the interaction between warfarin and rifampin, it is important for the nurse to assess the patient for which symptom?
    a. Abdominal pain
    b. Bleeding
    c. Confusion
    d. Oliguria

22. A patient has received instructions regarding TB therapy with rifampin. Which statement indicates the patient needs further teaching?
    a. "All of my providers should be told about my TB therapy."
    b. "I should call if I experience reddish-colored urine."
    c. "My contraceptives may not work; I should use condoms too."
    d. "Therapy with rifampin can stain my contact lenses."

►23. Several second-line agents for TB have the potential to damage the eighth cranial nerve. The nurse would assess for this damage by assessing for which symptom? **(Select all that apply.)**
    a. Dizziness
    b. Nystagmus
    c. Facial tic
    d. Tinnitus
    e. Loss of smell

✳24. It is priority to include which information when teaching a patient prescribed ethambutol?
    a. Call the provider if experiencing nausea.
    b. Contact the provider for any visual changes.
    c. Take the drug on an empty stomach.
    d. To avoid nausea, take the drug with food.

25. Which is true concerning rifampin therapy for leprosy?
    a. Is bactericidal to *M. leprae*.
    b. Eliminates drug resistance.
    c. Prevents nerve damage.
    d. Drug therapy is only short-term.

26. Which is true concerning multidrug therapy for TB?
    a. Broadens the spectrum of antimicrobial coverage
    b. Eliminates the need to determine drug sensitivity
    c. Does not create conditions leading to superinfection
    d. Is a major impediment to successful therapy

✳27. The nurse is caring for a patient prescribed bedaquiline. Which assessment finding is priority to report to the provider?
    a. Bruising
    b. Vomiting
    c. Fainting
    d. Discolored urine

DOSE CALCULATION QUESTIONS

28. The nurse is preparing to administer rifampin 420 mg intravenously. The solution was prepared by dissolving 600 mg of powdered rifampin in 10 mL of sterile water. Seven milliliters of the prepared solution were added to a 500-mL intravenous (IV) bag of 5% dextrose. The infusion is to run over 3 hours. What is the hourly rate of infusion that the nurse should program into the IV infusion pump?

29. The safe dose of cycloserine is 10–20 mg/kg per day. An 88-lb child is prescribed a 250-mg capsule twice a day. Is the dose safe?

CASE STUDIES

Case Study 1

A social worker who has sole custody of their two children is prescribed rifampin, isoniazid, ethambutol, and pyrazinamide after being diagnosed with active TB.

1. Why is therapy for active infection always initiated with at least two drugs?

2. What information should the nurse provide to ensure these medications are taken exactly as prescribed?

3. What obstacles might this patient face regarding adherence to drug therapy?

4. What will be necessary to determine the effectiveness of drug therapy?

5. The public health nurse is consulted regarding the need to identify all the people who share facilities with the patient to screen them for TB and prophylactically treat the individuals without active infection with isoniazid. Why is it essential to treat TB contacts prophylactically for TB?

6. When evaluating the contacts associated with an active TB patient, what considerations are made to determine whether they are candidates for isoniazid prophylactic therapy?

7. What is the drug of choice as the primary agent for treatment and prophylaxis of TB, and why is this true?

8. Two months into therapy, the nurse is reviewing laboratory results for the original patient, which include alanine aminotransferase (ALT) 65 IU/L, aspartate aminotransferase (AST) 80 units/L, total bilirubin 0.3 mg/dL, creatinine 0.8 mg/dL, and uric acid 12 mg/dL. What questions should the nurse ask this patient?

Case Study 2

A person who is homeless comes to the emergency department with weight loss, lethargy, a low-grade fever, and a productive cough streaked with blood. The chest X-ray indicates a suspicious area in the middle right lobe. They are hospitalized, and sputum cultures are ordered. The sputum cultures reveal *M. tuberculosis*. The patient's active TB is to be treated with a combination of drugs based on the sputum culture drug sensitivity. The patient is started on isoniazid, ethambutol, and pyrazinamide in the initial phase of therapy.

9. What organ function is the nurse most concerned about when a patient is taking this combination of drugs? What symptoms would suggest this adverse effect?

10. What are the benefits of directly observed therapy (DOT) for this patient?

11. What interventions could the public nurse implement to improve adherence to drug therapy with this patient?

12. If this patient were found to be HIV positive, what drug-drug interactions may occur between the TB drug regimen and HIV drug therapy?

13. The nurse is evaluating the patient when they come for DOT. The patient reports vision changes in which they feel like they are looking through a tunnel. What could be causing this visual change? What should the nurse do?

14. The nurse is writing a letter to a legislator because of proposed cuts to funding for health care that would affect patients with TB. What could the nurse include in the letter to justify the expense of the government aiding people who cannot afford TB treatment?

96 Miscellaneous Antibacterial Drugs: Fluoroquinolones, Metronidazole, Daptomycin, Rifampin, Rifaximin, and Fidaxomicin

STUDY QUESTIONS

Completion

1. An unusual adverse effect of fluoroquinolones is ________________ rupture.
2. Resistance has become common in ____________ ____________; therefore, fluoroquinolones are no longer recommended for this infection.
3. ________________ is resistant to ciprofloxacin.
4. Fluoroquinolones pose a risk of ______________.
5. Fluoroquinolones are ______________-spectrum agents.

CRITICAL THINKING, PRIORITIZATION, AND DELEGATION QUESTIONS

*6. The nurse is preparing to administer intravenous (IV) ciprofloxacin to a patient who developed septic arthritis following arthroscopic surgery of their right knee. It would be a priority to review which diagnostic test result as soon as it is available?
   a. Culture/sensitivity of wound drainage
   b. Magnetic resonance imaging of knee
   c. Blood culture and sensitivity
   d. X-ray of the right knee

*7. The nurse assesses a 6-year-old child who is receiving ciprofloxacin for a complicated urinary tract infection (UTI). Which is a priority patient problem?
   a. Pain
   b. Hypoglycemia
   c. Weight loss
   d. Hyponatremia

8. Which patients have an increased risk for tendon rupture when prescribed a fluoroquinolone? **(Select all that apply.)**
   a. Persons over the age of 60
   b. Patients with Type 2 diabetes
   c. Those who are taking statin drugs
   d. Individuals taking glucocorticoids
   e. Heart and kidney transplant recipients

►9. Which would be an indication that an infant prescribed ciprofloxacin has developed a *Candida* infection?
   a. Breast milk is supplemented with rice cereal.
   b. After every feeding, the infant has a stool.
   c. Each stool is mushy and seedy.
   d. Nursing is interrupted by crying.

►10. A consulting urologist orders ciprofloxacin 250 mg twice a day for an older adult with a UTI. The patient is also receiving ferrous sulfate 300 mg for anemia and calcium carbonate 400 mg four times a day for osteopenia. Which is the appropriate nursing action?
   a. Administer the drug 1 hour before other medications.
   b. The drug should be given 2 hours after other medications.
   c. Consult with the provider for administration guidance.
   d. Hold ferrous sulfate and calcium during drug therapy.

►11. The nurse is administering ciprofloxacin to a patient who receives theophylline for asthma. The nurse should monitor theophylline levels and assess for which symptoms?
   a. Constipation
   b. Drowsiness
   c. Tachycardia
   d. Weakness

12. Which is a common symptom that can occur with extended ciprofloxacin therapy?
   a. Circumoral cyanosis
   b. Peripheral edema
   c. Pinpoint maculopapular rash
   d. Sore patches on the tongue

►13. A patient has been prescribed moxifloxacin. Which assessment finding should be reported to the provider?
   a. Bradycardia
   b. Weakness
   c. Vomiting
   d. Headache

▶14. When a patient is prescribed a fluoroquinolone that is known to cause prolongation of the QT interval, the nurse should monitor for which laboratory result?
   a. Chloride
   b. Potassium
   c. Sodium
   d. Glucose

15. Which goal is most appropriate when a patient is prescribed metronidazole for *Clostridiodes difficile*?
   a. Clear lung sounds
   b. No burning on urination
   c. Soft, formed stool
   d. Normal temperature

16. The nurse is preparing to administer daptomycin to a patient with sepsis. Which situation would warrant the nurse withholding the medication and contacting the provider?
   a. Methicillin-resistant *Staphylococcus aureus* infection
   b. An international normalized ratio (INR) of 1.8
   c. Development of new-onset severe muscle pain
   d. Maintenance IV solution is Ringer lactate

17. Which nursing intervention is most appropriate when caring for a patient prescribed daptomycin?
   a. Increase fiber in the patient's diet.
   b. Dim the lights in the patient's room.
   c. Elevate the patient's IV site.
   d. Limit noise in the halls during the night.

18. Which isoenzyme of creatine phosphokinase (CPK) would be most helpful when monitoring for adverse effects if a patient is prescribed daptomycin and simvastatin?
   a. CPK
   b. CPK-1
   c. CPK-2
   d. CPK-3

19. The provider has asked the nurse to provide teaching to a patient who has requested a prescription for rifaximin before a trip to Central America. Teaching should include withholding the drug if the patient experiences which issue? **(Select all that apply.)**
   a. Amenorrhea
   b. Bloody stool
   c. Fever
   d. Flatulence
   e. Nausea

20. Following treatment ciprofloxacin, an older adult develops watery diarrhea, nausea, and abdominal tenderness. The patient's temperature is 101.5°F, and they do not feel like eating. The nurse knows which drugs are US Food and Drug Administration (FDA) approved to treat this condition? **(Select all that apply.)**
   a. Daptomycin
   b. Vancomycin
   c. Metronidazole
   d. Rifaximin
   e. Fidaxomicin

DOSE CALCULATION QUESTIONS

21. The drug handbook states that the maintenance dose of metronidazole is 7.5 mg/kg every 6 hours. A child is prescribed IV metronidazole 500 mg in 100 mL dextrose 5% in water (D_5W) every 6 hours. The child is 5′6″ and weighs 145 lb. Is the dose safe?

22. A loading dose of 1 g of metronidazole IV is ordered for a patient who weighs 176 lb. The recommended dose is 15 mg/kg. Is the dose safe?

CASE STUDIES

Case Study 1

An older adult patient returns to their provider after taking 10 days of ampicillin for upper respiratory infection. They continue with a low-grade fever and do not seem to have improved. The patient has a productive cough and thick secretions. The X-ray does not indicate pneumonia. The patient has a history of atrial fibrillation, for which they take an anticoagulant. Ciprofloxacin 250 mg, orally, two times a day for 7 more days is prescribed.

1. What in the patient's history may contribute to potential drug-drug interactions?

2. What foods should the patient avoid when taking oral ciprofloxacin?

3. The patient calls the provider's office in 2 days to report that they are much better and asks whether they can stop taking the medication, since it is so expensive and they are improving so much. How should the nurse respond?

4. What new problem might the patient develop while taking this antibiotic?

Case Study 2

An adolescent patient is admitted to the nursing unit after emergency surgery for a ruptured appendix. The patient is prescribed IV metronidazole 500 mg in 100 mL D_5W every 6 hours and ampicillin/sulbactam 1.5 g (in 50 mL normal saline) every 8 hours. Both are to run at a rate of 100 mL/h.

5. Metronidazole is scheduled at 0000, 0600, 1200, and 1800 at a rate of 100 mL/h. Ampicillin/sulbactam is scheduled at 0600, 1400, and 2200. Which would the nurse administer first at 0600, and when would the nurse start each drug?

6. What procedures need to be followed when administering these drugs?

7. Because the family delayed seeking treatment for their child's abdominal pain and gastrointestinal (GI) bacteria were expelled into the peritoneum, the nurse would monitor for what symptoms that suggest the bacteria have invaded the peritoneal cavity?

97 Antifungal Agents

STUDY QUESTIONS

Completion

1. The term for fungal disease is ____________ ____________________.
2. ______________________ infections can occur in any host.
3. Systemic antifungals fall into two major groups: drugs for __________ __________ and drugs for __________ __________.

True or False

For each of the following statements, enter T for true or F for false.

4. ___ Amphotericin B can bind to cholesterol in human cell membranes, causing toxicity.
5. ___ Amphotericin B damages the kidneys.
6. ___ Kidney damage can be minimized by infusing 1 L of saline on the days amphotericin is infused.
7. ___ Amphotericin B is rarely associated with fungal resistance.
8. ___ Amphotericin B has broad-spectrum bactericidal activity.
9. ___ Amphotericin B is only used for systemic fungal infections.
10. ___ Amphotericin B is the best drug for systemic fungal infections despite the potential for toxicity.
11. ___ Amphotericin B readily penetrates the central nervous system.
12. ___ Amphotericin B remains in human tissue more than a year after treatment is discontinued.

Matching

Match the fungal infection to its site of occurrence.

13. ___Body
14. ___Foot
15. ___Groin
16. ___Scalp
    a. Tinea capitis
    b. Tinea corporis
    c. Tinea cruris
    d. Tinea pedis

CRITICAL THINKING, PRIORITIZATION, AND DELEGATION QUESTIONS

17. When administering drugs that are potentially nephrotoxic, the nurse should consult the provider before administering which over-the-counter (OTC) drugs? **(Select all that apply.)**
    a. Dulcolax
    b. Acetaminophen
    c. Naproxen
    d. Aspirin
    e. Ibuprofen
18. At which point is the patient most likely to experience fever, chills, rigors, nausea, and headache when receiving amphotericin B?
    a. Immediately after the infusion begins
    b. 20–30 minutes after the infusion begins
    c. 1–3 hours after the infusion begins
    d. 3–6 hours after the infusion begins
19. A patient experiences sudden-onset shaking and chills after receiving a dose of amphotericin B. Which drug should the nurse administer?
    a. Acetaminophen
    b. Dantrolene
    c. Diphenhydramine
    d. Lorazepam

*20. Which laboratory results should the nurse review before administering a dose of amphotericin B?
    a. Creatinine levels
    b. Thyroid panel
    c. Liver function tests
    d. Platelet count

►21. Which laboratory results suggest bone marrow suppression caused by amphotericin B?
    a. Hemoglobin 10 g/dL
    b. Hematocrit 42%
    c. Platelet count 200 × 10^9/L
    d. White blood cells 4.5 × 10^9/L

22. A patient with a systemic fungal infection is prescribed amphotericin B and flucytosine. Which is the likely result?
    a. Decreased risk of amphotericin toxicity
    b. Increased risk of kidney dysfunction
    c. Increased risk of liver dysfunction
    d. Need a higher dose of amphotericin B

23. Which is true of itraconazole?
   a. The drug may cause neurologic toxicity.
   b. Food reduces the absorption of capsules.
   c. Itraconazole is a broad-spectrum antifungal.
   d. Can be used in patients with heart failure.

24. To achieve maximum absorption of itraconazole capsules, the nurse administers the drug with which liquid?
   a. Apple juice
   b. Milk
   c. Cola
   d. Water

*25. The nurse is reviewing test results for a patient who is prescribed itraconazole. Which result would warrant immediate consultation with the provider?
   a. Aspartate aminotransferase (AST) 35 IU/L
   b. Brain natriuretic peptide (BNP) 745 pg/mL
   c. Echocardiogram: ejection fraction 60%
   d. Serum potassium 3.8 mEq/L

26. The nurse is administering itraconazole to a patient who is also prescribed simvastatin. Because of the effect of itraconazole on hepatic isoenzyme CYP3A4, the combination increases the risk of rhabdomyolysis from simvastatin. The nurse should monitor the patient for which symptoms?
   a. Bleeding
   b. Hypoglycemia
   c. Hypotension
   d. Muscle pain

27. Which drug may prevent absorption of itraconazole, no matter when it is administered?
   a. Cyclosporin
   b. Digoxin
   c. Esomeprazole
   d. Ranitidine

*28. It would be a priority for the nurse to report which symptoms in a patient prescribed fluconazole?
   a. Diarrhea
   b. Mucositis
   c. Headache
   d. Nausea

29. The nurse reviews the laboratory results of a patient prescribed voriconazole 200 mg PO. Which laboratory result warrants withholding the drug and immediately notifying the provider?
   a. AST 37 IU/L
   b. Glucose 222 mg/dL
   c. Hgb 11.8 g/dL
   d. hCG 172 IU/mL

*30. A patient who has been receiving ketoconazole for 5 days experiences nausea and vomiting. Which is the priority nursing intervention?
   a. Administer the drug with food.
   b. Assess the skin and sclera.
   c. Consult the provider.
   d. Withhold the medication.

31. Which is the first action the nurse should take when preparing to administer IV caspofungin?
   a. Assess the IV site.
   b. Administer over 1 hour.
   c. Document administration.
   d. Prime the IV tubing.

32. The nurse would be concerned that a patient who is receiving micafungin is experiencing a histamine reaction and might have an anaphylactic reaction if the patient reports which symptoms?
   a. Bloating
   b. Headache
   c. Itching
   d. Nausea

33. The nurse reviews the complete blood count (CBC) of a patient who is prescribed flucytosine, and the nurse notes neutrophils at 27%. This patient is at risk for which patient problem?
   a. Fatigue
   b. Fluid volume deficit
   c. Impaired skin integrity
   d. Infection

34. The nurse is admitting a patient with oral candidiasis. They anticipate topical treatment with which drug? **(Select all that apply.)**
   a. Nystatin
   b. Fluconazole
   c. Ketoconazole
   d. Clotrimazole
   e. Miconazole

35. Griseofulvin is active against cells in which phase?
   a. In resting state
   b. During DNA synthesis
   c. During mitosis
   d. In premitotic period

DOSE CALCULATION QUESTIONS

36. The nurse is preparing to administer anidulafungin 100 mg IV to a patient with esophageal candidiasis. The drug books state a 100-mg vial is reconstituted with 30 mL sterile water, yielding a concentration of 3.33 mg/mL, and then further diluted in 100 mL of 0.9% normal saline. The infusion is to run over 90 minutes. The IV pump should be set to run at how many milliliters per hour?

37. The drug book recommends, after a successful test dose, that the first dose of amphotericin B deoxycholate should be 0.25 mg/kg of drug. The patient weighs 110 lb. The provider has ordered 12 mg. Is this a safe dose?

CASE STUDIES

Case Study 1

A young adult patient has been diagnosed with acute myelogenous leukemia (AML). They are admitted for chemotherapy. The patient's platelet count is low, and they have systemic mycoses requiring amphotericin B treatment. The patient's medications must be carefully evaluated to determine whether they are toxic.

1. What system is almost always damaged in some way by amphotericin B and can increase the risk of toxicity of other drugs?

2. What intervention can the nurse employ to reduce the risk of kidney damage by amphotericin B?

3. Why is it important for the provider to first order a 1-mg test dose of amphotericin B before starting full therapy?

4. What nursing measures should the nurse take when infusing amphotericin to prevent infusion-related adverse effects?

Case Study 2

A middle-aged truck driver has been prescribed voriconazole for esophageal candidiasis secondary to immune deficiency caused by HIV.

5. What teaching does the nurse need to provide this patient regarding drug therapy?

6. Why is this patient more at risk for hepatotoxicity and drug interactions than the average person?

98 Antiviral Agents I: Drugs for Non-HIV Viral Infections

STUDY QUESTIONS

True or False

For each of the following statements, enter T for true or F for false.

1. ___ It is hard to develop antiviral drugs that do not harm human tissue.
2. ___ Oral acyclovir will cure active herpes labialis.
3. ___ Oral therapy with acyclovir is only effective for varicella if dosing is begun within 24 hours of rash onset.
4. ___ Intravenous (IV) acyclovir should be administered slowly, and the patient should be well hydrated.
5. ___ It is possible to spread the infection when applying acyclovir ointment.
6. ___ Antivirals eliminate the risk of transmitting genital herpes between monogamous heterosexual partners.
7. ___ It is important to teach a patient who is prescribed valacyclovir to report unexpected bruising.
8. ___ Valganciclovir should not be administered to a person who is also prescribed a drug that causes bone marrow suppression.
9. ___ Famciclovir decreases the number of episodes of post–herpetic neuralgia associated with herpes zoster.
10. ___ Penciclovir and docosanol topical preparations decrease the duration of pain of cold sores by 50%.
11. ___ Palivizumab is a protease inhibitor indicated for preventing respiratory syncytial virus (RSV) infection in premature infants.
12. ___ Nirmatrelvir/ritonavir may lower the efficacy of oral contraceptives.

CRITICAL THINKING, PRIORITIZATION, AND DELEGATION QUESTIONS

13. A college student who has been diagnosed with their first genital herpes infection is discussing the condition and the prescribed topical acyclovir treatment with the college health center nurse. Which statement suggests that the patient needs teaching about this condition and drug therapy?
    a. "I need to clean with soap and water three to four times a day and dry carefully."
    b. "I should use gloves when applying the ointment and then immediately dispose of them."
    c. "I should not have sex when sores are present and always use a condom."
    d. "Using the ointment as soon as I get a sore will cure my herpes infection."

14. The nurse is teaching a patient who is prescribed continuous oral acyclovir therapy for recurrent genital herpes. The patient is currently in a long-term committed, monogamous relationship. Which information is important to include in the teaching?
    a. Condoms prevent the spread of herpes infection.
    b. You only need to use a condom when symptoms are present.
    c. Use a condom at all times, even when symptoms are absent.
    d. Your partner is already infected; condom use does not matter.

*15. Which is the priority nursing action to prevent the most common complications of IV acyclovir therapy?
    a. Assessing the IV site
    b. Ensuring fluid intake of 2.5 L/24 h
    c. Report vomiting to the provider
    d. Teaching careful perineal hygiene

*16. The nurse is preparing to administer IV acyclovir. Which is the priority assessment finding?
    a. BP 140/85 mm Hg
    b. Creatinine 0.9 mg/dL
    c. Dry oral mucous membranes
    d. Urine output 750 mL in 8 hrs

*17. It would be a priority to report which laboratory result to the provider if a patient is prescribed valacyclovir?
    a. CD4 less than $100/mm^3$
    b. Hemoglobin 11 g/dL
    c. Platelets $220,000/mm^3$
    d. White blood cells $12,800/mm^3$

18. The nurse is preparing to administer famciclovir 500 mg orally (PO) once a day to a patient who has developed shingles. The nurse reviews laboratory results that include estimated glomerular filtration rate (eGFR) of 35 mL/min. Which is the priority nursing action?
    a. Administer the drug.
    b. Consult the provider.
    c. Talk to the charge nurse.
    d. Withhold famciclovir.

19. The nurse would withhold ganciclovir and notify the provider if patient laboratory tests included which results?
    a. Blood urea nitrogen 20 mg/dL
    b. hCG 2775 mIU mL
    c. Neutrophils 2000/mm^3
    d. Platelets 75,000/mm^3

20. The nurse discusses care with the certified nursing assistant (CNA) assigned to a patient receiving ganciclovir. Which precaution would the nurse include regarding care?
    a. Monitor food intake and all output.
    b. Raise all four side rails and lower bed.
    c. Turn the patient at least every 2 hours.
    d. Use an electric razor to shave patient.

21. Which step is most important for a nurse who is trying to conceive to follow when administering valganciclovir?
    a. Administer with the patient in an upright position.
    b. Assess vital signs before administering the drug.
    c. Avoid touching or administering the drug.
    d. Dissolve the drug in 8 ounces of water or juice.

►22. Laboratory results for a patient who is prescribed foscarnet include fasting blood glucose (FBG) 90 mg/dL, aspartate aminotransferase (AST) 87 units/L, potassium 3.6 mEq/L, calcium 8.2 mg/dL, and magnesium 2 mEq/L. The nurse should assess for which symptom of electrolyte imbalance?
    a. Clammy skin
    b. Headache
    c. Muscle spasms
    d. Cracked lips

23. When administering adefovir, which assessment would suggest that therapy could be toxic?
    a. Constipation
    b. Vomiting
    c. Oliguria
    d. Yellow sclera

24. It is important for the nurse to assess for suicidal ideation if a patient is prescribed which drug?
    a. Interferon alfa
    b. Lamivudine
    c. Ribavirin
    d. Valacyclovir

*25. Which assessment finding would be priority to report to the provider if identified in a patient who is receiving lamivudine for hepatitis B (HBV)?
    a. Rapid breathing
    b. Bradycardia
    c. Poor appetite
    d. Vomiting

26. A patient is prescribed adefovir 10 mg PO once a day. Results of recent laboratory tests include CrCl 62 mL/min. Which is the priority nursing action?
    a. Administer the drug.
    b. Consult the provider.
    c. Withhold the drug.
    d. Request dose change.

27. Zanamivir is well tolerated by all patients with uncomplicated influenza except those with which condition? **(Select all that apply.)**
    a. Asthma
    b. Hypertension
    c. Heart failure
    d. Chronic bronchitis
    e. Emphysema

28. Which is the most significant factor in determining the effectiveness of oseltamivir when treating influenza?
    a. Administer oseltamivir with food.
    b. Causative organism is influenza A.
    c. Starting when symptoms begin.
    d. Has had the influenza vaccine.

29. Which new assessment finding would be most significant if noted in an infant who is receiving inhaled ribavirin for RSV?
    a. Coarse rhonchi in upper airways
    b. Pulse 120 beats/minute
    c. Respirations 30 breaths/minute
    d. Wheezing throughout lungs

30. A patient on amiodarone for hypertrophic cardiomyopathy and self-medicating with St. John wort has recently been diagnosed with the hepatitis C genotype 2. They ask why they can't take one of the combination NS5A or -5B inhibitors. Which is the appropriate nursing response? **(Select all that apply.)**
    a. "You may develop symptomatic bradycardia."
    b. "NS5A inhibitors are not effective for your genotype."
    c. "St. John wort is contraindicated with these drugs."
    d. "Resistance can build easily to both of these drugs."
    e. "Hepatitis C resolves spontaneously; you don't need treatment."

DOSE CALCULATION QUESTIONS

31. The recommended dose of acyclovir for an immunocompromised child with chicken pox is 30 mg/kg per day in divided doses every 8 hours for 7–10 days. What is the safe dose for a child who weighs 44 lb?

32. Foscarnet 40 mg/kg IV every 12 hours is prescribed for a patient weighing 95 kg. How many mg will be in each dose? Foscarnet is available as 24 mg/mL. How many mL will be administered each dose?

CASE STUDY

A patient comes to the clinic to establish care, as they recently moved to the area. They report a history of multiple blood transfusions resulting from an auto accident many years ago. The nurse documents multiple tattoos on the patient's bilateral upper arms that were placed during the patient's tours of duty in Afghanistan. The patient reports fatigue and loss of appetite, along with occasional nausea. They noticed their stool has gotten pale and their urine is tea colored. When labs are drawn, HBsAg is positive, as well as the patient's total antibody to HBV core antigen (anti-HBC). The patient's aminotransferase levels are elevated. Following a liver biopsy and further lab work demonstrating active disease, the patient was prescribed entecavir 0.5 mg daily.

1. Entecavir is a nucleoside analog. How does it work to treat HBV?

2. Even though entecavir is well tolerated, which side effects may occur?

3. Due to the development of hepatomegaly in patients taking other nucleoside analogs, what would the nurse monitor after treatment has begun?

99 Antiviral Agents II: Drugs for HIV Infection and Related Opportunistic Infections

STUDY QUESTIONS

Matching

Match the drug to its mechanism of action.

1. ___ Efavirenz
2. ___ Enfuvirtide
3. ___ Maraviroc
4. ___ Raltegravir
5. ___ Ritonavir
6. ___ Abacavir
7. ___ Ibalizumab
8. ___ Fostemsavir

   a. Binds with CCR5, thereby blocking viral entry into CD4 cells.
   b. Prevents the HIV envelope from fusing with the cell membrane of CD4 cells, thereby blocking viral entry and replication.
   c. Prevents HIV from attaching to CD4 receptors.
   d. Causes premature termination of growing viral DNA strands.
   e. Binds directly to HIV reverse transcriptase, disrupting the active center of the enzyme, thereby suppressing enzyme activity.
   f. Stops HIV replication by terminating the integration of HIV into DNA.
   g. Binds with domain 2 of CD4 receptors, thereby blocking a postattachment step that is necessary for HIV to enter the host cell.
   h. Inhibits HIV protease, thereby preventing the maturation of HIV.

CRITICAL THINKING, PRIORITIZATION, AND DELEGATION QUESTIONS

9. The nurse is teaching a patient about the need for multidrug therapy for HIV. Which statement, if made by the patient, would indicate a need for further teaching?
   a. "If I don't take the drugs as prescribed, the virus is likely to become resistant."
   b. "The higher the viral load, the greater the chance for drug resistance."
   c. "The virus recognizes the drug and is able to change to prevent destruction."
   d. "When RNA changes to DNA within the host cell, genetics change spontaneously."

10. During teaching, a patient prescribed nucleoside/nucleotide reverse transcriptase inhibitor (NRTI) asks the nurse, "What is hepatic steatosis?" Which is the appropriate nursing response?
    a. "Fatty degeneration of the liver."
    b. "Increased secretions of glands."
    c. "Infection of the liver."
    d. "Stools that are foamy and float."

11. Single Episode: Extended Multiple Response

Military Time: 0830 Received patient from emergency department. Patient is HIV-1 positive. Admit to unit with PCP infection. Most recent CD4 count (1 month ago) was 200 cells/mm^3, and their HIV viral load was 10,000 copies/mL. Patient is taking Bictegravir/emtricitabine/tenofovir alafenamide (Biktarvy) 1 tab PO daily at 0700 hrs. Alert and oriented x 4. Responds to questions appropriately. Cleanly dressed. Patient states they feel worn out. Lungs with diminished breath sounds throughout, dry cough. Becomes short of breath with activity. Heart with regular rate and rhythm. Skin cool and dry; patient is pale. No edema. Blood pressure 142/88, respirations 18, heart rate 95, temperature 102.5°F. Oxygen saturation 92% on room air. Patient is 5′8″ and weighs 150 pounds. Orders received for trimethoprim-sulfamethoxazole 340 mg IV every 8 hours for 21 days. Discussed therapy with patient including drug dosing, actions, and side effects. All patient questions answered.	Which laboratory tests should the nurse monitor during drug therapy? **Select all that apply.** a. Aspartate aminotransferase b. Alanine aminotransferase c. Blood urea nitrogen d. Complete blood count e. Creatinine f. Lipid profile g. Prothrombin time h. Total bilirubin

12. Which nursing assessment finding would be most significant in a patient receiving didanosine?
    a. Sweating
    b. Headache
    c. Sleepiness
    d. Vomiting

*13. A patient who is prescribed rilpivirine reports loss of interest in usual activities. Which is the priority nursing action?
    a. Asking about difficulties with therapy
    b. Assessing thoughts of harming self
    c. Identifying reasons for loss of interest
    d. Providing a safe environment

►14. When planning nursing interventions and teaching for the most common adverse effects of efavirenz, which is the priority patient problem?
    a. Liver dysfunction
    b. Hypercholesterolemia
    c. CNS symptoms
    d. Mild to severe rash

*15. Which is the priority assessment finding in a patient receiving nevirapine? **(Select all that apply.)**
    a. Dizziness
    b. Nausea
    c. Paresthesia
    d. Rash
    e. Conjunctivitis
    f. Muscle pain

16. A patient who is HIV positive has recently been prescribed efavirenz. They call the provider's office and report experiencing drowsiness and dizziness. Which is an appropriate recommendation by the telephone triage nurse?
    a. Make an appointment ASAP.
    b. Discontinue taking efavirenz.
    c. Take efavirenz at bedtime.
    d. Take efavirenz with food.

17. Weight-bearing exercise and adequate calcium intake are most important if antiretroviral therapy includes which drug?
    a. Zidovudine
    b. Abacavir
    c. Rilpivirine
    d. Tenofovir

*18. The nurse is teaching a patient about antiviral drugs. The patient indicates body image is important to them. Adherence could be a problem for which class of drugs?
    a. Integrase strand transfer inhibitors
    b. Nucleoside reverse transcriptase inhibitors
    c. Non-nucleoside reverse transcriptase inhibitors
    d. Protease inhibitors

19. Patients who are prescribed efavirenz should be instructed to not self-prescribe the herbal product St. John wort. Which is the possible effect of this combination?
    a. Increased NNRTI metabolism
    b. Suicidal ideation
    c. Efavirenz toxicity
    d. Synergistic effect

20. A patient taking lopinavir/ritonavir oral solution should not be prescribed which drug? **(Select all that apply.)**
    a. Methadone
    b. Metronidazole
    c. Disulfiram
    d. Oral contraceptives
    e. Ketoconazole

►21. The nurse is caring for a patient who is HIV positive and taking indinavir. The patient reports sharp, colicky flank pain. Before notifying the provider, which nursing action would be most appropriate?
    a. Assess bowel sounds.
    b. Raise head of the bed.
    c. Check vital signs.
    d. Strain urine.

22. Which are known adverse effects of raltegravir? **(Select all that apply.)**
    a. Insomnia
    b. Oral lesions
    c. Headache
    d. Malaise
    e. Ecchymosis

*23. The nurse is caring for a patient prescribed enfuvirtide. Which symptom would be priority to consult with the provider?
    a. Headache
    b. Pruritus
    c. Ecchymosis
    d. Cough

24. Which action, when administering enfuvirtide, increases the risk of a severe injection-site reaction?
    a. Injecting the drug deep into a muscle
    b. Not adequately cleaning the injection site
    c. Reconstituting the drug in sterile water
    d. Refrigerate the solution reconstituting

25. A patient receiving maraviroc calls to report that they have vomited and have severe abdominal pain, and have developed a pruritic rash. Which is the appropriate nursing advice while waiting to be seen by the provider?
    a. Administer acetaminophen.
    b. Discontinue maraviroc.
    c. Withhold all food and fluids.
    d. Call emergency services.

26. Which is the most important role of the nurse when antiviral treatment failure occurs?
    a. Identifying contributing factors
    b. Identifying the patient's immune status
    c. Supporting the patient emotionally
    d. Teaching the new drug regimen

27. Principles of treating HIV-seropositive pregnant women include: **(Select all that apply.)**
    a. Prophylaxis for the infant/neonate.
    b. Benefits outweigh the risks.
    c. Do not treat during pregnancy.
    d. The drugs are not teratogenic.
    e. Only include one drug at a time.

►28. When emptying a urinal of a patient who is HIV seropositive, the nurse splashes urine on intact skin. Which is the appropriate nursing action?
    a. Go to the emergency department (ED).
    b. Begin postexposure prophylaxis.
    c. Carefully cleanse the exposed area.
    d. Report incident immediately to a supervisor.

29. Which assessment finding would best indicate that antiretroviral therapy is currently effective?
    a. CD4 T count 400 cells/mm^3
    b. Neutrophils 2750/mm^3
    c. Plasma HIV RNA below 20 copies/mL
    d. White blood cell (WBC) 5000/mm^3

DOSE CALCULATION QUESTIONS

30. Intravenous (IV) zidovudine 120 mg is to be diluted to 4 mg/mL. How much 5% dextrose for injection should be added to the drug?

31. An 8-year-old child is prescribed enfuvirtide. The recommended dose is 2 mg/kg subcutaneously (subQ) twice a day. How much will the nurse administer twice a day if the child weighs 44 lb?

CASE STUDY

A young adult patient has been HIV seropositive for 12 years. Their antiretroviral therapy includes zidovudine. When being interviewed by the nurse during a routine clinic appointment, the patient reports declining vision, headaches, and daily temperature elevations. Physical examination findings include multiple enlarged lymph nodes and several white retinal patches.

1. What complications of HIV are likely to be occurring?

2. What concerns does the nurse have about treatment for the likely complication?

3. The provider wants to begin with IV therapy. What strategies can the nurse employ when administering IV ganciclovir to reduce the risk of, and identify possible damage to, the patient's renal system?

4. The patient tells the nurse that they have no job or insurance at present. What would the nurse be concerned about?

100 Drug Therapy for Sexually Transmitted Infections

STUDY QUESTIONS

True or False

For each of the following statements, enter T for true or F for false.

1. ___ Annual screening for *Chlamydia trachomatis* is recommended for all sexually active women younger than 25 years.
2. ___ Gonorrhea is often asymptomatic in women.
3. ___ Flulike symptoms are common during the primary stage of syphilis.
4. ___ Clue cells are typically found on microscopic examination in cases of bacterial vaginosis.
5. ___ Trichomoniasis is the most common viral sexually transmitted infection (STI) in the United States.
6. ___ Anogenital infections may be caused by HSV-1, the herpesvirus that causes cold sores.

CRITICAL THINKING, PRIORITIZATION, AND DELEGATION QUESTIONS

7. Which is the most accurate resource about nursing care for sexually transmitted infections?
   a. The Centers for Disease Control and Prevention
   b. Drug manufacturers
   c. The US Food and Drug Administration
   d. Nursing textbooks

*8. A neonate was delivered vaginally to a mother with an active *C. trachomatis* infection. Which is the priority system to monitor when caring for this infant?
   a. Gastrointestinal
   b. Ophthalmic
   c. Renal
   d. Respiratory

9. Which is the reason doxycycline would not be prescribed for a female patient for whom pregnancy status is unknown?
   a. Damage to fetal bones
   b. Candidiasis
   c. Hepatotoxicity
   d. Loss of sense of taste

10. A friend tells the nurse that a sexual partner has informed them that they have gonorrhea. The patient has a refillable prescription of ciprofloxacin for recurrent cystitis and tells the nurse they know they have used this drug in the past for gonorrhea. Which is the most important reason why the nurse should discourage using this ciprofloxacin?
    a. The patient is likely to develop an allergic reaction.
    b. Law requires reporting of gonorrhea infections.
    c. Cipro is no longer effective against *Neisseria gonorrhoeae.*
    d. Dosing of Cipro is too low to treat *N. gonorrhoeae.*

11. A patient who is receiving intramuscular ceftriaxone 250 mg × 1 plus azithromycin 1 g by mouth for disseminated gonococcal infection reports a stiff neck. Which is the primary nursing action?
    a. Assess for history of arthritis.
    b. Complete nursing assessment.
    c. Consult the provider.
    d. Document the finding.

*12. The throat culture of a 6-year-old boy is positive for *N. gonorrhoeae.* Which is the nursing priority in this situation?
    a. Assessing for eye exudate
    b. Calculating the dose of ceftriaxone
    c. Ensuring the safety of the child
    d. Removing the child from his home

13. A patient is admitted to the hospital with a diagnosis of pelvic inflammatory disease (PID). She asks the nurse why her provider has recommended hospitalization and intravenous (IV) antibiotics instead of oral antibiotic therapy at home. Which is the basis of the nurse's response?
    a. Inadequately treated PID is likely to cause fallopian tube scarring.
    b. PID is very contagious, and the patient needs to be in isolation.
    c. The recommended antibiotic for PID is available only by IV route.
    d. Insufficiently treated PID increases the risk of cervical cancer.

14. A middle-aged adult develops septic arthritis. When obtaining a history, it is important to evaluate for which previous infection?
    a. *C. trachomatis*
    b. *N. gonorrhoeae*
    c. *Treponema pallidum*
    d. *Trichomonas vaginalis*

*15. The nurse is caring for a neonate whose mother has an active infection with *N. gonorrhoeae.* Which is a priority nursing outcome for the neonate?
    a. Blinks in response to light shone in the eyes
    b. Breastfeeds every 3 hours without dyspnea
    c. Clear breath sounds throughout on auscultation
    d. No conjunctival discharge experienced

16. Which is the reason for differing treatment recommendations for acute epididymitis based on the patient's age?
    a. The organism in older males is resistant to the antibiotic used in younger males.
    b. The infecting organism is different in young males compared to older males.
    c. Younger males have better kidney functioning than do older males.
    d. Adherence is an issue with multidose therapy in young males.

17. Which is the cause of recurrent STIs?
    a. Prescribing the incorrect antibiotic
    b. Seeking treatment early in the disease
    c. Taking the medication as prescribed
    d. Failure to treat the sexual partner

18. A 35-year-old female reports a yellow-green vaginal discharge. She is diagnosed with trichomoniasis and prescribed metronidazole. It is important for the nurse to teach the patient the importance of not consuming which item?
    a. Alcohol
    b. Antacids
    c. Grapefruit juice
    d. Milk

19. The nurse sees a patient in the clinic who reports thin, foul-smelling vaginal discharge. On microscopic examination, the provider identifies clue cells. The nurse understands the patient has developed which vaginal infection?
    a. Chlamydial infection
    b. Trichomoniasis
    c. Bacterial vaginosis
    d. Gonococcal infection

20. Which is a major goal of therapy with famciclovir for genital herpes?
    a. Providing analgesia for painful lesions
    b. Decreasing the length of active episodes
    c. Eradication of the virus in nerve endings
    d. Prevention of superinfections during outbreaks

DOSE CALCULATION QUESTIONS

21. A 7-lb neonate develops *C. trachomatis* pneumonia following intrapartal exposure. The recommended safe dose of erythromycin ethylsuccinate for neonates is 50 mg/kg daily divided every 6 hours × 14 days. What is the safe dose of this drug?

22. Ceftriaxone, 1 g every 24 hours, is prescribed IV for a patient with disseminated gonococcal infection. It is available to be mixed with 50 mL of D_5½ NS to be administered over 30 minutes. What is the rate of infusion in mL/h?

CASE STUDY

A sexually active 19-year-old female presents to the emergency department with a 2-week history of dull bilateral abdominal pain, low back pain, and mucopurulent vaginal discharge with increased pain today. She denies fever, nausea, vomiting, diarrhea, and urinary symptoms. She reports irregular periods since age 13 years. Her last menstrual period was 2 months ago. She does not use any measure of birth control. She was treated at the health department 3 months ago for an "infection" and states that she took the medication when she remembered and did not return for a follow-up examination. She has had two sexual partners in the past 6 months, one of whom was also treated for an infection 3 months ago at the health department. She is unsure whether he was adherent to his treatment plan or whether he is symptomatic at this time. She has no known medication allergies and takes no medication on a regular basis.

Her vital signs are blood pressure (BP) 110/72 mm Hg, pulse 88 beats/min, respirations 20/min, and temperature 99.4°F. The physician orders a complete blood count (CBC), sedimentation rate, rapid plasma reagin, serum pregnancy, and a catheterized urinalysis. The physician performs abdominal and pelvic examinations and obtains cervical cultures for gonorrhea and chlamydia and specimens for saline and KOH wet preps. The physical examination reveals a soft abdomen, right and left lower quadrant tenderness without rebound, and normal bowel sounds. The pelvic exam reveals mucopurulent vaginal discharge and mild right and left adnexal tenderness with bimanual exam. The laboratory results reveal Hgb 11.1, WBC 7.0, and negative results for urinalysis and pregnancy tests.

After reviewing the medical history, physical exam, and laboratory results (excluding the cultures), the physician makes a diagnosis of PID. Orders include administering ceftriaxone 250 mg intramuscularly (IM) × 1 and prescriptions for doxycycline 100 mg twice a day for 14 days, metronidazole 500 mg twice a day for 14 days, and acetaminophen 300 mg and codeine 60 mg 1 tablet every 4 hours as needed for pain. The patient is told that she will be notified regarding the results of the cultures.

1. Why is it important to determine whether the patient is pregnant before administering doxycycline or tetracycline?

2. The patient is to be observed for 30 minutes after administration of the cephalosporin injection and then discharged home. She is given instructions for bed rest for 2 days with a reexamination in 24–48 hours if the signs and/or symptoms increase or persist. What teaching regarding the prescribed medication and follow-up care should the nurse provide to this patient?

3. Why is it important for the patient to avoid all forms of alcohol?

4. The patient is instructed to inform her sexual partners of the need for examination. The patient's phone number and address are verified for notification purposes. She is also advised that the culture results will be reported to the health department if they are positive, and the health department will then follow up with her. The patient states that she does not understand why she has to inform her sexual partners of her infection and why she has to take all of the medication if she is feeling better in a couple of days. What information and instructions can the nurse provide to the patient to help her understand the importance of adherence to her treatment plan?

5. After completing the teaching, the patient's verbalizations reflect that she still does not recognize the significance of her infection or importance of adhering to therapy. How might this alter the plan of care for this patient?

101 Antiseptics and Disinfectants

STUDY QUESTIONS

Matching

Match the term with its description.

1. ___ Anything used to prevent spread or occurrence of an infection or disease
2. ___ Preparation applied to objects
3. ___ Kills microorganisms
4. ___ Suppresses the growth and replication of microorganisms but does not kill them
5. ___ Reduction of contamination to a level compatible with public health standards
6. ___ Agent applied to living tissue
7. ___ Complete destruction of all microorganisms
   a. Antiseptic
   b. Disinfectant
   c. Germicide
   d. Germistatic
   e. Prophylactic
   f. Sanitization
   g. Sterilization

True or False

For each of the following statements, enter T for true or F for false.

It is acceptable to use an alcohol-based sanitizer to cleanse the hands instead of soap and water in which of the following situations?

8. ___ After contact with an unknown powder present on a patient
9. ___ Before eating
10. ___ After removing gloves
11. ___ After setting up a patient for lunch who is in isolation for vancomycin-resistant enterococci (VRE)
12. ___ After setting up a patient for lunch who is in isolation for tuberculosis (TB)
13. ___ After taking linens into a patient's room
14. ___ After using the restroom
15. ___ Before taking a pulse
16. ___ When the hands have been exposed to wound drainage

CRITICAL THINKING, PRIORITIZATION, AND DELEGATION QUESTIONS

17. Which are properties of an ideal antiseptic?
   a. Germicidal
   b. Broad spectrum
   c. Germistatic
   d. Low microbial resistance
   e. Short duration of action

18. Which is least significant in preventing a surgical incision site infection?
   a. Cleaning surgical site with antiseptic
   b. Preoperative hand scrubbing of nurses
   c. Rigorous disinfection of operating room
   d. Sterilization of surgical instruments

19. To ensure effectiveness of ethyl alcohol as an antiseptic, which action should the nurse take?
   a. Apply ethyl alcohol directly to open wounds.
   b. Combine alcohol with other microbial agents.
   c. Alcohol concentration should be greater than 75%.
   d. Use a gel that prolongs evaporation of the alcohol.

*20. Which is the priority reason for not wiping a subcutaneous heparin injection site with an isopropyl alcohol pad immediately after drug injection?
   a. Bruising at injection site
   b. Neutralization of heparin
   c. Reduced drug absorption
   d. Significant injection pain

21. Alcohol hand sanitizers are not effective against which organisms? **(Select all that apply.)**
   a. *Bacillus anthracis*
   b. *Clostridium difficile*
   c. Methicillin-resistant *Staphylococcus aureus* (MRSA)
   d. *Mycobacterium tuberculosis*
   e. VRE

22. When the nurse is preparing to cleanse a wound, which preparation would be most appropriate and effective?
   a. Glutaraldehyde
   b. Iodine solution
   c. Iodine tincture
   d. Povidone-iodine

23. Which surgical scrub is fast-acting and antibacterial and remains active on the skin after rinsing?
   a. Benzalkonium chloride
   b. Chlorhexidine
   c. Hexachlorophene
   d. Povidone-iodine

24. The operating room nurse is preparing to apply benzalkonium chloride as a surgical scrub. Before applying the solution, which is the priority nursing action?
   a. Clean skin with 70% alcohol.
   b. Shave the operative area.
   c. Wash the skin with soap.
   d. Warm the solution.

25. The nurse should scrub their hands and forearms with an antimicrobial soap for surgical scrub asepsis for which length of time?
   a. 1–2 minutes
   b. 2–6 minutes
   c. 6–8 minutes
   d. 8–10 minutes

26. The nursing professor is orienting student nurses to the intensive care unit. Hygiene instructions should include which directive? **(Select all that apply)**.
   a. Use foam sanitizer for dirty hands.
   b. No type of jewelry is allowed.
   c. Do not wear artificial nails.
   d. Keep nail tips under ¼ inch.
   e. Remove gloves after patient care.

CASE STUDY

The delivery room nurse needs to prepare used instruments for disinfection with glutaraldehyde before being sent for sterilization.

1. What steps should the nurse take before soaking the instruments?

2. How long do the instruments need to soak?

3. What precautions does the nurse need to take when disinfecting with glutaraldehyde?

4. Describe the handwashing technique the nurse would use after completing this disinfection process.

102 Anthelmintics

STUDY QUESTIONS

True or False

For each of the following statements, enter T for true or F for false.

1. ___ Helminthiasis is the most common affliction of humans.
2. ___ Anthelmintics treat parasitic worm infestations.
3. ___ Parasitic worm infestation always causes symptoms.
4. ___ When individual treatment is impractical, improved hygiene may be the most valuable intervention.
5. ___ The sooner drug treatment is started after infestation, the less reproduction of the worm occurs in the body.
6. ___ Helminthiasis can involve the liver, lymphatic system, and blood vessels.
7. ___ Treatment may be deemed not needed if there is a high probability of reinfestation or the patient cannot afford the drug.
8. ___ Roundworms can cause pancreatitis by blocking the pancreatic duct.
9. ___ Pinworms live in the human body for 7–10 days.

CRITICAL THINKING, PRIORITIZATION, AND DELEGATION QUESTIONS

▶10. The nurse is caring for a patient who has started therapy with mebendazole for hookworm infestation. It is important for the nurse to assess for which common complication of hookworm infestation?
   a. Vomiting
   b. Anemia
   c. Pruritis
   d. Diarrhea

11. A patient who has been treated with albendazole for trichinosis is now prescribed prednisone. Which is the purpose of this medication?
   a. Kill larvae that have migrated.
   b. Prevent calcification of dead larvae.
   c. Inhibit migration of larvae.
   d. Reduce inflammation during larval migration.

12. Nursing examination of a missionary who was admitted after becoming ill in Haiti reveals severe scrotal and peripheral edema. Which other assessment findings suggest possible nematode infestation?
   a. Limited range of motion
   b. Multiple bruises
   c. Swollen lymph nodes
   d. Weak hand grasps

13. A patient who works for the World Health Organization (WHO) and whose job duties include worldwide travel reports a recent change in visual acuity and the development of subcutaneous nodules with associated pruritus. The nurse should assess for recent travel to which area? (**Select all that apply.**)
   a. Argentina
   b. Guatemala
   c. Kenya
   d. Mexico
   e. Peru
   f. Rwanda
   g. Venezuela

*14. The nurse is caring for a patient with intestinal roundworms. It would be a priority to report which diagnostic test result to the provider?
   a. Aspartate aminotransferase (AST) 5 IU/L
   b. Blood urea nitrogen (BUN) 15 mg/dL
   c. Human chorionic gonadotropin (hCG) 3400 IU/L
   d. International normalized ratio (INR) 1

15. To prevent complications from therapy with praziquantel, which should be included in patient teaching?
   a. Avoid hazardous activity.
   b. Chew tablet before swallowing.
   c. Monitor daily urine output.
   d. Take on an empty stomach.

16. The nurse is administering albendazole to an older adult patient who has been diagnosed with the larval form of the pork tapeworm. Which laboratory result would warrant consultation with the prescriber regarding administration of the medication?
    a. Alanine aminotransferase (ALT) 175 IU/L
    b. BUN 25 mg/dL
    c. Creatinine 1.4 mg/dL
    d. Potassium 3.8 mg/dL

*17. The nurse is caring for a patient with *Wuchereria bancrofti* infection who has just begun therapy with diethylcarbamazine. Which symptom would be a priority concern?
    a. Dizziness
    b. Headache
    c. Nausea
    d. Confusion

DOSE CALCULATION QUESTIONS

18. Mebendazole 500 mg × 1 is prescribed. How many 100-mg tablets should be administered at each dose?

19. Praziquantel 600 mg × 1 is prescribed for a 165-lb male with beef tapeworm infection. Is this dose safe?

CASE STUDY

The parent of a 2½-year-old child who attends daycare notices that their child has been restless, not sleeping well, has been scratching the perineal area, and has been wetting the bed. The parent calls the pediatric office and is told by the nurse to put transparent tape in the child's anal area as soon as the child wakes up. The nurse further instructs the parent to remove the tape, put it in a plastic bag, and bring it to the office. On examination of the tape sample, the pediatric nurse practitioner (PNP) diagnoses enterobiasis.

1. What is the probable mode of transmission of this parasite?

2. The PNP prescribes mebendazole for the entire family. What did the prescriber need to determine before prescribing the drug for the entire family?

3. How could the pinworm infestation have been transmitted from the child to other family members?

4. What teaching can the nurse provide these family members to prevent future infestation and spread of pinworms?

5. The entire family is adherent to the prescribed therapy. Why is there little problem with adherence with this therapy?

6. The parents are embarrassed and do not want to notify the daycare of the child's infection. How should the nurse respond?

103 Antiprotozoal Drugs I: Antimalarial Agents

STUDY QUESTIONS

Completion

1. Malaria deaths in sub-Saharan Africa are most likely in __________________ children.
2. Malaria is transmitted by the __________________ __________________.
3. Infection in the human begins with sporozoites invading the __________________.
4. The liver releases merozoites that infect ______ ____________.
5. __________________ malaria is the most common form.
6. Falciparum malaria does not __________________ because it does not form hypnozoites that remain in the liver.
7. __________________ __________________ __________________ is the term for dark urine associated with falciparum malaria.

Matching

Match the type of treatment with its definition.

8. ___ Prophylaxis
9. ___ Prevention of relapse
10. ___ Treatment of an acute attack

a. Clinical cure
b. Radical cure
c. Suppressive therapy

CRITICAL THINKING, PRIORITIZATION, AND DELEGATION QUESTIONS

11. The repeating episodes of fever, chills, and profuse sweating that are characteristic of malaria are due to which factor?
    a. Infection at the site of the mosquito bite
    b. Ingestion of blood by the mosquito
    c. Red blood cell (RBC) rupture
    d. Toxicity of the suppressant drugs

✳12. Prompt treatment of suspected cases of falciparum malaria is most urgent if the patient experiences which symptom?
    a. Chills
    b. Dark urine
    c. High fever
    d. Sweating

✳13. To prevent a serious complication, which is the priority nursing intervention when caring for a patient who has malaria caused by *Plasmodium falciparum*?
    a. Checking for respiratory distress
    b. Assessing vital signs every 4 hours
    c. Blood glucose checks every 2 hours
    d. Monitoring liver function studies

✳14. A patient with falciparum malaria is at risk for hypoglycemia. It is a priority to assess the patient for which signs and symptoms?
    a. Cold, clammy skin
    b. Hot, dry skin
    c. Hunger and thirst
    d. Nausea and vomiting

15. Which is the reason primaquine is not used for relapse prevention of infection with malaria caused by *P. falciparum*?
    a. Primaquine is not used prophylactically.
    b. *P. falciparum* is resistant to primaquine.
    c. Relapses disappear without drug treatment.
    d. *P. falciparum* does not form hypnozoites.

✳16. The nurse should monitor urine color during treatment with primaquine if laboratory results which results?
    a. Hemoglobin 8 g/dL
    b. Hematocrit 40%
    c. RBC 4.9 × 10^6/mcL
    d. Reticulocytes 2%

✳17. It is a priority to teach patients who are prescribed quinine for malaria to report which effect?
    a. Fatigue
    b. Headache
    c. Palpitations
    d. Pallor

18. Which is the reason primaquine and quinine should not be administered to persons with glucose-6-phosphate dehydrogenase (G6PD) deficiency?
    a. Causes cinchonism
    b. Increases hemolysis
    c. Postural hypotension
    d. Drug neutralization

19. Which nursing action is appropriate concerning quinine administration to pregnant females?
   a. Administer the drug as ordered.
   b. Consult with the pharmacist.
   c. Assess for any adverse effects.
   d. Do not administer the drug.

*20. Which is the priority assessment when administering proguanil?
   a. Bleeding gums
   b. Headache
   c. Hair loss
   d. Insomnia

►21. Which change is a reason for the nurse to withhold mefloquine and contact the provider?
   a. Headache
   b. Heartburn
   c. Apathy
   d. Nausea

22. Tetracycline is prescribed for a female patient who has chloroquine-resistant malaria. Which laboratory test result would warrant withholding the drug and contacting the provider?
   a. Alanine aminotransferase 60 IU/L
   b. Estimated glomerular filtration rate 75 mL/min
   c. Human chorionic gonadotropin 90 mIU/mL
   d. RBC count 4.2 million cells/mcL

23. Tafenoquine is active against both *Plasmodium vivax* and *P. falciparum*. Prior to initiation of therapy, which test should be performed on all potential recipients? (**Select all that apply.**)
   a. CBC
   b. hCG
   c. ECG
   d. G6PD
   e. Chest X-ray (CXR)

DOSE CALCULATION QUESTIONS

24. Artesunate 2.4 mg/kg per minute continuous infusion is ordered for a patient who weighs 165 lb. Following dilution, the concentration of artesunate is 10 mg/mL. How many mL will the nurse administer?

25. Clindamycin 20 mg/kg per day in three divided doses is recommended for a child with malaria. What is acceptable dosing for a child who weighs 55 lb?

CASE STUDY

A middle-aged adult has just returned from Africa after 4 years of service with the World Health Organization (WHO). During that time, they had been taking chloroquine prophylactically to prevent malaria in case they were bitten by a mosquito infected with *Anopheles*.

1. What does this treatment accomplish?

2. What other measures should the patient have been taught to decrease the risk of malarial infection?

3. Before service in Africa was completed, the patient quit taking chloroquine because they were experiencing nausea and vomiting. Soon after, they started experiencing episodes of high fever followed by chills and then diaphoresis occurring every 2 days. The patient was diagnosed with vivax malaria and was unable to work due to the frequency and intensity of the symptoms. The patient is prescribed a three-dose treatment of chloroquine for the acute attack of malaria. What teaching could the nurse provide to decrease adverse effects and prevent serious effects?

4. The patient tells the nurse that they know that missionaries took IV quinine in the past and asks why they weren't prescribed that drug. What information can the nurse share about the decrease in use of quinine?

5. The patient was advised that they should return home for treatment with primaquine to prevent relapse. Why was the patient not treated in Africa where they could continue to work?

6. When the patient completes their acute treatment, they ask why they cannot continue taking the chloroquine to prevent the recurrence of the malaria symptoms. What is the basis of the nurse's response to this question?

104 Antiprotozoal Drugs II: Miscellaneous Agents

STUDY QUESTIONS

Matching

Match the term with its description.

1. ___ Cryptosporidiosis
2. ___ Giardiasis
3. ___ Toxoplasmosis
4. ___ Trichomoniasis

   a. Infection is acquired most commonly by eating undercooked meat.
   b. Transmission is fecal-oral, often by ingesting water contaminated with livestock feces.
   c. Usual site of infestation is the genitourinary tract.
   d. Infestation usually occurs by drinking contaminated water.

CRITICAL THINKING, PRIORITIZATION, AND DELEGATION QUESTIONS

*5. A farmer is hospitalized after developing cryptosporidiosis. The patient is currently being treated with prednisone for an exacerbation of chronic obstructive pulmonary disease. Which is the priority patient problem?
   a. Decreased functional ability
   b. Fatigue
   c. Disrupted fluid balance
   d. Nausea

6. It is important to teach a patient who is prescribed metronidazole that it is very important to report which possible adverse effect to the provider?
   a. Dark urine
   b. Metallic taste
   c. Mouth ulcers
   d. Paresthesias

7. An emergency department nurse is providing discharge teaching to a patient who is prescribed metronidazole for giardiasis. The patient is breastfeeding her infant. It is important for the nurse to teach this patient to feed her baby formula and discard her pumped breast milk throughout the time the medication is taken and for which time after?
   a. 1 day
   b. 3 days
   c. 1 week
   d. 3 weeks

8. A patient who has been taking tinidazole asks what side effects they can expect. The nurse provides information on the most common side effects and tells the patient they should call the provider if which occur(s)?
   a. Palpitations
   b. Nausea
   c. Seizures
   d. Depression

9. The nurse notes yellowish discoloration of the sclera of an immunocompetent 7-year-old who is receiving nitazoxanide for giardiasis. Which is the appropriate nursing action?
   a. Administer the drug.
   b. Call the pharmacy.
   c. Withhold the drug.
   d. Contact the provider.

10. A kidney transplant recipient comes to the clinic reporting symptoms of body aches, swollen lymph nodes, headache, and fatigue. When vital signs are taken, the patient is found to have a temperature of 101.4°F. When questioned by the healthcare provider, it is discovered that the patient adopted a kitten from the shelter about a month ago. The kitten sleeps with them but is not yet litter box trained. Based on this information, the nurse would expect the patient to be started pyrimethamine plus which other drug? (**Select all that apply.**)
   a. Atovaquone
   b. Clindamycin
   c. Nitazoxanide
   d. Paromomycin
   e. Sulfadiazine

11. A college student comes to the health center with symptoms of penile discharge, burning after urination, and itching. The student also reports discomfort with sexual intercourse. Upon questioning, the patient reports having had sexual intercourse with multiple partners. The nurse would prepare to teach the patient about which drug?
   a. Sulfadiazine
   b. Tinidazole
   c. Clindamycin
   d. Penicillin

DOSE CALCULATION QUESTION

12. An immunocompromised patient is prescribed nitazoxanide suspension 750 mg every 12 hours for 14 days. Available is nitazoxanide suspension 100 mg/5 mL. How many milliliters will the patient take at each dose?

CASE STUDY

The nurse works in a busy family practice. A 17-year-old female patient presents to the office with complaints of stabbing right upper quadrant pain, anorexia, chills, and diarrhea for 10 days.

1. What subjective information would be helpful to collect before the primary care practitioner (PCP) sees the patient?

   The patient was on a camping trip in the White Mountains of New Hampshire a few weeks ago. She experienced nausea and fatigue toward the end of trip, and the symptoms have gotten worse since coming home. She denies alcohol and tobacco use and sexual activity and is currently experiencing menses. She has lost 4 lb in the last 2 weeks. Assessment findings include temperature 102.7°F, pulse 98 beats/min, blood pressure (BP) 100/64 mm Hg, dry mucous membranes, abdominal guarding, and weakness. The PCP orders a complete blood count (CBC) and differential, electrolytes, and a computed tomography (CT) scan of the abdomen. The PCP diagnoses giardiasis. Because the patient states that she will have difficulty being adherent with three-times-a-day dosing with metronidazole, the PCP prescribes tinidazole 2 g once a day for 3 days.

2. During teaching regarding the adverse effects of this drug, the nurse should explain the importance of contacting the provider if what symptoms occur?

3. Based on the patient's exposure to the organism, symptoms, and developmental considerations, what other teaching should the nurse provide?

4. One duty is to review laboratory tests and notify the PCP of results. The nurse is reviewing laboratory results for the patient with giardiasis. Abnormal results include white blood cell (WBC) 12,800/mm^3, sodium 137 mEq/L, potassium 3.6 mEq/L, and multiple small abscesses in the liver on CT scan. Which test result is most important to promptly review with the PCP and why?

5. The PCP asks the nurse to have the patient come in immediately. After explaining the laboratory test results, the patient agrees to be faithful for a course of metronidazole followed by iodoquinol. What teaching should the nurse provide?

105 Ectoparasiticides

STUDY QUESTIONS

Matching

Indicate if the statement applies to pediculosis (P), scabies (S), or both (B).

1. ___ Do not live on pets
2. ___ Burrows visible as dotted lines on skin
3. ___ Common site of adult infestation is in webs between fingers
4. ___ Intense pruritis
5. ___ Lice infestation
6. ___ Mite infestation
7. ___ Scratching may result in secondary infection
8. ___ Transmission possible via contact with inanimate objects
9. ___ Treatment differs by site of infestation
10. ___ Usually treated with topical drugs

CRITICAL THINKING, PRIORITIZATION, AND DELEGATION QUESTIONS

11. Which is the proven mode of transmission of head lice?
    a. Jump between people
    b. Head-to-head contact
    c. Sharing personal hats
    d. Sharing hairbrushes
12. Which patient should not receive lindane? (**Select all that apply.**)
    a. Previous adverse reaction
    b. History of acne vulgaris
    c. Has not tried safer drug
    d. Recent use of lindane
    e. Weighs 115 pounds
13. Which treatment for head lice must be applied at least twice to be effective?
    a. Benzyl alcohol
    b. Ivermectin
    c. Lindane
    d. Permethrin
14. Which is the drug of choice for head lice?
    a. Lindane
    b. Ivermectin
    c. Spinosad
    d. Permethrin

DOSE CALCULATION QUESTIONS

15. A child with resistant scabies is prescribed permethrin lotion 1% and ivermectin 200 mcg/kg x one today and repeat in 7 days. The child weighs 65 pounds. Available are 3 mg tablets. How much ivermectin will be administered in each dose?

CASE STUDY

A second-grade teacher consults the school nurse about a child in their class. The child is one of three siblings attending the elementary school. The child has long hair, and over the past week the child has been constantly scratching their head. They have scratched their head so much that their hair is tangled and almost impossible to brush, and the child's scalp is bleeding. The school nurse notes small white spots on the hair shaft close to the scalp. Examination under the microscope reveals nits. The nurse contacts the child's parents to report these nits, telling them that it is probably head lice.

1. How should the school nurse handle the possibility that other children in the school may be infested?
2. The child's parents are quite upset about the lice. They want to know how their child could have gotten "these bugs" and how to tell whether others in the family have them. How should the nurse respond?

3. The parents were told by a friend to cut all their child's hair off to get rid of the lice. What are the reasons why the nurse would not want the parents to do this?

4. The parents contact the pediatrician, who orders permethrin 1% shampoo. What should the office nurse include in the explanation for using this product?

5. What is the purpose of the fine-toothed comb in head lice treatment?

6. The child's parent tells the nurse that when they had head lice as a child, their prescriber had their parents apply lindane shampoo. The parent wants to know why that is not used anymore. What would the nurse tell him?

106 Basic Principles of Cancer Chemotherapy

STUDY QUESTIONS

Completion

1. Death due to cancer has dropped _______________ over the past 25 years.
2. The treatment of choice for disseminated cancer is ____________.
3. _______________ cancer is one of the most common locations of cancer in males.
4. The most common treatment for solid tumors is _______________.
5. _______________ uses the body's natural defense system to kill cancerous cells.
6. ______________________ drugs are the class of anticancer drugs used most often.
7. Telomerase permits repeated cell _______________.

CRITICAL THINKING, PRIORITIZATION, AND DELEGATION

8. Which characteristic best describes cancer cell reproduction?
   a. Abnormal behavior
   b. Rapid cell division
   c. Aberrant growth
   d. Persistent proliferation
9. A patient is admitted for surgical removal of a cancerous tumor of the colon. They are concerned about the prospect of living with a colostomy and ask the nurse why the provider cannot just give them some drugs to kill the cancer. Which is the basis of the nurse's response concerning solid tumors? (**Select all that apply.**)
   a. They are disseminated.
   b. Fewer actively dividing cells.
   c. Have fewer cells in the G_0 phase.
   d. Poor blood supply at the core.
   e. Have normal DNA sequence.
10. The partner of a cancer patient asks why some tumors become resistant to chemotherapy. Which is the appropriate explanation?
    a. "One mechanism of drug resistance is increased repair of the damage to DNA caused by chemotherapy drugs."
    b. "A mechanism of drug resistance is decreased efflux of chemotherapy drugs by the cancer cells."
    c. "Drug resistance can be caused by cancer cells increasing the uptake of chemotherapy drugs."
    d. "Destruction of the P-glycoprotein transport molecule can result in resistance to chemotherapy drugs."
11. The parent of a child with leukemia is concerned about their child's fear and discomfort during chemotherapy. They ask the nurse why the child cannot receive one large dose of a single powerful drug instead of multiple doses of different drugs. After teaching, which statement suggests that this parent needs further explanation?
    a. "Different chemotherapy drugs kill the cancer cells in different ways."
    b. "Each drug only kills cancer cells at a particular point of cell reproduction."
    c. "Using multiple drugs is less likely to result in drug resistance to all of them."
    d. "Adverse effects are reduced if multiple drugs are administered at different times."
12. The nurse would expect which action when two or more chemotherapeutic drugs are used together?
    a. If selected carefully, no overlapping toxicities.
    b. When used alone, the drugs are less effective.
    c. Can mix the drugs in the same IV solution.
    d. The drugs have the same mechanism of action.
13. A patient with brain cancer asks the nurse why they are putting the drug into their back instead of infusing it into a vein. Which is the basis of the nurse's response?
    a. Allows higher doses of chemotherapy
    b. Enables the drug to get to the tumor cells
    c. Prevents many of the adverse effects
    d. Avoids development of drug resistance

►14. The nurse is caring for an older adult patient who developed pancreatitis during chemotherapy. Laboratory results include red blood cell (RBC) 2.8×10^6/mL, white blood cell (WBC) 4100/mm^3, neutrophils 18,000/mm^3, and platelets 147,000/mm^3. Which is the priority patient problem?
   a. Reduced motor function
   b. Low blood pressure
   c. Decreased gas exchange
   d. Decreased level of consciousness

15. The nurse is caring for a patient receiving chemotherapy who is on neutropenic precautions. The nurse washes their hands and puts on gloves before entering the patient's room. The patient refuses care by the nurse until the nurse washes their hands at the sink in the room and puts on new gloves. Which is the appropriate nursing action?
   a. Explain the increased risk for infection by removing clean gloves.
   b. Discuss that they washed their hands just before entering the room.
   c. Rewash their hands in the room and put on new gloves as requested.
   d. Rewash hands, but do not put on gloves, as they might tear from moisture.

16. For a patient with cancer who is receiving chemotherapy, which food would be least likely to cause an infection if the patient develops neutropenia?
   a. Commercially canned fruit
   b. Lettuces from the garden
   c. Meat cooked rare
   d. Organic goat yogurt

►17. The nurse is administering subcutaneous insulin to a patient receiving chemotherapy who is experiencing bone marrow suppression. Which is the appropriate technique?
   a. Administer via an existing intravenous (IV) port.
   b. Apply pressure to the site following injection.
   c. Delay administration until after the patient has eaten.
   d. Wipe the injection site with Betadine after injection.

*18. A patient receiving chemotherapy develops hyperuricemia. Nursing interventions address the effects of hyperuricemia on which organ or body system?
   a. Blood
   b. Joints
   c. Kidneys
   d. Liver

►19. When administering a known vesicant, which is priority nursing information?
   a. If the patient has been premedicated with an antiemetic.
   b. Stop infusion immediately if extravasation occurs.
   c. Understand the mechanism of action of the drug.
   d. Wear gloves during drug administration.

CASE STUDY

A young adult patient is admitted to the oncology unit with a diagnosis of Hodgkin disease, confirmed by biopsy. The patient is started on therapy, which consists of external radiation treatments and chemotherapy. The patient asks the nurse, "How does cancer spread?"

1. What information can the nurse provide about the characteristics of cancer cells that promote growth and metastasis?

2. The patient asks why people are more likely to get cancer if they have a family history of cancer. How are genetics linked to cancer?

3. The nurse is discussing strategies to minimize the adverse effects of chemotherapy, including stomatitis. The patient asks why these drugs cause mouth ulcers if they are given intravenously. How should the nurse respond?

4. What interventions can the nurse suggest to minimize the effects of chemotherapy on the patient's gastrointestinal (GI) tract?

107 Anticancer Drugs I: Cytotoxic Agents

STUDY QUESTIONS

True or False

For each of the following statements, enter T for true or F for false.

1. ___ Cytotoxic cancer drugs kill cancer cells and healthy cells.
2. ___ Cells in the G_0 phase are most likely to be killed by cytotoxic drugs.
3. ___ It is critical that phase-specific cytotoxic drugs be administered on a specific schedule.
4. ___ Cell cycle phase–nonspecific drugs are equally effective during any phase of the cell cycle.
5. ___ Bifunctional alkylating agents are more effective than monofunctional agents.
6. ___ Alkylating agents are considered cell cycle phase nonspecific.
7. ___ Most antimetabolites are M-phase specific.
8. ___ Folic acid analogs are effective because folic acid is toxic to cancer cells.
9. ___ Failure to administer leucovorin in the right dose at the right time can be fatal.
10. ___ Antitumor antibiotics are used to treat infections associated with neutropenia caused by cancer drugs.

CRITICAL THINKING, PRIORITIZATION, AND DELEGATION QUESTIONS

►11. Which teaching would be appropriate relating to a common, serious adverse effect of every category of cytotoxic drugs?
   a. "Change positions slowly to prevent dizziness."
   b. "Do not drive at night; it may not be safe."
   c. "It's important to perform weight-bearing exercise."
   d. "Use an electric razor to avoid cutting yourself."

✳12. Which diagnostic test result would be priority when a patient is receiving cytotoxic drugs for cancer?
   a. Absolute neutrophil count 476/mm^3
   b. Platelets 130,000/mm^3
   c. Reticulocytes 3.2%
   d. White blood cell (WBC) 11,000/mm^3

13. Which administration strategy is most likely to ensure that cell cycle phase–specific drugs are present when cancer cells are going through the specific phase? (**Select all that apply**.)
   a. Combined with other drugs
   b. Administered at frequent intervals
   c. Infused over a prolonged time
   d. Rapid infusion of large doses
   e. Small doses infused frequently

14. Which is the reason cell cycle phase–nonspecific drugs may not kill cells in the G_0 phase?
   a. The cells have time to repair damage.
   b. The cells are not cancerous in the G_0 phase.
   c. The cell is reproducing.
   d. The cell's DNA is not harmed.

15. The nurse is teaching a patient who has been prescribed oral cyclophosphamide. Which statement suggests a need for further teaching?
   a. "I need to call my provider if I develop a fever higher than 100.4°F."
   b. "This drug should be taken 1 hour before or 2 hours after meals."
   c. "Drinking at least 65 ounces of fluids every day is important."
   d. "If my skin color changes, I should call my health care provider."

16. Mesna is prescribed with high-dose cyclophosphamide for which reason?
   a. Decreases nausea
   b. Inhibits DNA repair
   c. Potentiates drug action
   d. Prevents bleeding

✳17. It is priority for the nurse to consult with the oncologist before administering cisplatin if the patient reports which symptom since the last infusion?
   a. Headache
   b. Nausea
   c. Tinnitus
   d. White blood cell count 10 × 109/L

18. Which is a symptoms of bone marrow suppression associated with oxaliplatin?
   a. Platelets 450 × 10^9/L
   b. Hematocrit 30%
   c. Hemoglobin 14 g/dL
   d. White blood cell count 10 × 10^9/L

19. A female patient of childbearing age should be instructed to use two reliable forms of birth control during therapy and for which length of time after therapy when prescribed methotrexate?
   a. 2 weeks
   b. 2 month
   c. 6 weeks
   d. 6 months

✳20. The nurse is caring for a patient prescribed methotrexate. Which diagnostic test result is a priority to report to the provider?
   a. Alanine aminotransferase (ALT) 55 IU/L
   b. Blood urea nitrogen (BUN) 22 mg/dL
   c. Creatinine clearance 45 mL/min
   d. Hemoglobin 10.8 g/dL

✳21. A patient with laryngeal cancer is receiving large doses of methotrexate and leucovorin. Which is the priority nursing action?
   a. Give ondansetron 30 min before infusion.
   b. Infuse leucovorin exactly as prescribed.
   c. Administer methotrexate after leucovorin.
   d. Monitor the patient's serum electrolyte levels.

►22. A patient has been taught about the adverse effects of methotrexate therapy. Which patient statement suggests understanding of the teaching?
   a. "I should report a new cough to the doctor immediately."
   b. "Drinking cranberry juice protects my kidneys from damage."
   c. "Drinking grapefruit juice prevents drug breakdown."
   d. "I should increase my fluid intake to four glasses each day."

23. The nurse teaches a patient that dexamethasone is used as a premedication for patients who are treated with paclitaxel to prevent which condition?
   a. Bradycardia
   b. Hypotension
   c. Swelling of tongue
   d. Fluid retention

✳24. Which indicates symptoms of cytarabine syndrome? (**Select all that apply**.)
   a. Fever
   b. Headache
   c. Stomatitis
   d. Bone pain
   e. Conjunctivities

25. Which is a symptom of hand-foot syndrome associated with administration of fluorouracil?
   a. Palm tingling
   b. Bone pain
   c. Diarrhea
   d. Loss of hair

✳26. Which symptom, if occurring in a patient receiving mercaptopurine, would be priority to the nurse?
   a. Constipation
   b. Diarrhea
   c. Hair loss
   d. Petechiae

27. Which is a harmless side effect of doxorubicin?
   a. Transient dysrhythmias.
   b. Alopecia.
   c. Conjunctivitis.
   d. Red color to sweat.

28. The nurse should warn patients that they may experience a blue-green discoloration of their urine and the whites of their eyes if they receive which antitumor antibiotic?
   a. Epirubicin
   b. Idarubicin
   c. Liposomal daunorubicin
   d. Mitoxantrone

✳29. The nurse is preparing to administer bleomycin to a patient with testicular cancer. It would be priority to report which diagnostic test result to the provider?
   a. Erythrocyte sedimentation rate (ESR) 10 mm/h
   b. Estimated glomerular filtration rate (eGFR) 75 mL/min
   c. Peak expiratory flow (PEF) 54% of best
   d. Brain natriuretic peptide (BNP) 125 pg/mL

✳30. An adolescent patient is scheduled to receive vincristine for Hodgkin lymphoma. Developmentally, which adverse effect is a priority concern for this patient?
   a. Alopecia
   b. Constipation
   c. Nausea
   d. Paresthesias

✳31. Which nursing action would be priority when administering an infusion of paclitaxel?
   a. Monitor urine output.
   b. Monitor vital signs.
   c. Prepare for vomiting.
   d. Reposition every 2 hours.

✳32. Which assessment finding is most significant if a patient is receiving docetaxel?
   a. Blood pressure 147/90 mm Hg
   b. 8-hr output of 850 mL
   c. Expiratory wheezing
   d. 2+ pitting edema

33. The partner of a patient who received cabazitaxel reports that the patient has been up all night with diarrhea. The patient is currently in bed and too weak to stand up. The partner asks the nurse what to do. Which is the appropriate nursing response?
    a. Give 1 tsp Pepto Bismol.
    b. Allow the patient to rest.
    c. Take frequent sips of Sprite.
    d. Seek medical care now.

DOSE CALCULATION QUESTIONS

34. Filgrastim is prescribed 5 mcg/kg per day. The patient weighs 132 lb. What dose should be administered?

35. What is the maximum recommended lifetime dose of doxorubicin for a patient who is 72″ tall and weighs 220 lb, when the cumulative lifetime dose should be kept below 550 mg/m^2?

CASE STUDIES

Case Study 1

A patient is admitted to the outpatient area for their first course of intravenous fluorouracil chemotherapy for metastatic breast cancer.

1. What techniques should the nurse use when administering this drug to prevent personal harm?

2. What administrative techniques should the nurse use to prevent patient injury from this drug?

Case Study 2

The nurse is preparing to administer doxorubicin to a patient with ovarian cancer.

3. Developmentally, what effect of this drug would be a priority for the nurse to prepare this patient to experience?

4. What things should the nurse assess and teach the patient to report relating to the risk of cardiotoxicity?

5. Ramipril 2.5 mg daily is prescribed. What should the nurse include in teaching about this drug?

108 Anticancer Drugs II: Hormonal Agents, Targeted Drugs, and Other Noncytotoxic Anticancer Drugs

STUDY QUESTIONS

True or False

For each of the following statements, enter T for true or F for false.

1. ___ Hormonal agents lack serious adverse effects.
2. ___ Chemotherapy and hormonal therapy are adjuvant treatments to improve the response to other treatment modalities.
3. ___ For hormonal agents to be effective, the tumor must have receptors for the hormone being blocked.
4. ___ Tamoxifen is not recommended for breast cancer prevention for females older than 60 years because they have a lower incidence of breast cancer than females of ages 40–59 years.
5. ___ Antidepressant drugs fluoxetine, paroxetine, and sertraline slow the metabolism of tamoxifen by the liver, causing tamoxifen toxicity.
6. ___ The likelihood of infusion reactions to trastuzumab increases with each subsequent dose of the drug.

CRITICAL THINKING, PRIORITIZATION, AND DELEGATION QUESTIONS

*7. A 58-year-old patient has been taking tamoxifen to prevent breast cancer. Which question would be priority for the nurse to ask?
   a. "Has anyone in your family ever had breast cancer?"
   b. "Have you ever been told that your cholesterol is high?"
   c. "Have you experienced a broken wrist, hip, or backbone?"
   d. "Have you had vaginal bleeding after the drug was started?"

8. Which teaching would be appropriate for the most common adverse effect of tamoxifen?
   a. Adequate hydration
   b. Dress in layers
   c. Use of OTC drugs
   d. Small, frequent meals

*9. The nurse is caring for a patient prescribed a selective estrogen receptor modulator. Which adverse effect would be priority to report to the provider?
   a. Calf pain and swelling
   b. Hot flashes and night sweats
   c. Longer menstrual cycles
   d. Nausea without vomiting

10. The nurse is caring for a patient prescribed tamoxifen. The patient reports feeling like they want to cry all the time. They state their best friend in the support group takes sertraline, and they ask if they can take it too. Which is the appropriate nursing response?
   a. "That drug will increase side effects of tamoxifen."
   b. "Let's talk to the provider about putting you on it."
   c. "Sertraline reduces the effectiveness of tamoxifen."
   d. "Have you tried St. John wort? It might be better."

*11. In a patient prescribed toremifene which would be priority to report to the provider?
   a. 1+ periferal edema
   b. Menstrual irregularities
   c. Hot flashes
   d. Tenderness in right leg

12. A 38-year-old patient with breast cancer asks why she has been prescribed tamoxifen instead of anastrozole. Which is the appropriate nursing response? **(Select all that apply.)**
   a. Only postmenopausal females receive anastrozole.
   b. Anastrozole can cause endometrial and other cancers.
   c. Tamoxifen is more effective and has fewer adverse effects.
   d. Both pre- and postmenopausal females can take tamoxifen.
   e. Females taking tamoxifen should avoid becoming pregnant.

*13. The nurse is caring for a patient prescribed trastuzumab. The nurse would consult the provider immediately if the patient suddenly developed which symptom?
   a. Crackles throughout the lung fields
   b. Generalized weakness and fatigue
   c. Headache and sensitivity to light
   d. Temperature of 100.4°F (38°C)

14. Which is the primary nursing action when caring for a patient receiving their first dose of trastuzumab who reports shortness of breath?
    a. Assess lung sounds.
    b. Elevate the head of the bed.
    c. Notify the provider.
    d. Stop the drug infusion.

15. Which suggests possible cardiotoxicity from trastuzumab? (**Select all that apply.**)
    a. Brain natriuretic peptide (BNP) 850 pg/mL
    b. Echocardiogram with ejection fraction of 60%
    c. Diminished breath sounds bilateral lung bases
    d. Left shift of point of maximal impulse (PMI)
    e. Slight increase in pulse with deep inspiration

16. The provider of a potentially cardiotoxic drug asks the nurse, "What is the patient's weight?" Which information is the provider seeking?
    a. Actual weight in kilograms
    b. Body mass index (BMI)
    c. Change in weight in the past 24 hours
    d. How weight relates to ideal body weight

17. Which herb has been known to increase metabolism of imatinib and possibly decrease effectiveness?
    a. Echinacea
    b. Feverfew
    c. Garlic
    d. St. John wort

►18. Which symptom suggests hypercalcemia from metastasis of breast cancer to bone?
    a. 4+ deep tendon reflexes (DTRs)
    b. Bilateral weak hand grasps
    c. Negative Babinski reflex
    d. Positive Homans sign

19. A patient who is receiving leuprolide for advanced prostate cancer is at risk for new-onset diabetes. Which symptom suggests that the patient is experiencing hyperglycemia?
    a. Anorexia
    b. Diaphoresis
    c. Frequent urination
    d. Xeroderma

20. Which injection interval should the nurse question if a patient is prescribed leuprolide depot injection?
    a. Once a month
    b. Once every 4 months
    c. Once every 6 months
    d. Once every 12 months

►21. Teaching for a patient prescribed nilutamide should include instructions to call the provider for which symptom?
    a. Hypertension.
    b. Palpitations.
    c. Dry, hacking cough.
    d. Muscle weakness.

22. Which would be an indication to either discontinue or reduce the dose of abiraterone? (**Select all that apply.**)
    a. Alanine aminotransferase (ALT) 196 μ/L
    b. Beta-human chorionic gonadotropin (β-hCG) 32 mIU/mL
    c. Prostate-specific antigen (PSA) 7.2 mg/mL
    d. Total bilirubin 1.0 mg/dL
    e. Aspartate aminotransferase (AST) 160 μ/L

23. Which drugs are commonly used for premedication before infusing sipuleucel-T? (**Select all that apply.**)
    a. Acetaminophen
    b. Aspirin
    c. Diphenhydramine
    d. Epinephrine
    e. Ibuprofen

*24. Which value should be reported to the provider immediately when a patient is prescribed docetaxel or cabazitaxel?
    a. Absolute neutrophil count (ANC) 875/mm^3
    b. Hemoglobin/hematocrit (Hb/Hct) 13.2/37%
    c. Platelets 400,000/mm^3
    d. White blood cell (WBC) 11,000/mm^3

25. The teaching plan for patients receiving cetuximab should include the importance of immediately reporting the sudden onset of which symptom?
    a. Fever
    b. Irritability
    c. Nausea
    d. Dyspnea

26. Which assessment finding suggests that a patient who is receiving panitumumab is experiencing hypomagnesemia?
    a. Constipation
    b. Muscle cramps
    c. Fever
    d. Hypotension

*27. The nurse notes a 2-lb weight gain in 24 hours when assessing a hospitalized patient who has been receiving imatinib for chronic myeloid leukemia. It is priority for the nurse to assess which body system?
    a. Cardiopulmonary status
    b. Gastrointestinal status
    c. Musculoskeletal status
    d. Neurologic status

28. Which is the most common symptom of QT prolongation and should be reported to the provider of nilotinib?
    a. Dizziness
    b. Palpitations
    c. Shortness of breath
    d. Sudden fainting

*29. Which assessment finding would be of concern to the nurse caring for a patient who is prescribed sunitinib for advanced renal cell carcinoma?
a. 10-mm Hg increase in blood pressure
b. Large bruises at venipuncture sites
c. Dizziness with position changes
d. Hb 13.2 g/dL

30. Which symptom, if occurring 12–24 hours after the first infusion of rituximab, suggests possible drug-induced tumor lysis syndrome (TLS)?
a. Constipation
b. Nausea
c. 3+ Edema
d. Weakness

▶31. A patient is receiving rituximab. The nurse should teach the patient to report which symptoms?
a. Dizziness and throat tightness
b. Muscle aches and pains
c. Stomatitis and widespread rash
d. Vomiting and diarrhea

32. Which is true about the drug Zevalin?
a. Binds to receptors on T cells
b. Cell kill results largely from immune attack
c. The drug is linked with a radioactive isotope
d. Delivers a toxin that causes DNA damage

▶33. Teaching should include prompt reporting of abdominal pain, chest pain, shortness of breath, change in mental status, and blood in sputum when a patient is receiving which drug?
a. Bevacizumab
b. Bortezomib
c. Carfilzomib
d. Rituximab

34. Which is a symptom of the most common serious adverse effect of vorinostat?
a. Anorexia
b. Fatigue
c. Diarrhea
d. Dyspnea

35. The nurse is caring for a patient prescribed ipilimumab. The patient is now reporting weight gain, fatigue, and cold intolerance. Which adverse effect of ipilimumab is the patient likely experiencing?
a. Hypothyroid
b. Hyperthyroid
c. Cushing disease
d. Diabetes

36. To prevent some of the most common adverse effects of interferon alfa-2b, the nurse teaches the patient about administering which drugs?
a. Acetaminophen
b. Dexamethasone
c. Diphenhydramine
d. Ondansetron

*37. The oncology nurse has just completed infusing aldesleukin when the patient suddenly becomes short of breath. Which is the priority nursing action?
a. Assess the patient's vital signs.
b. Flush the intravenous (IV) line.
c. Elevate the head of the bed.
d. Notify the oncologist.

38. Which nursing action is included in preparation for administering bacillus of Calmette and Guérin (BCG) vaccine?
a. Accessing a central venous line
b. Assessing the IV site for patency
c. Inserting a urethral catheter
d. Identifying landmarks for intramuscular (IM) injection

39. The nurse teaches a patient receiving BCG vaccine to use precautions to protect from contamination with excreted urine for 6 hours following therapy, including cleaning the toilet with which solution?
a. Alcohol
b. Ammonia
c. Hypochlorite
d. Peroxide

*40. Which is the nursing priority when a patient is experiencing neuropsychiatric effects from interferon alfa-2b?
a. Completing drug therapy
b. Adherence with antidepressants
c. Establishing a support system
d. Preventing injury

DOSE CALCULATION QUESTION

41. A loading dose of cetuximab 800 mg via IV infusion is prescribed for a patient who is 5′10″ and 180 lb. The recommended dose is 400 mg/m^2. Is the prescribed dose safe and therapeutic?

CASE STUDY

Abiraterone and prednisone are prescribed for a patient with metastatic castration-resistant prostate cancer who was previously treated with docetaxel.

1. The nurse should teach the patient to report what symptoms of possible electrolyte imbalance?

2. What foods should the patient consume to avoid the risk of these imbalances?

3. What are possible effects of a decrease in glucocorticoid production?

4. What symptoms should the nurse teach the patient to report because they suggest possible liver damage from the abiraterone?

5. What OTC drug can rise to toxic levels if taken when prescribed this therapy? What are the possible effects?

109 Drugs for Eye Conditions and Diseases

STUDY QUESTIONS

Matching

Match the term or drug with its description.

1. ___ Produces mydriasis and cycloplegia
2. ___ Progressive optic nerve damage with eventual impairment of vision
3. ___ Contracts the ciliary muscle facilitating outflow of aqueous humor
4. ___ Decreases production of aqueous humor
5. ___ Dilates pupil by activating α_1-adrenergic receptors on the radial muscle of the iris
6. ___ Facilitates outflow of aqueous humor in part by relaxing the ciliary muscle; may increase pigmentation of the eyelid
7. ___ Maximally effective doses in systemic therapy reduce aqueous flow by 50%
8. ___ Inhibits the breakdown of acetylcholine, causing miosis and reduction of intraocular pressure (IOP)
9. ___ Paralysis of ciliary muscle
10. ___ Constriction of the pupil
11. ___ Widening of the pupil
12. ___ Administered intravenously (IV), in combination with other drugs, to produce rapid lowering of IOP in patients with acute angle-closure glaucoma
13. ___ May delay optic nerve degeneration and may protect retinal neurons from death
14. ___ May increase IOP rapidly and to dangerous levels
    a. Phenylephrine
    b. Brimonidine
    c. Anticholinergic drugs
    d. β-Adrenergic blocker
    e. Carbonic anhydrase inhibitor
    f. Muscarinic agonist
    g. Cholinesterase inhibitor
    h. Acute angle-closure glaucoma
    i. Cycloplegia
    j. Miosis
    k. Mydriasis
    l. Acetazolamide
    m. Primary open-angle glaucoma (POAG)
    n. Prostaglandin analog

Completion

15. Age-related macular degeneration (ARMD) causes blurring of ____________________ vision.
16. ____________________ are yellow deposits under the retina.
17. Vision loss occurs in advanced ______________ ARMD and ____________________ ARMD.
18. Patients who take vitamins to slow progression of ARMD should also ensure adequate intake of copper to prevent copper deficiency ____________.

CRITICAL THINKING, PRIORITIZATION, AND DELEGATION QUESTIONS

*19. Which is the priority nursing action for the prevention of blindness from POAG?
    a. Administer eye medications as ordered.
    b. Explain the importance of eye screening.
    c. Identify individuals at high risk for glaucoma.
    d. Teach the common symptoms of glaucoma.

*20. The nurse works in emergency department triage. Which patient would be priority for receiving care?
    a. Seeing halos around lights
    b. Experiencing itching eyes
    c. Sensitivity to bright sunlight
    d. Sudden onset severe eye pain

21. Even though systemic effects of topical timolol, echothiophate, and pilocarpine eye drops are uncommon, which finding would be a reason for the nurse to contact the provider before administering the drops? (**Select all that apply.**)
    a. Wheezing bilateral lung fields
    b. Blood pressure 170/100 mm Hg
    c. Clouding of lens of right eye
    d. Keyhole appearance to pupil
    e. Pulse 50 beats/min apically

22. Which is the priority nursing action if a brown discoloration of the iris is noted on a patient who has hazel eyes and is receiving latanoprost?
    a. Administer the medication.
    b. Assess for migraine symptoms.
    c. Teach proper contact hygiene.
    d. Withhold the medication.

23. It is important for the nurse to teach orthostatic precautions when a patient is prescribed which drug for POAG?
    a. Apraclonidine
    b. Bimatoprost
    c. Brimonidine
    d. Latanoprost

24. The nurse determines that the patient needs more teaching related to pilocarpine eye drops if the patient includes which issue in the list of things to be reported immediately to the ophthalmologist?
    a. Floaters in vision
    b. Halos around lights
    c. Flashes of light
    d. Painless loss of vision

25. The nurse is caring for a patient who is prescribed echothiophate. Which symptom would suggest possible development of cataracts? (**Select all that apply.**)
    a. Difficulty reading small print
    b. Eye pain when reading
    c. Floaters in visual field
    d. Halos around lights
    e. Discharge from eyes

26. A patient has been prescribed oral acetazolamide for refractory POAG; after starting the drug, they are experiencing the adverse effects of severe vomiting and diarrhea. Which is the priority nursing assessment?
    a. Hypercalcemia
    b. Hyperglycemia
    c. Hypokalemia
    d. Hypernatremia

►27. Which adverse effects of mydriatic drugs warrant withholding the drug and consulting the provider? (**Select all that apply.**)
    a. Blurred vision
    b. Headache
    c. Palpitations
    d. Sensitivity to light
    e. Sudden eye pain

28. The nurse can help decrease the progression of ARMD by providing which teaching to patients who are at risk?
    a. Have preventive iridectomy or laser iridotomy surgery.
    b. Use adequate lighting and assistive glasses when reading.
    c. Take high doses of vitamins C and E, beta-carotene, and zinc.
    d. Wear sunscreen and ultraviolet (UV)-protective sunglasses outdoors.

✳29. It is priority for the nurse to teach a patient who had a vitreous humor injection of ranibizumab to immediately seek medical care if which occurs?
    a. Blurred vision
    b. Conjunctival redness
    c. Halos around lights
    d. Light sensitivity

30. Patients who are prescribed verteporfin should be taught which information?
    a. Protect skin from sunlight.
    b. Assess for fever daily.
    c. Report eye discharge.
    d. Expect some ocular pain.

31. A patient asks the nurse what they might experience using the ocular decongestant tetrahydrozoline for allergic conjunctivitis. Which would be included in the nurse's explanation?
    a. Takes days to start to work.
    b. Eyes burn with overuse.
    c. It can cause cataracts.
    d. IOP can elevate with use.

DOSE CALCULATION QUESTIONS

32. Aflibercept 2 mg will be administered intravitreally every 8 weeks for your patient with neovascular ARMD. Available is 40 mg/mL. How much do you anticipate will be injected each week?

33. Acetazolamide 225 mg IV every 4 hours is ordered for your patient with acute angle closure. Available is 500 mg/5 mL. How many milliliters will be administered IV?

CASE STUDY

An older adult is seen by their ophthalmologist at the direction of their primary care provider. They have a history of chronic obstructive pulmonary disease, psoriasis, and colon cancer. The patient is accompanied by their adult child and is reluctant to seek care because their eyes are "fine." A topical anesthetic is placed in the eye, and the ophthalmologist measures IOP. It is 23 mm Hg. Tropicamide drops are applied, and the patient is sent to wait until mydriatic and cycloplegic effects occur.

1. What are mydriatic and cycloplegic effects, and what are their purposes in this situation?

2. After further examination, the patient is diagnosed with POAG. The adult child asks how their parent could have glaucoma and not be aware of it. How should the nurse respond?

3. The patient is prescribed latanoprost 1 drop to each eye at bedtime. The prescription is denied by the patient's insurer. The provider changes the order to betaxolol 1 drop in each eye twice a day. Why had the provider originally chosen latanoprost instead of betaxolol for this patient?

4. What teaching should the nurse provide the patient regarding the betaxolol prescription and their glaucoma?

5. The patient returns to the ophthalmologist to have their IOP checked. The IOP is at 25 mm Hg. The provider adds brimonidine 1 drop instilled in each eye three times a day and dorzolamide 1 drop three times a day. The patient asks why the provider did not just order the additional drops of latanoprost. How should the nurse respond?

6. What teaching should the nurse provide about therapy with brimonidine and dorzolamide?

110 Drugs for Skin Conditions

STUDY QUESTIONS

Completion

1. The ____________________ is the outermost layer of the skin.
2. All cells of the epidermis arise from the ________ ____________________.
3. The cytoplasm of dead epidermal cells is converted to ____________________.
4. The outer layer of the epidermis is called the stratum ____________________.
5. ____________________ determines skin color and protects the skin from damage from ultraviolet (UV) rays.
6. Blood vessels and nerves are found in the ____________________.
7. Sebaceous glands secrete an oily composite known as ____________________.
8. Subcutaneous tissue is primarily composed of ____________________.

Matching

Match the topical drug vehicle with its description

9. Good for inflamed or dry skin
10. Some may contain acids, which can cause burning
11. Provide highest medication absorption
12. Liquefy on contact and often have cooling effect as they dry
13. Can be used safely in areas that are occluded
14. Reduce friction between surfaces
15. Good choices for oily skin and large or hairy areas
    a. Pastes
    b. Powders
    c. Foams
    d. Gels
    e. Lotions
    f. Creams
    g. Ointments

CRITICAL THINKING, PRIORITIZATION, AND DELEGATION QUESTIONS

16. The nurse is teaching the parents of a 2½-year-old child about the administration of topical glucocorticoid therapy prescribed for their child's eczema. Which statement would suggest the need for further teaching?
    a. "Apply a thick film when using the cream."
    b. "I should not cover cream once applied."
    c. "Only apply cream to areas with the rash."
    d. "The cream can help stop the itching."

*17. A patient who was admitted for a knee replacement asks the nurse to get an order for "cortisone cream" because they have an irritated area of skin in their groin. Which is the priority nursing action?
    a. Explain proper use of cortisone.
    b. Apply the cream as requested.
    c. Keep area covered with cloth.
    d. Fully assess the area indicated.

*18. The nurse is teaching an adolescent about expected and adverse effects of applying salicylic acid. It is priority to teach the patient to report which symptom?
    a. Tinnitus
    b. Dry skin
    c. Headache
    d. Itching

19. A patient who has recently been prescribed benzoyl peroxide calls the telephone triage nurse in a dermatology office because they have begun experiencing scaling and swelling at the site of application. Which is the expected nursing response?
    a. Continue to use the benzoyl peroxide.
    b. Use the drug less often than before.
    c. Decrease amount of drug used.
    d. Stop using the benzoyl peroxide.

*20. When taking a history from a patient being seen for the first time for acne, it is a priority to alert the provider if the adolescent has a history of which condition?
    a. Asthma
    b. Obesity
    c. Diabetes
    d. Tendonitis

21. A late-middle-aged adult patient asks what the nurse can tell them about using tretinoin to prevent wrinkles. Which is true about tretinoin?
    a. Benefits in patients over 50 have not been established.
    b. It eliminates deep, coarse wrinkles caused by sun exposure.
    c. It enhances the gene that codes for collagen breakdown.
    d. It repairs damage to skin caused by chronic sun exposure.

22. A patient has been prescribed adapalene for acne. Which statement would the nurse include in teaching? (**Select all that apply.**)
    a. An increase in acne lesions is common early in therapy.
    b. Apply a sunscreen before applying adapalene cream.
    c. Expect a decrease in blackheads and inflamed lesions.
    d. Stop the drug if a burning sensation in the skin occurs.
    e. Use a sunscreen and wear protective clothing outdoors.

23. It is important to teach patients who have been prescribed azelaic acid to follow which directions when applying the cream? (**Select all that apply.**)
    a. Rub in until it disappears.
    b. Avoid contact with eyes.
    c. Apply only to affected areas.
    d. Use on every area that is red.
    e. Cover with transparent dressing.

24. A patient has been prescribed an oral contraceptive and spironolactone for treatment of acne that has been resistant to topical treatments. It is important to instruct the patient to report which symptom?
    a. Weakness and nausea
    b. Bone pain and constipation
    c. Cool, clammy skin
    d. Thirst and flushed skin

25. Which is the reason to use sunscreens that contain avobenzone?
    a. They are effective on prominent body parts such as the nose.
    b. They contains the only ingredient that absorbs UVA1 rays.
    c. They are currently available in a clear dry spray formula.
    d. They are most efficient in reflecting the sun's UV rays.

26. Which is the underlying causative factor of psoriasis?
    a. Autoimmune inflammatory disorder
    b. Excessive production of sebum
    c. Excessive production of keratinocytes
    d. Chronic exposure to excess sunlight

27. A patient asks the nurse why they should not use a high-potency glucocorticoid on their face. The basis of the nurse's response is that the face is especially prone to which effect of topical glucocorticoids?
    a. Acne-like eruptions
    b. Changes in pigmentation
    c. Sensitivity to sunlight
    d. Atrophy of the skin

28. A patient is admitted with fatigue, nausea, vomiting, and constipation. Lab test results include Na^+ 136 mEq/L, K^+ 3.5 mEq/L, and Ca^{++} 12 mg/dL. The nurse notes red patches with silvery, flaking scales on the patient's knees, elbows, and scalp. If treated with calcipotriene, it is important for the nurse to teach which point?
    a. Long-term use can cause hypernatremia.
    b. It may take a month for response to occur.
    c. There is no risk to fetal development.
    d. Calcipotriene also prevents sunburn.

29. A patient is prescribed anthralin. Which statement suggests a need for additional teaching?
    a. "I need to wash my hands after application."
    b. "It is best if I put the cream on at bedtime."
    c. "I need to cover the cream with a bandage."
    d. "If the area becomes red, I need to call my PCP."

30. Which laboratory result for a patient who is receiving methotrexate as treatment for psoriasis would be of most concern to the nurse?
    a. Alanine aminotransferase (ALT) 35 IU/L
    b. Hemoglobin (Hgb) 12 g/dL
    c. Platelet count $2000/mm^3$
    d. White blood cell (WBC) count $9000/mm^3$

31. Ustekinumab should be used with caution in a person with a history of which condition?
    a. Bipolar disorder
    b. Osteoarthritis
    c. Hypothyroidism
    d. Latent tuberculosis

*32. Which is the priority nursing education to prevent squamous cell carcinoma?
    a. Avoid chronic exposure of the skin to sunlight.
    b. Examine moles for irregular borders.
    c. Report rough, scaly, red-brown papules.
    d. Use sunscreen when out in sunlight.

33. The nurse in a long-term care facility is administering topical fluorouracil to actinic keratosis lesions. Which assessment suggests that therapy has achieved the desired effect and treatment can be stopped?
    a. Burning and vesicle formation
    b. Complete healing of lesion
    c. Erosion, ulceration, and necrosis
    d. Severe inflammation and stinging

34. Which is an important teaching point for patients using diclofenac gel?
   a. Minimize exposure to sunlight.
   b. Cover area with occlusive dressing.
   c. Discontinue treatment if redness occurs.
   d. The medications may stain clothing.

*35. Which laboratory result for a 27-year-old patient, who has an appointment to receive podophyllum for genital warts, would be most important for the nurse to report to the gynecologist administering the treatment?
   a. ALT 35 IU/L
   b. hCG positive
   c. Hgb 14 g/dL
   d. WBC $5000/mm^3$

36. Which is the principle of seborrheic dermatitis treatment?
   a. Cessation of microbial cellular reproduction
   b. Treatment of inflammation caused by yeast
   c. Reduction of cellular histamine release
   d. Increased scalp oil production soothing dry skin

DOSE CALCULATION QUESTIONS

37. Infliximab 150 mg is prescribed. The drug is diluted in 250 mL of 0.9% NaCl to be infused over 3 hours. What is the rate of infusion in milliliters per hour?

38. Ustekinumab is supplied in a solution of 45 mg/0.5 mL. Prescribed is 90 mg. What is the correct dosage?

CASE STUDIES

Case Study 1

The nurse identifies that body image is a priority concern when collecting data from a patient who is being seen in the dermatology practice. The patient has heard of using tretinoin to prevent aging of the skin. The patient asks if this drug really works.

1. What information can the nurse provide?

2. The patient is concerned about cost and asks if tretinoin is better than face creams that you can buy in the drugstore. What does research suggest on this topic?

3. The patient and provider agree that tretinoin is appropriate for this patient. What information can the nurse provide when the patient asks how this differs from the tretinoin prescribed for their child's acne?

4. What teaching should the nurse provide about use of tretinoin products?

5. The patient reports that they have always used a sunscreen of at least SPF 30 and reapply it regularly because they enjoy activities out in the sun. What teaching about skin protection should the nurse provide to this patient?

Case Study 2

A high school senior is being seen at the dermatology office after treatment with antibiotics, benzoyl peroxide, tretinoin, and adapalene over the past 2 years has failed to provide acceptable control of acne.

6. What data needs to be collected when the provider is considering treatment with isotretinoin?

7. The dermatologist has decided to prescribe isotretinoin and has asked the office nurse to reinforce teaching regarding this drug. What are some patient problems that should be included when planning teaching relating to this patient, diagnosis, and treatment?

8. How should the nurse respond to the patient's question of how isotretinoin therapy differs from tretinoin?

9. Because patients do not always remember what is explained to them, what teaching methods besides oral explanation should the nurse provide to this patient?

10. What teaching must the nurse provide this patient regarding the iPLEDGE program?

111 Drugs for Ear Conditions

STUDY QUESTIONS

Completion

1. The visible outside part of the ear is called the __________________ or __________________.

2. The auditory canal and auricle make up the __________________ __________________.

3. The malleus, incus, and stapes transmit sound vibrations from the __________________ to the __________________ ear.

4. The __________________ __________________ allows air pressure within the middle ear to equalize with air pressure in the environment.

5. The __________________ __________________ provide our sense of balance.

True or False

For each of the following statements, enter T for true or F for false.

6. ___ Cerumen should be removed from the auditory canal every time we bathe.

7. ___ Acute otitis media (AOM) can be caused by blockage of the eustachian tube.

8. ___ Presence of ear pain (otalgia) suggests serious complications have occurred.

9. ___ In an otherwise healthy child with AOM, it is more important to treat the pain than the infecting microbe.

10. ___ AOM primarily occurs in children aged 5–12 years.

CRITICAL THINKING, PRIORITIZATION, AND DELEGATION QUESTIONS

11. The nurse is caring for a 2-year-old child. When bathing the child, the nurse notes sticky, crusting exudate filling the right external ear canal. The nurse would use which term when documenting this finding?
    a. Otalgia
    b. Otitis media
    c. Otorrhea
    d. Otosclerosis

12. Which assessment finding in a child receiving amoxicillin would be a reason for the parent to contact the provider?
    a. Allergy to clarithromycin
    b. Frequent brown diarrhea
    c. Maculopapular facial rash
    d. Multiple intensely itchy hives

13. Which is the most significant reason why prophylactic antibiotic therapy for recurrent otitis media is not currently recommended?
    a. Antibiotic resistance
    b. Adverse drug effects
    c. Cost of antibiotics
    d. Parenteral choice

14. Which is recommended for acute otitis externa?
    a. Tartaric acid
    b. Citric acid
    c. Salicylic acid
    d. Acetic acid

15. The nurse works telephone triage in a primary care office. A patient calls reporting ear pain. Which information would warrant the patient being seen immediately? (**Select all that apply.**)
    a. Elderly diabetic patient
    b. Immunocompromised patient
    c. Pain when touching the outer ear
    d. Purulent otic discharge
    e. Cleans ear canal with cotton swabs

16. Which vaccination has been shown to decrease the risk of AOM?
    a. Diphtheria and tetanus toxoids and acellular pertussis (DTaP) vaccine
    b. Mumps, measles, rubella (MMR) vaccine
    c. Oral polio vaccine (OPV)
    d. Pneumococcal conjugate vaccine (PCV)

17. Amoxicillin-clavulanate is used for antibiotic-resistant AOM because the clavulanate
    a. Allows for a lower dose of amoxicillin.
    b. Decreases incidence of adverse effects.
    c. Increases antibacterial action against *Streptococcus pneumoniae.*
    d. Prevents destruction of the antibiotic by bacterial enzymes.

DOSE CALCULATION QUESTIONS

18. A child who was born prematurely and weighs 10 lb at 3 months is prescribed amoxicillin 200 mg to be administered twice a day for AOM. The pharmacy supplies an oral suspension of 250 mg/mL. How much amoxicillin should be administered?

19. Amoxicillin 750 mg is prescribed for a 38-kg child. How many milliliters should be administered if the drug is available as 500 mg/10 mL?

NEXT-GENERATION NCLEX SINGLE-EPISODE CASE STUDY

Health History	Nurse's Notes	Physician's Orders	Laboratory Profile

Time, military: 1045

Parent brings 6-month-old to the pediatric clinic for evaluation of fever. When the infant was picked up from daycare yesterday, they were fussy and difficult to feed and put down for the night. They woke up frequently during the night but wanted comforting more than feeding. The parent states the infant kept tugging their left ear. This morning, the infant was more groggy than usual and refused to eat. The parents took a temperature, which read 102.5°F rectally. They did not treat and immediately called for an appointment at that time.

Further questioning reveals the infant came home from daycare 2 weeks ago with a cough and runny nose with clear drainage. Symptoms resolved in a little over 24 hours with acetaminophen elixir. Additionally, during that same time, the infant's grandparent had come for a short visit, and the grandparent smokes about two packs per day. The infant has had no vomiting or diarrhea. They have not been on any recent antibiotics and have not had any ear surgeries or frequent ear infections.

On exam, the infant is lethargic but does arouse to tactile stimuli and become fussy and begin pulling on left ear. Lungs are clear to auscultation. Heart with regular rate and rhythm. Abdomen soft and nontender. There is no lymphadenopathy. Sclera are clear, and eyes are without crusting or drainage. Nose without crusting. Septum midline. Clear drainage present. Oropharynx with pink mucus membranes. Right ear canal free of erythema or edema, tympanic membrane without edema or redness, light reflex present. Left ear canal with erythema present, no edema. Tympanic membrane dull red with mild bulging. No light reflex. Infant cries when pinna is pulled down.

Vital signs: rectal temperature 103.0°F, heart rate 160 beats per minute, respirations 40 breaths per minute, blood pressure 65/45 mm Hg, oxygen saturation 98% on room air. Height is 26.5 inches, and weight is 16 pounds.

The nurse anticipates which treatment, adhering to the American Academy of Pediatrics guidelines? (Select all that apply. One, some, or all may apply).

a. Topical 2% lidocaine eardrops, 3 drops left ear 4 times a day for 7 days
b. Acetaminophen 72.5 mg every 4 hours as needed for pain
c. Begin amoxicillin 290 mg every 12 hours for 10 days
d. Recommend annual influenza vaccination
e. Recommend the pneumococcal conjugate vaccine
f. Call if symptoms persist or worsen in 48 hours
g. Clindamycin 60.5 mg every 8 hours
h. Antipyrine-benzocaine otic 3 drops every 2 hours for 3 days

112 Management of Poisoning

STUDY QUESTIONS

Matching

Match the chelating agent and the metal(s) it binds with. (**Select all that apply.**)

1. ___ Arsenic
2. ___ Copper
3. ___ Ethylene glycol
4. ___ Gold
5. ___ Iron
6. ___ Lead
7. ___ Mercury

a. Deferoxamine
b. Dimercaprol
c. Edetate calcium disodium
d. Fomepizole
e. Penicillamine
f. Succimer

CRITICAL THINKING, PRIORITIZATION, AND DELEGATION QUESTIONS

*8. Which is the priority nursing intervention for a patient with a suspected ingestion of a poison?
a. Administering an antidote
b. Supporting respirations
c. Identifying the poison
d. Preventing drug absorption

9. A person with an unknown medical history arrives at the emergency department (ED) after ingesting an unidentified poison. The patient is comatose when arriving at the ED. An intravenous (IV) line of normal saline is infusing, respirations are unlabored at 17 breaths per minute, and blood pressure (BP) is 118/72 mm Hg. Which assessment findings suggest hypoglycemia? (**Select all that apply.**)
a. Capillary refill 2–3 seconds
b. Diaphoresis
c. Deep tendon reflex (DTR) 2+
d. Dry mucous membranes
e. Pulse 115 beats/min

10. The nurse knows which is the most accurate and efficient method of identifying the poison?
a. Analysis of gastric contents
b. Assessment of symptoms
c. Examining the container
d. Interviewing the caregiver

11. Which is the purpose of an antidote to a poison?
a. Increase renal excretion of the poison.
b. Prevent absorption of the poison.
c. Remove residual poison from stomach.
d. Counteract the effects of a poison.

12. Activated charcoal is most effective in binding with poisons in the gastrointestinal (GI) tract and preventing absorption when administered in which manner?
a. After the patient has vomited
b. Only with fat-soluble poisons
c. Within 30 minutes of poison ingestion
d. With milk or other lactose product

►13. The nurse is assessing a 3-year-old patient who is receiving 0.5 L/h of polyethylene glycol via a nasogastric tube after having ingested 60 tablets of an adult iron supplement. Which is the most concerning assessment finding?
a. BP 80/52 mm Hg
b. Dark brown emesis
c. Pulse 120 beats/min
d. 475 mL of liquid stool

14. A child has ingested several bottles of 81-mg chewable aspirin. The ED resident informs the nurse that treatment will include enhancing renal excretion of the drug. The nurse would question all but which order?
a. Acetic acid
b. Ammonium chloride
c. Citric acid
d. Sodium bicarbonate

▶15. A patient has been placed on hemoperfusion to remove poison from their body. The nurse should monitor the patient for which symptom?
   a. Bleeding
   b. Dehydration
   c. Hyperglycemia
   d. Seizures

16. Which is the mechanism of action of deferoxamine?
   a. Binds to iron in the blood
   b. Accelerates iron metabolism
   c. Facilitates excretion of iron
   d. Reverses effects of iron toxicity

▶17. A nurse assesses the vital signs of a patient who is being treated for ferric iron poisoning with IV deferoxamine. Which finding suggests that the administration rate of the drug might be too rapid?
   a. BP 150/85 mm Hg
   b. Pulse 112 beats/min
   c. Respirations 15/min
   d. Temperature 100.4°F (38°C)

18. The nurse is teaching a patient who has been prescribed deferasirox for iron overload associated with β-thalassemia. Which statement suggests a need for additional instruction?
   a. "I need to have bloodwork done to ensure my kidneys are okay."
   b. "I need to crush the tablet and mix it with a full glass of juice."
   c. "I should stop taking this drug if I have a fever higher than 99°F."
   d. "If I take this with a drug for heartburn, it won't be absorbed."

19. Which would be an appropriate technique when the nurse is administering dimercaprol?
   a. Deep injection into the dorsogluteal muscle
   b. Subcutaneous injection into abdominal fat
   c. Subcutaneous injection above the vastus lateralis
   d. Deep injection into the ventrogluteal muscle

20. The nurse is caring for a 3-year-old child who weighs 15 kg and is scheduled to receive an intramuscular dose of calcium EDTA for lead poisoning. The child's urinary output has averaged 15 mL/h for the last 4 hours. Which is the appropriate nursing action?
   a. Administer the drug.
   b. Consult the provider.
   c. Withhold the medication.
   d. Assess for kidney failure.

21. The nurse would withhold calcium EDTA and contact the provider for which laboratory result?
   a. Albumin 5 g/dL
   b. Amylase 190 IU/L
   c. Protein total 8.3 g/dL
   d. Protein in urine 287 mg/dL

▶22. It is most important for the nurse to monitor the results of which laboratory test when caring for a patient with Wilson disease who is receiving penicillamine?
   a. Alanine aminotransferase
   b. Blood urea nitrogen
   c. Complete blood count
   d. Total bilirubin

23. A child who was admitted after ingesting antifreeze is treated with fomepizole. Which symptom suggests that the child's body is attempting to compensate for metabolic acidosis?
   a. Decreased urine output
   b. Increased urine output
   c. Rapid, deep respirations
   d. Shallow breathing

24. The nurse teaches parents that dialing 1-800-222-1222 will connect them with which service?
   a. A local poison center
   b. The national poison center
   c. A pharmacist
   d. A specially trained nurse

DOSE CALCULATION QUESTIONS

25. Your 56-kg patient is receiving a 15 mg/kg loading dose of fomepizole. How many milligrams should be administered? How many milliliters should be withdrawn and diluted with 100 mL normal saline? How many milliliters per hour should be programmed into the infusion pump?

26. Calcium EDTA 1 ampule is diluted in 500 mL of normal saline solution. It is to be infused in 90 minutes. What rate in milliliters per hour should be programmed into the IV pump?

CASE STUDY

A 4-year-old who has been playing outside in their yard comes into the house and says they do not feel well. The parents notice a purple stain on their child's face. Knowing that they do not have any grape juice in the house, the parents ask their child what they have eaten. The child tells them about some berries they found in the yard. The parents call the poison control center, and the child is rushed to the ED.

1. When the nurse questions the parents, they describe "weeds" growing at the back of the yard with blueberry-size purple berries that their child may have ingested. What should be done to identify the ingested substance?

2. The stomach contents contain a neurotoxin. What data can the nurse collect to assist the emergency physician with deciding if charcoal, gastric lavage, or whole-bowel irrigation is the best approach for this poisoning?

3. The parents are sure that the ingestion of the poison occurred less than 30 minutes ago. Gastric lavage and aspiration are ordered. What is the nurse's role?

4. Why is the child positioned on the left side with their head down?

5. The child is stabilized and observed overnight. What instruction should the nurse provide this family before discharge?

113 Potential Weapons of Biologic, Radiologic, and Chemical Terrorism

STUDY QUESTIONS

True or False

For each of the following statements, enter T for true or F for false.

1. ___ Anthrax spores can live outside of a host for many years.
2. ___ Inhalation anthrax can cause hemorrhage and inflammation of the meninges of the brain.
3. ___ Approximately 20% of patients who contract cutaneous anthrax die despite antibiotic therapy.
4. ___ Raxibacumab neutralizes deadly anthrax toxins in humans.
5. ___ Antibiotic treatment of cutaneous anthrax is not likely to prevent cutaneous lesions.
6. ___ Anthrax vaccination can be administered before and immediately after exposure.
7. ___ Bubonic plague is not transmitted from person to person.
8. ___ Smallpox vaccine involves pricking the skin with the live virus.
9. ___ Early treatment with antibiotics is often effective when treating smallpox.

CRITICAL THINKING, PRIORITIZATION, AND DELEGATION QUESTIONS

*10. Which symptom would be a priority to report to the provider if a patient is suspected of being exposed to *Bacillus anthracis?*
   a. Blurred vision
   b. Diarrhea
   c. Hemoptysis
   d. Malaise

11. Which statement, if made by a patient receiving ciprofloxacin for cutaneous anthrax, would indicate understanding of drug therapy teaching?
   a. "I must take all of the drug as directed or I could die."
   b. "I should take the antibiotic until the scabs fall off."
   c. "If I start the drug now, I will not have itchy vesicles."
   d. "My prescription needs to be changed if I get pregnant."

12. The community health nurse, who works in areas known to have *B. anthracis*, promotes routine vaccination with anthrax vaccine for people with which occupation?
   a. Police officer
   b. Postal worker
   c. Receptionist
   d. Sheep farmer

▶13. Intramuscular streptomycin 0.5 g twice a day is prescribed for a 150-lb male who has been diagnosed with tularemia. Nursing assessments before administration of the drug include blood pressure (BP) 140/72 mm Hg, pulse 88 beats/min, respirations 24/min, moist cough, and end-inspiratory crackles in upper lobes. Which intervention should the nurse implement?
   a. Call the provider about the low dose.
   b. Administer the drug as ordered.
   c. Wear a high-efficiency particulate mask.
   d. Inject drug in the dorsogluteal muscle.

14. A patient is admitted with a diagnosis of pneumonic plague. Which precaution would be best to prevent spread of this infection?
   a. Contact precautions
   b. Droplet precautions
   c. Universal precautions
   d. Airborne precautions

15. Which symptoms suggest a smallpox infection?
   a. Headache, high fever, chills, and rigors
   b. Multiple red spots on tongue and buccal mucosa
   c. Painless ulcers with necrotic core and eschar
   d. Tender, enlarged, inflamed lymph nodes

16. The public health nurse is administering smallpox vaccine to police officers. Which statement would indicate a need for further teaching?
   a. "I should keep the site covered to avoid spreading the live vaccine."
   b. "I should seek medical care if any drainage occurs from the site."
   c. "I should not get pregnant for at least 4 weeks after vaccination."
   d. "This vaccination is effective even if I was exposed yesterday."

17. The Department of Health and Human Services has contracted to buy the modified vaccinia virus Ankara (MVA) instead of ACAM2000 in case of a terrorist attack with smallpox. Which is the reason MVA has been chosen?
    a. It is safe for immunocompromised people.
    b. It does not have a risk of postvaccine encephalitis.
    c. It is the only drug approved by the FDA.
    d. It is less expensive and more effective than Dryvax.

18. The nurse is preparing to vaccinate a patient who has been exposed to the smallpox virus. The patient states that she is pregnant. Which is the appropriate nursing action?
    a. Administer the vaccine.
    b. Administer cidofovir first.
    c. Assess risk versus benefits.
    d. Withhold the vaccine.

▶ 19. Which is the priority patient problem when caring for a patient with botulism poisoning?
    a. Decreased gas exchange
    b. Decreased mobility
    c. Aspiration
    d. Altered vision

20. The nurse is providing emergency care after a disaster at a nuclear power plant that caused the release of radioactive material. Which dose of potassium iodide should be administered to a patient who breastfeeds her infant?
    a. None
    b. 65 mg daily
    c. 130 mg daily
    d. 195 mg daily

21. Which statement, if made by a patient who has been prescribed pentetate calcium trisodium therapy for americium poisoning, would suggest understanding of teaching?
    a. "I can't take these drugs if my kidneys don't work."
    b. "I need to take a pill daily for at least 2 months."
    c. "I should drink 100 ounces of fluid each day."
    d. "I should try to empty my bladder every 8 hours."

22. The nurse knows that adverse effects of Prussian blue increase the risk of toxicity of which medication?
    a. Acetaminophen
    b. Atenolol
    c. Digoxin
    d. Furosemide

DOSE CALCULATION QUESTIONS

23. A female has potassium iodide 65-mg tablets. Their 2½-year-old daughter is exposed to radiation. How many tablets should she administer if the recommended dose is 32 mg?

24. A 47-lb 6-year-old child requires treatment with pentetate zinc trisodium. The provider orders 300 mg intravenous (IV) daily. Is this dose safe and effective?

NEXT-GENERATION NCLEX SINGLE-EPISODE CASE STUDY

A military nurse is participating in a drill imitating exposure to mustard gas released into the air over an Army camp. The nurse assesses three patients as they arrive to assign treatment categories.

Patient 1:

HEALTH HISTORY	NURSE'S NOTES	PHYSICIAN'S ORDERS	LABORATORY PROFILE

1450:

Patient 1 received via litter. Exposure is reported to have occurred 3 hours ago. Medics reported the patient is incontinent of stool and has repeatedly vomited during transport. Patient went through decontamination outside facility.

Patient is lying on their side in fetal position, grimacing and rocking back and forth. Patient is alert and oriented. Erythema visible on neck. Sclera clear. Lungs clear to auscultation. Heart regular rate and rhythm without murmur. Abdomen with diffuse tenderness and pain with deep palpation. Hyperactive bowel sounds throughout.

Patient takes no routine medications.

Vital signs: BP 102/66, heart rate 108 beats per minute, respirations 12 breaths per minute, temperature 102°F, oxygen saturation 98% on room air. Pain, 9 out of 10 on a scale of 0 to 10.

Patient 2:

HEALTH HISTORY	NURSE'S NOTES	PHYSICIAN'S ORDERS	LABORATORY PROFILE

1455:

Patient 2 received via litter. Exposure is reported to have occurred 3 hours ago. Medics reported the patient has been rubbing their eyes and crying during transport. Patient went through decontamination outside facility.

Patient is lying on their side with pillow covering their face.

Patient is alert and oriented. Eyes begin to water copiously when pillow is removed, and patient immediately covers eyes with hands. Refuses ocular examination. Reports blurred vision. Lungs clear to auscultation. Heart regular rate and rhythm without murmur. Abdomen soft and nontender; normoactive bowel sounds throughout.

Vital signs: BP 122/76, heart rate 115 beats per minute, respirations 14 breaths per minute, temperature 99.2°F, oxygen saturation 98% on room air. Pain, 8 out of 10 on a scale of 0 to 10.

Patient 3:

HEALTH HISTORY	NURSE'S NOTES	PHYSICIAN'S ORDERS	LABORATORY PROFILE

1500:

Patient 3 received via litter. Exposure is reported to have occurred a little over 3 hours ago. Medics reported the patient has been sneezing and coughing during transport. Patient went through decontamination outside facility.

Patient is lying in bed, alert and oriented. Voice is hoarse. Becomes dyspneic when answering questions.

Eyes are watery, sclera are clear. Lungs with expiratory wheezing throughout on auscultation. Heart regular rate and rhythm without murmur. Abdomen soft and nontender; normoactive bowel sounds throughout.

Vital signs: BP 135/76, heart rate 110 beats per minute, respirations 18 breaths per minute, temperature 99.5°F, oxygen saturation 93% on room air. Pain, 4 out of 10 on a scale of 0 to 10.

For each patient finding below, mark to specify if the finding is consistent with dermal contact, respiratory exposure, or ingestion of mustard gas.

ASSESSMENT FINDING	DERMAL CONTACT	RESPIRATORY EXPOSURE	INGESTION
Wheezing			
Photophobia			
Fever			
Vomiting			
Blurred vision			

Answer Key

Answers to the Case Studies can be reviewed online at http://evolve.elsevier.com/Lehne/.

CHAPTER 1

1. b
2. d
3. c
4. a
5. Selectivity
6. Low cost
7. Reversible action
8. Freedom from interactions
9. Possession of a simple generic name
10. Effectiveness
11. Ease of administration
12. Safety
13. Chemical stability
14. Predictability
15. c (Tingling around the mouth indicates allergic reaction, which is the priority over all the other patients.)
16. a (While all actions help to meet the therapeutic objective in some way, the BEST is to assess a patient for adverse drug reactions when taking a new drug.)
17. c

CHAPTER 2

1. d
2. b
3. f
4. h
5. c
6. a
7. e
8. g
9. b
10. d (Suggests possible anaphylactic reaction.)
11. c
12. d (This is the priority nursing diagnosis based on safety factors.)
13. b (These assessments are a priority, as well as being needed to determine if prescribed pain medication can safely be administered.)
14. d

CHAPTER 3

1. a
2. h
3. e
4. c
5. g
6. f
7. b
8. d
9. Generic
10. Chemical
11. Generic
12. Brand
13. Generic
14. Generic

Next-Generation NCLEX Item Type: Matrix Multiple Choice

Cognitive Skill: Recognize Cues

The nurse admits a patient with a history of hypertension, coronary artery disease, diabetes, and osteoporosis. While completing drug reconciliation, the nurse notes the patient's drug list has some drugs by generic name and others by brand name. The nurse knows this is a problem and can lead to drug duplication.

Click to specify which drug is listed by its generic name and which is listed by its brand name.

DRUG	GENERIC NAME	BRAND NAME
Diovan		x
simvastatin	x	
hydrochlorothiazide	x	
Plavix		x
aspirin	x	
Glucophage		x
Aleve		x

Rationale: simvastatin, hydrochlorothiazide, and aspirin are generic names (note: they all begin with lowercase letters); Diovan, Plavix, Glucophage, and Aleve are brand names (note: they all begin with uppercase letters).

15. d
16. b, c
17. a
18. c
19. b, c, d, e

CHAPTER 4

1. e
2. c
3. b
4. f
5. a
6. d
7. c
8. a
9. b
10. T
11. F
12. T
13. T
14. F
15. T
16. F
17. F
18. T
19. F
20. T
21. F
22. T
23. T
24. T
25. F
26. T
27. d (Continued administration of morphine would lead to respiratory arrest.)
28. b (Since the nurse has realized the error just after administration, assessment for excessive bleeding is not a priority as of yet; the incident report would be completed after provider notification; routine assessment for deep vein thrombosis [DVT] would continue as scheduled.)
29. a (Insulin administered into the muscle will be absorbed faster, leading to a more rapid drop in blood glucose.)
30. c (An estimated glomerular filtration rate [eGFR] at 30 mL/min suggests kidney disease; normal eGFR is 60 mL/min or higher.)
31. a (Most general anesthetics are excreted by exhalation.)
32. b, c, d
33. b
34. d

CHAPTER 5

1. T
2. F
3. T
4. T
5. T
6. T
7. F
8. F
9. T
10. T
11. F
12. T
13. F
14. T
15. a
16. a, d
17. b, d, e (Morphine can cause respiratory depression, confusion, dizziness, and constipation.)
18. b
19. a

NGN Stand-Alone Item Type: Bowtie

HEALTH HISTORY	NURSE'S NOTES	PHYSICIAN'S ORDERS	LABORATORY PROFILE

Time: 1040 hrs
A patient comes to the emergency department with decreased level of consciousness and severely depressed respirations. The person accompanying the patient reported finding an empty bottle of methadone HCL, an opiate, next to the patient. The patient has a history of heroin use disorder and is treated at a nearby rehabilitation center. They also have a history of alcohol use disorder and vape. Vital signs: temperature 97.6°F, pulse 48, blood pressure 92/60, respirations 6 and shallow, and oxygen saturation 80% on room air. Pupils are pinpoint. Skin is pale and clammy. Glucose level 154.

After reviewing the electronic health record (EHR), complete the Bowtie chart, selecting the nursing actions to take, the potential condition, and parameters to monitor.

Action to Take: Administer naloxone	Potential Condition: Overdose	Parameter to Monitor: Level of consciousness
Action to Take: Place on Oxygen at 2–4 liters per nasal canula		Parameter to Monitor: Respirations

NURSING ACTIONS	POTENTIAL CONDITIONS	PARAMETERS TO MONITOR
Position on left side	Alcohol intoxication	Pain
Administer naloxone	Overdose	Blood pressure
Elevate head of bed	Hypoglycemia	Level of consciousness
Place on oxygen at 2–4 L per NC	Hypoxia	Respirations
Perform CPR	Head injury	Heroin drug level

Rationale: The patient is experiencing a methadone overdose. The actions to take are to administer an agent that blocks receptors for morphine and related opioids (naloxone). Additionally, due to the low oxygen saturation, O_2 should be administered. Following the administration of naloxone, patients should be monitored for recurrent symptoms (altered mental status, respiratory depression, and shock).

The patient is not experiencing alcohol intoxication, and their blood sugar is high, not low, while they are experiencing hypoxia; their overall condition, based on presented symptoms, is overdose; there is no overt history to suggest a head injury.

Placing the patient on their left side is not priority during overdose, and neither is elevating the head of bed (HOB); the patient has a pulse of 48, so CPR is not indicated. The parameters to monitor should relate to the nursing actions taken. Monitoring pain, BP, and heroin levels do not.

CHAPTER 6

1. T
2. F
3. T
4. T
5. T
6. T
7. a (Combining metronidazole and alcohol leads to acetaldehyde syndrome manifested by nausea, copious vomiting, flushing, palpitations, headache, sweating, thirst, chest pain, weakness, blurred vision, and hypotension; blood pressure may ultimately decline to shock levels.)
8. b
9. c
10. d (By inhibiting the effects of clopidogrel, the use of omeprazole can lead to reduced antiplatelet effects and increase the risk of recurrent myocardial infraction [MI].)
11. d (Levels of phenytoin may increase, leading to toxicity.)
12. c
13. c
14. a

CHAPTER 7

1. c
2. e
3. b
4. f
5. a
6. d
7. Physically dependent
8. Allergic
9. Carcinogenic
10. Teratogenic
11. Side effects
12. Idiosyncratic
13. Iatrogenic
14. Toxicity
15. d
16. a, d, e
17. c (Suggests possible anaphylactic reaction; need order for epinephrine.)
18. d
19. c (Statins can cause hepatotoxicity; liver injury is evidenced by elevations in serum transaminase levels [levels presented are roughly threefold increased].)
20. a
21. d
22. b
23. c
24. b
25. a
26. d

CHAPTER 8

1. Body surface area
2. Increase
3. Bioavailability
4. Tachyphylaxis
5. Bleeding
6. Intense; longer
7. d
8. d (Tolerance to nitroglycerin-induced vasodilation can develop over the course of a single day; the provider must be contacted to determine when the patch should be reapplied once the previous patch has been removed.)
9. a (Acidic drugs ionize in alkaline media.)
10. c (This is a sign of hypokalemia.)
11. d
12. b

CHAPTER 9

1. F
2. T

3. F
4. T
5. T
6. F
7. T
8. T
9. a, b, d, e
10. c
11. c
12. c
13. b
14. d
15. b

CHAPTER 10

1. F
2. T
3. T
4. T
5. T
6. F
7. T
8. T
9. F
10. T
11. e
12. c
13. b
14. a
15. d
16. b
17. a, b, e
18. a, b, d
19. c
20. b, c

CHAPTER 11

1. T
2. F
3. T
4. F
5. T
6. F
7. T
8. T
9. F
10. T
11. d
12. f
13. a
14. g
15. b
16. c
17. h
18. e
19. d
20. a, b
21. b
22. c
23. c

CHAPTER 12

1. F
2. T
3. T
4. F
5. T
6. F
7. d
8. f
9. a
10. c
11. b
12. e
13. a, c, d
14. c (Normal respiratory rate for a newborn is 30–60 respirations per minute; a respiratory rate of 22/min is depressed.)
15. a
16. a
17. b
18. a
19. 227 mg is calculated safe dose. Yes, 225 mg is safe.
20. 4.5 mL

CHAPTER 13

1. F
2. T
3. F
4. F
5. T
6. T
7. F
8. T
9. T
10. c (Creatinine clearance is a more precise test used to help detect and diagnose kidney dysfunction.)
11. a
12. d (Increased risk of GI bleeding with long-term use in the geriatric patient.)
13. b (Prazosin can cause orthostatic hypotension and falls in older adults.)
14. c (Is an indicator of severe urinary retention requiring catheterization.)
15. b
16. a, b, c
17. b

CHAPTER 14

1. i
2. f
3. b
4. c
5. d
6. a

7. e
8. h
9. g
10. T
11. F
12. T
13. F
14. F
15. T
16. b
17. d
18. a, c, d
19. b

CHAPTER 15

1. e
2. b
3. d
4. c
5. a
6. Skeletal muscle
7. Pupillary constriction; focuses eye
8. Bronchodilation; respiratory rate
9. Slowing
10. Motility (peristalsis); digestion
11. Emptying (voiding)
12. Skeletal muscle
13. Baroreceptor reflex
14. Parasympathetic nervous system
15. c (Compensatory sympathetic nervous system response.)
16. b
17. a (Inhaled cholinesterase inhibitors cause wheezing and chest tightness and increased nasal and pulmonary secretions, causing cough.)
18. d (Anticholinergic side effects include urinary retention.)
19. b (All of the options are side effects of doxazosin; however, the priority is dizziness—it is a sign of hypotension; doxazosin has a significant side effect of orthostatic hypotension, which can lead to falls.)
20. c (While norepinephrine does bind to B2 receptors, it does so very poorly.)
21. a (Tamsulosin may increase the risk of cataract surgery-related complications due to relaxation of the smooth muscles of the iris.)
22. b (While all options are a side effect of monoamine oxidases [MAOs], monitoring blood pressure is the priority, as failure to adhere to dietary restrictions can trigger a hypertensive crisis.)

CHAPTER 16

a. Administer
b. Consult
c. Consult
d. Consult
e. Administer
f. Consult
g. Administer
h. Administer
i. Consult
j. Consult
2. c, e
3. b (Prominent symptoms of muscarinic poisoning are profuse salivation, lacrimation [tearing], visual disturbances, bronchospasm, diarrhea, bradycardia, and hypotension. Severe poisoning can produce cardiovascular collapse.)
4. b
5. c, d, e
6. c
7. 4 tablets

CHAPTER 17

a. Consult
b. Consult
c. Administer
d. Consult
e. Consult
f. Consult
g. Consult
2. a (Treatment consists of [1] minimizing intestinal absorption of the antimuscarinic agent, and [2] administering an antidote. Minimizing absorption is accomplished by administering activated charcoal, which will absorb the poison within the intestine, thereby preventing its absorption into the blood.)
3. b, d, e
4. d
5. a
6. d (Compared with other drugs for overactive bladder, trospium is notable for its low bioavailability, lack of central nervous system effects, and lack of metabolism-related interactions with other drugs.)
7. c (The combination of these drugs alters drug metabolism, increasing darifenacin and nevirapine levels, increasing the risk of adverse effects.)
8. b, c, d
9. a, c
10. a
11. a, e
12. c
13. b (Patients should wash their hands immediately after application of oxybutynin topical.)
14. 5-mL dose
    a. 0.1 mg is safe dose
    b. 0.2 mL dose

CHAPTER 18

1. f
2. e
3. b
4. g
5. a
6. d
7. c
8. h
9. b

10. a, e
11. a, b
12. a (Neuromuscular blockade decreases protective reflexes [coughing, gagging]; in the period after surgery, the loss of muscle strength resulting from blockade can lead to aspiration.)
13. a
14. d
15. 3.5 tablets per dose
16. 4.2 mL of neostigmine

CHAPTER 19

1. c
2. b
3. e
4. d
5. a
6. a
7. d
8. b, d, e
9. c
10. c
11. a
12. d (Succinylcholine produces a state of flaccid paralysis; respiratory depression secondary to neuromuscular blockade is the major concern.)
13. 250 mg

CHAPTER 20

1. e
2. a
3. c
4. b
5. d
6. T
7. F
8. T
9. F
10. T
11. T
12. b, c, d
13. a (Stop infusion and then infiltrate the site with phentolamine.)
14. c, d
15. c, d
16. a
17. b, d
18. d
19. a
20. 22.5 mL/h
21. Dilute the vial in at least 50 mL of diluent and infuse at a rate of 3 mL/h.

CHAPTER 21

1. b
2. c
3. a
4. T
5. T
6. F
7. F
8. F
9. F
10. F
11. T
12. a, c, d, e
13. a, b
14. b
15. c (Terazosin can cause orthostatic hypotension [a drop in SBP of >20 mm Hg] and reflex tachycardia [increased heart rate in response to stimulus conveyed through the cardiac nerves].)
16. a
17. c
18. c (Prazosin can cause first-dose hypotension. To minimize the risk, advise patients to take the first dose at bedtime.)
19. b
20. a (Blockade of cardiac β_1 receptors can produce bradycardia.)
21. a (Adverse neonatal effects have been observed with betaxolol. It crosses the placenta and may lead to bradycardia in the neonate; the normal pulse for a newborn is 100–160 bpm.)
22. c (While metoprolol is approved for treating heart failure, it can also cause heart failure if used incautiously.)
23. a, b, d
24. b (Patients should be informed about the early signs of heart failure (shortness of breath on mild exertion or when lying supine, night coughs, swelling of the extremities, weight gain from fluid retention) and instructed to notify a nurse or the provider if these occur.)
25. d (Blockade of β_2 receptors in the lung can cause bronchoconstriction.)
26. b, c
27. d (Combining a β-blocker with a calcium channel blocker can produce excessive cardiosuppression.)
28. 0.4 mL
29. 150 mL/h

CHAPTER 22

1. Peripheral adrenergic
2. Hypertension
3. Direct-acting adrenergic receptor blockers
4. Drowsiness, xerostomia, rebound hypertension
5. Vasodilation
6. b, c, e
7. b
8. c (Clonidine is embryotoxic in animals. Because of the possibility of fetal harm, clonidine is not recommended for pregnant females. Pregnancy should be ruled out before clonidine is given.)
9. b
10. a, b
11. c (If Coombs is going to turn positive, then it will be between 6 and 12 months; 5% of patients develop

hemolytic anemia. If hemolytic anemia develops, then methyldopa should be withdrawn immediately.)
12. b
13. 2 tablets
14. 200 mL/h

CHAPTER 23

1. a, d, e
2. a
3. c
4. c

CHAPTER 24

1. Dopamine agonists
2. Catechol-*O*-methyltransferase (COMT) inhibitors
3. Anticholinergic agents
4. MAOB inhibitors
5. Levodopa
6. Amantadine
7. c
8. b
9. b
10. c (Postural hypotension is common early in treatment. The underlying mechanism is unknown. Hypotension can be reduced by increasing intake of salt and water. An alpha-adrenergic agonist can help too.)
11. b
12. a (Rasagiline may increase the risk of malignant melanoma.)
13. c
14. a (Ropinirole may cause increased hepatic enzymes.)
15. b
16. d (Ergot derivatives have been associated with valvular heart injury.)
17. a (Tolcapone is potentially dangerous; deaths from liver failure have been reported.)
18. c
19. b, d, e
20. 6 tablets
21. 2 orally disintegrating tablets

CHAPTER 25

1. F
2. F
3. T
4. F
5. F
6. T
7. T
8. F
9. F
10. T
11. F
12. T
13. T
14. d
15. a (With oral dosing, the most common cholinergic effects are nausea, vomiting, diarrhea, abdominal pain, and anorexia. Weight loss [7% of initial weight] occurs in 18% to 26% of patients.)
16. c (Cholinesterase inhibitors can cause diarrhea; fiber helps control this issue.)
17. a, b, c
18. d
19. c
20. b, c
21. d
22. 2 capsules
23. 2.5 mL—use 3-mL syringe

CHAPTER 26

1. T
2. F
3. T
4. F
5. T
6. T
7. T
8. T
9. T
10. F
11. F
12. c, e
13. c
14. b
15. c (Interferon β can suppress bone marrow function, thereby decreasing production of all blood cell types, including platelets.)
16. d (Mitoxantrone can cause serious toxicity, including heart damage.)
17. d, e
18. c, e
19. a, b, c
20. b
21. d
22. c
23. 0.2 mL/dose
24. 16.66 gtt/min = 17 gtt/min

CHAPTER 27

1. e
2. m
3. a
4. k
5. g
6. n
7. j
8. c
9. f
10. h
11. i
12. b
13. l

14. d
15. a, b, d, e
16. a
17. b
18. c, e
19. d
20. a (Small changes in dosage can produce disproportionally large changes in serum drug levels.)
21. b (Phenytoin is a teratogen.)
22. a (Between 2% and 5% of patients develop a morbilliform [measles-like] rash. Rarely, morbilliform rash progresses to toxic epidermal necrolysis or Stevens-Johnson syndrome, an inflammatory skin disease characterized by red macules, papules, and tubercles. If a rash develops, phenytoin should be stopped.)
23. b (The drug should be administered with a medication syringe; a "teaspoon" is inexact)
24. b
25. a (To avoid transmitting infections, wash hands frequently with soap and water.)
26. a (Carbamazepine can cause vertigo. These reactions are common during the first weeks of treatment. Fortunately, tolerance usually develops with continued use. These effects can be minimized by initiating therapy at low doses and giving the largest portion of the daily dose at bedtime [safety measures to prevent falls].)
27. a, b, d, e
28. d (A major risk factor for severe skin reactions is a genetic variation known as human leukocyte antigen [HLA]-B * 1502, which occurs primarily in people of Asian descent.)
29. c
30. a (Valproic acid has been associated with fatal liver failure; inform patients about signs and symptoms of liver injury [reduced appetite, malaise, nausea, abdominal pain, jaundice] and instruct them to notify the provider if these develop.)
31. b
32. a
33. a (Severe overdose produces generalized CNS depression; death results from depression of respiration. Assessing vital signs evaluates respiratory status.)
34. d, e
35. c
36. c (Angioedema is a life-threatening swelling of the face, tongue, lips, throat, and larynx.)
37. a
38. d (Topiramate can cause metabolic acidosis.)
39. b
40. c
41. d
42. c (Zonisamide belongs to the same chemical family as sulfonamide antibiotics.)
43. Yes. Calculated safe/effective dose is 19.88 mg.
44. 0.16 mL

CHAPTER 28

1. T
2. F
3. F
4. F
5. T
6. F
7. F
8. F
9. F
10. T
11. d (Centrally acting muscle relaxants can produce generalized depression of the CNS. Drowsiness, dizziness, and lightheadedness are common. Patients should be warned not to participate in hazardous activities [e.g., driving] if CNS depression is significant. In addition, they should be advised to avoid alcohol and all other CNS depressants.)
12. c
13. a
14. a, b, e
15. 0.4 mL
16. No. The safe dose is 168 mg

CHAPTER 29

1. T
2. T
3. T
4. F
5. F
6. T
7. F
8. F
9. T
10. T
11. F
12. a (Hypersensitivity reactions, from dermatitis to anaphylaxis, can be triggered by local anesthetics.)
13. c (Anesthetics can reach systemic circulation, resulting in neonatal respiratory depression; normal respiratory rate for a newborn is 30–60 breaths per minute.)
14. d (When spinal anesthesia is used, the provider should be notified if the patient fails to void within 8 hours of the end of surgery; spinal anesthesia frequently causes headache. These "spinal" headaches are posture dependent and can be relieved by having the patient assume a supine position. Due to headaches, asking the patient to sit up to attempt to void or having them go to the bathroom to void may not be possible.)
15. b
16. a (Systemic absorption of epinephrine can result in systemic toxicity [e.g., palpitations, tachycardia, nervousness, hypertension].)
17. d
18. b, d

19. c (When the tourniquet is loosened at the end of surgery, about 15–30% of administered anesthetic is released into the systemic circulation; it is at this point that systemic adverse events can occur.)
20. c

CHAPTER 30

1. f
2. d
3. b
4. e
5. g
6. c
7. a
8. c
9. b
10. a (Depression of respiratory and cardiac function is a concern with virtually all inhalation anesthetics.)
11. d
12. c (With an illicit drug, it is important to determine both duration of use and amount used per day. Drugs that act on the respiratory and cardiac systems can affect response to anesthesia and increase risk of adverse interactions.)
13. b (Return of CNS function is gradual; precautions are needed until recovery is complete.)
14. c (Opioid-induced respiratory depression is added with anesthetic-induced respiratory depression, thereby increasing risk of postoperative respiratory distress.)
15. d (The risk of malignant hyperthermia is greatest when an inhalation anesthetic is combined with succinylcholine.)
16. a (Isoflurane causes hypotension; hypotension results from vasodilation. Amlodipine lowers blood pressure through peripheral arterial dilation.)
17. b
18. d
19. a, b, d

CHAPTER 31

1. T
2. F
3. T
4. T
5. F
6. F
7. T
8. a, b, c
9. a (Nausea and vomiting can be reduced by pretreatment with an antiemetic (e.g., prochlorperazine) and by having the patient remain still.)
10. a, c, d
11. c (Signs of withdrawal include excessive crying, sneezing, tremor, hyperreflexia, fever, and diarrhea; fever and diarrhea may result in hypovolemia.)
12. d
13. b (Dosage must be carefully titrated when treating toxicity in opioid addicts because the degree of physical dependence in these individuals is usually high, and hence an excessive dose of naloxone can transport the patient from a state of poisoning to one of acute withdrawal.)
14. d
15. a, d
16. c
17. a (The dose of fentanyl in the lozenge on a stick is sufficient to kill nontolerant individuals—especially children.)
18. a, b, c, d
19. d (Repeated dosing can result in normeperidine, a toxic metabolite that can cause dysphoria, irritability, tremors, and seizures.)
20. b
21. a (By activating μ-receptors in the gut, opioids inhibit secretion of fluids into the intestinal lumen. Principal nondrug measures include increased fiber and fluids.)
22. b
23. d
24. 0.6 mL. Push one line (0.2 mL) every 10 seconds. Total liquid is 5.6 mL; 5 lines/mL = 30 lines ("pushes") over 5 minutes (300 seconds). Push one line (0.2 mL) every 10 seconds.
25. 0.08 mL

CHAPTER 32

1. c
2. a
3. d
4. b
5. a, b, d
6. d
7. c (The objective of treatment is to reduce pain to an agreed-upon level and lower if possible.)
8. b
9. c (For patients undergoing chemotherapy, inhibition of platelet aggregation by nonsteroidal antiinflammatory drugs [NSAIDs] is a serious concern [e.g., bleeding or bruising].)
10. c
11. a (Respiratory depression is greatest at the outset of treatment.)
12. d
13. c (Primary adverse effects of NSAIDs include gastric ulceration.)
14. b
15. d (Carbamazepine is myelosuppressive.)
16. d (Severe respiratory depression can be reversed with naloxone; however, caution is required. Excessive dosing will reverse analgesia, thereby putting the patient in great pain.)
17. a
18. d (Respiratory depression is increased by concurrent use of other drugs that have CNS-depressant actions [e.g., alcohol, barbiturates, benzodiazepines].)
19. At 4 mg/min = 0.68 mL per 15 seconds or 0.55 mL per 5 mg/min. Since the dose can be pushed over 4–5 minutes, round down to 0.6 mL rather than up to 0.7 mL

CHAPTER 33

1. c
2. e
3. f
4. d
5. a
6. b
7. g
8. b, d, e
9. d
10. b, c
11. b (While all of these are a concern with a patient receiving meperidine, breathing [safety] is the priority.)
12. c (Ergotamine can cause peripheral vasoconstriction.)
13. a
14. a, c
15. d
16. b (Coronary vasospasm is the biggest concern in patients taking sumatriptan; however, about 50% of patients experience unpleasant chest symptoms, usually described as "heavy arms" or "chest pressure," rather than pain. These symptoms are transient and not related to ischemic heart disease.)
17. a (Confusion may be an indicator of serotonin syndrome.)
18. c
19. b (Propranolol can exacerbate symptoms of asthma.)
20. c
21. b, c, d
22. b
23. 1 mL
24. 2 tablets

CHAPTER 34

1. F
2. T
3. F
4. T
5. T
6. T
7. F
8. F
9. c
10. a
11. a (Laryngeal dystonia can impair respiration.)
12. d (Acute dystonia can be both disturbing and dangerous. Typically, the patient develops severe spasms of the muscles of the tongue, face, neck, or back.)
13. b (Dantrolene can reduce rigidity and hyperthermia associated with neuroleptic malignant syndrome.)
14. c
15. d (First-generation agents produce varying degrees of muscarinic cholinergic blockade, thus eliciting the full spectrum of anticholinergic responses. Monitoring intake and output is one means of assessing urinary retention.)
16. c
17. a, e
18. a, b, e
19. a
20. c
21. a
22. c (Haloperidol should be used with caution in patients with dysrhythmia risk factors, including long QT syndrome, hypokalemia or hyperkalemia, or a history of dysrhythmias, heart attack, or severe heart failure.)
23. b, d, e
24. c (Clozapine produces agranulocytosis in 1–2% of patients. The overall risk of death is about 1 in 5000. The usual cause is Gram-negative septicemia; high fever would be an indicator of such infection.)
25. a, b, c, d (Risperidone can cause metabolic effects, including diabetes and dyslipidemia. Dosage requires adjustment with kidney and liver dysfunction.)
26. Total of 4 mL - 2 mL in 2 sites because the fluid volume should not exceed 2–3 mL per IM injection site.

CHAPTER 35

1. Little interest; pleasure
2. Dosage change
3. 1; 3
4. 4; 9
5. More adverse effects
6. Stimulating; insomnia
7. Heart
8. Monoamine oxidase inhibitor (MAOI)
9. Antihistamines; sleep aids
10. impotence, orgasm, ejaculation, sexual interest
11. Tyramine
12. b (Patients with depression often think about or attempt suicide. During treatment with antidepressants, especially early on, the risk of suicide may increase. If mood deteriorates, or if thoughts of suicide intensify, the patient should see his or her provider immediately.)
13. a, c, e
14. c (If mood deteriorates, or if thoughts of suicide intensify, the patient should see their provider immediately; the answer "provide a safe environment" assumes the patient is in the hospital, which may not be the case.)
15. a, c, d
16. c (Because fluoxetine is highly bound to plasma proteins, it can displace other highly bound drugs. Displacement of warfarin [an anticoagulant] is of particular concern. Monitor responses to warfarin closely.)
17. a (The most common side effects are sexual dysfunction, nausea, headache, and manifestations of CNS stimulation, including nervousness, insomnia, and anxiety.)
18. c
19. d (Selective serotonin reuptake inhibitors [SSRIs] used in late pregnancy can cause persistent pulmonary hypertension in the neonate. Flaring nostrils and grunting are signs of respiratory distress.)
20. b (SNRIs can result in neonatal withdrawal syndrome, characterized by irritability, abnormal crying, tremor, respiratory distress, and possibly seizures.)
21. b

22. a
23. b (The combination of a tricyclic antidepressant [TCA] with an MAOI can lead to severe hypertension, owing to excessive adrenergic stimulation of the heart and blood vessels.)
24. a, b, c, e
25. b
26. c (Tranylcypromine is an MAOI and symptoms of hypertensive crisis, which include headache, tachycardia, palpitations, nausea, and vomiting.)
27. c, e
28. b
29. d
30. c (Patients should not take bupropion if they have seizures; the most serious adverse effect of bupropion is seizures.)
31. a (Mirtazapine can cause agranulocytosis – which occurs when the ANC drops below 100 cells/mcL)
32. d
33. a
34. 2 controlled-release (CR) tablets of 25 mg each
35. 2 capsules

CHAPTER 36

1. F
2. T
3. T
4. F
5. F
6. T
7. F
8. F
9. c (In a mixed episode, patients experience symptoms of mania and depression simultaneously. Patients may be agitated and irritable [as in mania] but may also feel worthless and depressed. The combination of high energy and depression puts them at significant risk for suicide.)
10. a (Evaluate the patient for absence of manic symptoms [flight of ideas, pressured speech, hyperactivity].)
11. b (Chronic lithium use has been associated with degenerative changes in the kidney.)
12. a, b, c, e (Diuretics, NSAIDs, anticholinergic drugs, and tricyclic antidepressants can increase the risk of lithium toxicity.)
13. c (Diuretics promote sodium loss and can thereby increase the risk of lithium toxicity.)
14. a, b, d (All of these are possible signs of liver failure.)
15. a (Administer the drug; a serum level at 6 mcg/mL is within the target range of 4–12 mcg/mL.)
16. a (These labs are normal.)
17. d (Lamotrigine can cause life-threatening rashes, including Stevens-Johnson syndrome and toxic epidermal necrolysis; typical presentation includes blistering of mucous membranes, typically in the mouth.)
18. 2 capsules
19. 7.5 mL

CHAPTER 37

1. a
2. c
3. d
4. b
5. T
6. T
7. F
8. F
9. T
10. T
11. T
12. F
13. T
14. F
15. a, b, e
16. b
17. b (Triazolam has rapid onset to promote falling asleep. However, because it has a short half-life, it *may* not be a good choice for patients who have difficulty maintaining sleep. Document the patient's statement and call the provider to request a medication to prevent waking later in the night such as estazolam, a benzodiazepine with a slower onset).
18. b (Flumazenil can reverse the sedative effects of benzodiazepines but may not reverse respiratory depression.)
19. d (Safety is paramount, as patients taking benzodiazepines in sleep-inducing doses may carry out complex behaviors and then have no memory of their actions. Reported behaviors include sleep driving, preparing and eating meals, making phone calls, and having sexual intercourse. Additionally, when employed to treat anxiety, benzodiazepines sometimes cause paradoxical responses, including insomnia, excitation, euphoria, heightened anxiety, and rage.)
20. a
21. b, d
22. d
23. b
24. d (Severe barbiturate overdose produces generalized CNS depression; death results from depression of respiration.)
25. b, e
26. a
27. a (If therapy is to succeed, the underlying reason for sleep loss must be determined.)
28. b
29. 2 tablets
30. First dose 2 mL, second dose 3 mL

CHAPTER 38

1. T
2. F
3. T
4. T
5. F
6. F
7. F

8. T
9. F
10. T
11. Agoraphobia
12. Generalized anxiety disorder (GAD)
13. Social anxiety disorder
14. Obsessive-compulsive disorder (OCD)
15. Posttraumatic stress disorder (PTSD)
16. Panic disorder
17. d (An intoxicated person is considered legally incapable of consent.)
18. c (The anesthesiologist should be notified of all medications taken by a patient due to potential drug interactions.)
19. c, e (Antidepressants do a better job at decreasing cognitive symptoms of anxiety but are not as good at decreasing somatic symptoms.)
20. a (Alprazolam should be used with caution in those with pulmonary impairment, as it is a CNS depressant.)
21. c
22. d (Overdose with a TCA can cause fatal dysrhythmias)
23. a
24. b
25. 1 1/2 (1.5) tablets
26. 1.1–3.3 mg

CHAPTER 39

1. c
2. f
3. b
4. e
5. g
6. a
7. d
8. T
9. F
10. T
11. T
12. F
13. F
14. T
15. a, d
16. a (Normal range of blood pressure for a 5-year-old is 89–112/46–72.)
17. c
18. a (Chronic amphetamine use produces physical dependence. If abruptly withdrawn, abstinence syndrome occurs.)
19. b
20. b
21. d
22. a
23. b
24. d
25. d (Because clonidine can lower blood pressure (and slow heart rate too), blood pressure and heart rate should be measured at baseline, after each dose increase, and periodically thereafter.)
26. 60 mg is a safe dose.
27. 6 gtt/min

CHAPTER 40

1. Tolerance
2. Physically dependent
3. Psychological dependence
4. Withdrawal syndrome
5. Cross tolerance
6. Cross dependence
7. Dopamine
8. Chronic; relapsing
9. a, b, c, d
10. a, b, c, d
11. b
12. c
13. a

CHAPTER 41

1. T
2. F
3. F
4. F
5. T
6. T
7. F
8. F
9. T
10. F
11. F
12. T
13. b
14. e
15. a
16. c
17. d
18. a, c, e
19. d
20. b
21. a (Approximately 35% of cases of acute pancreatitis can be attributed to alcohol, making alcohol the second most common cause of the disorder. Symptoms of pancreatitis include severe abdominal pain radiating to the back; amylase is used to diagnose pancreatitis. Normal amylase ranges from 25 to 85 units/L.)
22. a, c, d
23. b, c, d, e
24. a
25. c
26. c
27. d
28. a
29. d (Acamprosate is used along with counseling and social support to help people who have stopped drinking large amounts of alcohol to avoid drinking alcohol again.)
30. 1/2 tablet
31. 1 mL (2 mL of drug + 1 mL diluent = 3 mL)

CHAPTER 42

1. T
2. T
3. F
4. T
5. T
6. F (10 seconds)
7. T
8. F
9. F
10. T
11. T
12. T
13. T
14. F
15. T
16. F
17. T
18. T
19. c
20. c
21. c
22. a
23. a, b
24. a
25. a
26. a, b, c, d
27. 2 extended-release (ER) tablets
28. 1 tablet

CHAPTER 43

1. F
2. T
3. T
4. T
5. F
6. T
7. F
8. T
9. T
10. F
11. F
12. F
13. T
14. F
15. T
16. F
17. F
18. T
19. F
20. T
21. F
22. T
23. c (The desire to avoid symptoms of withdrawal may be sufficient to promote continued drug use.)
24. d (Following IV injection, effects of naloxone begin almost immediately and persist for about 1 hour; respiratory depression will return when the effects of naloxone have worn off.)
25. b (Symptoms of opioid withdrawal include abdominal cramping, diarrhea, nausea, and vomiting.)
26. d
27. d
28. b (Barbiturates reduce ventilation; doses only three times greater than those needed to induce sleep can cause complete suppression of the neurogenic respiratory drive. With severe overdose, barbiturates can cause apnea and death.)
29. a (Severe overdose can produce hyperpyrexia, convulsions, ventricular dysrhythmias, and hemorrhagic stroke. Diazepam can reduce anxiety, suppress seizures, and alleviate hypertension and dysrhythmias. IV nitroprusside can be used to correct severe hypertension.)
30. c
31. a, b, c, d
32. d (The most pronounced effect of volatile nitrates is venodilation, which causes a profound drop in systolic blood pressure.)
33. b
34. 2 sublingual tablets
35. 4 mL

CHAPTER 44

1. b
2. e
3. d
4. a
5. c
6. T
7. F
8. F
9. F
10. T
11. F
12. T
13. T
14. F
15. 180,000
16. 99
17. Sodium; chloride
18. Thick segment of the ascending limb of the loop of Henle
19. Acids, bases, calcium, chloride, glucose, lipids, magnesium, potassium, sodium, uric acid, water (fluid)
20. c
21. c (1000 mL of water is approximately 1 kg. 1 kg = 2.2 lb; 176 - 2.2 lb = 173.8, rounding to 174 lbs.).
22. a
23. a, b, d, e
24. c (Loop diuretics [which act early in the nephron] are ideal for patients with congestive heart failure [HF].)

25. c (Although uncommon, furosemide can cause hyperglycemia due to inhibition of insulin release; symptoms of hyperglycemia include frequent urination, increased thirst, blurred vision, and feeling weak or unusually tired.)
26. a (This selection has the 20-mm Hg drop in SBP associated with orthostatic hypotension.)
27. a, b, c, d
28. c (Muscle weakness and cramping are symptoms associated with hypokalemia.)
29. b
30. d
31. c
32. d (A low sodium level can lead to lithium toxicity due to alterations in sodium/hydrogen exchange and decreased excretion of lithium.)
33. b
34. b
35. b (Thiazides can elevate plasma levels of glucose particularly in patients with diabetes, resulting in significant hyperglycemia.)
36. b (Adolescents and young adults are particularly concerned about body image, perceived flaws, and appearing different from their peers.)
37. c, d
38. c (Some water-softening systems replace calcium and magnesium ions with sodium ions. The higher the concentration of calcium and magnesium, the more sodium needed to soften the water. Patients on a very low-sodium diet who are concerned about the amount of sodium in softened water may want to consider a water purification system that uses potassium chloride instead.)
39. 0.5 (1/2) tablet
40. 330/2.2 = 150 kg; 150 × 0.1 mg/kg = 15 mg; 15 mg/40 mg in 5 mL = 1.875 (1.9) mL. Push over 1 to 2 minutes.

CHAPTER 45

1. Volume expansion
2. Hypotonic contraction
3. Hypertonic contraction
4. Isotonic contraction
5. Sodium
6. Metabolic alkalosis
7. Respiratory alkalosis
8. Metabolic acidosis
9. a
10. b
11. c
12. d
13. a (In isotonic contraction, volume should be replenished slowly to avoid pulmonary edema.)
14. d
15. b (Laxative abuse can lead to hypokalemia [potassium < 3.5 mEq/dL]; treatment is potassium.)
16. c (Except for the sustained-release tablets, solid formulations of KCl can produce high local concentrations of potassium, resulting in severe intestinal injury; notify provider and change formulation [e.g., effervescent tablets or powder, which can be diluted].)
17. a (Except for the sustained-release tablets, solid formulations of KCl can produce high local concentrations of potassium, resulting in severe intestinal injury [ulcerative lesions, bleeding, perforation]; death has occurred.)
18. b (Serum levels of potassium are regulated primarily by the kidneys; normal creatinine ranges from 0.5 mg/dL to 1.2 mg/dL.)
19. a (Excess insulin drives potassium into cells.)
20. d, e
21. b (The most serious consequence of hyperkalemia is disruption of the electrical activity of the heart.)
22. b (In the heart, excessive magnesium can suppress impulse conduction through the atrioventricular [AV] node. Accordingly, magnesium sulfate is contraindicated for patients with AV heart block.)
23. a
24. 110 lb = 50 kg; 2 mg/kg/h = 100 mg/h; 3 vials of NaBicarb is 150 mEq in 150 mL added to 850 mL dextrose 5% in water [D_5W] (total 1000 mL); yields a concentration of 0.15 mEq/mL. 100 mEq/hr divided by 0.15 mEq = 15 mL/hr x 4 hours.

CHAPTER 46

1. F
2. T
3. T
4. T
5. T
6. F
7. F
8. T
9. T
10. F
11. F
12. f
13. b
14. g
15. l
16. a
17. h
18. e
19. k
20. i
21. j
22. d
23. c
24. b
25. a, b, c
26. d (Cardiac output = heart rate × stroke volume; 90 × 55 mL = 4950 mL—a normal cardiac output.)
27. a (Afterload is arterial pressure that the left ventricle must pump against; blood pressure [BP] reflects the force of blood moving through the arteries.)
28. b, d, e
29. a, b, c, f (All of these are signs of therapeutic response to vasodilator administration.)
30. a (≥20 mm Hg systolic and ≥10 mm Hg diastolic after standing for 1 minute are indicators of orthostatic hypotension.)

CHAPTER 47

1. d
2. e
3. g
4. f
5. b
6. a
7. i
8. h
9. c
10. d
11. c
12. a
13. a, b, d, e
14. b, c, e
15. a, c, d (Side effects of angiotensin-converting enzyme inhibitors [ACEIs] include hyperkalemia, renal insufficiency, and first-dose hypotension in patients who are sodium depleted.)
16. d (A precipitous drop in BP may occur following the first dose of an ACEI. This reaction is caused by widespread vasodilation secondary to abrupt lowering of angiotensin II levels. First-dose hypotension is most likely in patients with severe hypertension, in patients taking diuretics, and in patients who are sodium depleted or volume depleted.)
17. c
18. a (Angioedema is a potentially fatal reaction that develops in up to 1% of patients. Symptoms, which result from increased capillary permeability, include giant wheals and edema of the tongue, glottis, and pharynx. Severe reactions should be treated with subcutaneous [subQ] epinephrine.)
19. d
20. a
21. d (Aspirin, ibuprofen, and other nonsteroidal antiinflammatory drugs [NSAIDs] may reduce the antihypertensive effects of ACEIs.)
22. b
23. a, d, e
24. b
25. d (Severe hyperkalemia can occur in patients prescribed these drugs. Salt substitutes are high in potassium.)
26. 2 tablets

CHAPTER 48

1. blood vessels, heart
2. peripheral arterioles, arteries, arterioles
3. Arterioles (blood vessels)
4. Vasodilation; reduced arterial pressure; increased coronary perfusion.
5. -ine
6. b (In the sinoatrial [SA] node, calcium channel blockade can cause bradycardia; in the AV node, blockade can cause partial or complete atrioventricular (AV) block; and in the myocardium, blockade can decrease contractility.)
7. b
8. a, c, e (Verapamil can exacerbate cardiac dysfunction in patients with bradycardia, sick sinus syndrome, heart failure [HF], and AV block. Beta-blockers can intensify the adverse cardiac effects of verapamil.)
9. b
10. b (Extended-release formulations should not be crushed.)
11. d (Blockade of cardiac calcium channels can cause bradycardia, AV block, and HF.)
12. b (CCBs have been associated with chronic eczematous eruptions typically starting 3 to 6 months after treatment onset. If the reaction is mild, switching to a different CCB may help. If the condition is severe, use of verapamil and other CCBs should stop.)
13. a, b, c, d
14. b
15. a
16. c (Sustained release [SR] is taken twice daily; long acting [LA] is administered once daily.)
17. d
18. c
19. b
20. a, c, d (When taken in excessive dosage, nifedipine loses selectivity. Hence, toxic doses affect the heart in addition to blood vessels, resulting in palpitations, syncope and other symptoms of reflex tachycardia, including dyspnea).
21. 11 mL/h
22. 20 mg is the safe dose for this patient.

CHAPTER 49

1. T
2. F
3. F
4. T
5. F
6. T
7. F
8. T
9. T
10. c (Principal adverse effects of hydralazine are hypotension and tachycardia.)
11. b
12. a (About 80% of patients taking minoxidil for 4 weeks or more develop hypertrichosis [excessive growth of hair])
13. a (Fluid retention is both common and serious with minoxidil. Volume expansion may be so severe as to cause cardiac decompensation.)
14. c
15. d (If a systemic lupus erythematosus (SLE)–like reaction occurs, hydralazine should be withdrawn. Approximately 50% of patients have constitutional symptoms of fever, weight loss, and fatigue. Reporting fever as a priority over fatigue is important, as those with an SLE-like reaction may also develop pericarditis, of which low-grade fever is a sign.)

16. a (Oral antihypertensives should be initiated simultaneously.)
17. c (Nitroprusside is used to lower blood pressure rapidly in hypertensive emergencies. Oral antihypertensive medication should be initiated simultaneously.)
18. d (This rate may precipitate a drop in BP; additionally, prolonged infusions or rapid infusions may increase risk for cyanide or thiocyanide poisoning, which involve the central nervous system [CNS].)
19. 72 mL/h

CHAPTER 50

1. n
2. m
3. j
4. d
5. b
6. k
7. l
8. o
9. g
10. h
11. a
12. i
13. c
14. f
15. e
16. c
17. d
18. a (Antihypertensive drugs can cause a number of adverse effects, ranging from sedation to sexual dysfunction; it is hard to convince people who feel well to take drugs that may make them feel worse.)
19. a, b, c, e
20. b
21. c (Principal adverse effect of thiazides is hypokalemia.)
22. d
23. a
24. c (The most disturbing side effect of α-blockers is orthostatic hypotension. Hypotension can be especially severe with the initial dose. Significant hypotension continues with subsequent doses but is less profound. Hypotension puts the patient at risk of falling.)
25. c
26. a (The major cause of treatment failure in patients with chronic hypertension is lack of adherence to the prescribed regimen.)
27. b
28. c
29. b
30. a
31. a
32. c
33. b (β-Blockers can suppress glycogenolysis and mask early signs of hypoglycemia and therefore must be used with caution.)

CHAPTER 51

1. e
2. d
3. c
4. b
5. a
6. c
7. f
8. e
9. b
10. h
11. a
12. i
13. d
14. g
15. j
16. k
17. c
18. b
19. a, c, d (The combination of increased venous tone plus increased blood volume found in heart failure [HF] causes pulmonary edema, peripheral edema, hepatomegaly, and increased jugular venous distention [JVD]; weight gain results from fluid retention.)
20. b
21. c (Weakness is a symptom of hyperkalemia.)
22. d (Dopamine is administered by continuous infusion. Constant monitoring of BP, electrocardiogram [ECG], and urine output are required.)
23. c
24. a
25. a, c, d (All of these are signs and symptoms of drug-induced lupus-like syndrome.)
26. b, c, d
27. a (Anorexia, nausea, and vomiting are the most common gastrointestinal [GI] side effects of digoxin and may signal the onset of more serious toxicity.)
28. b (The optimal range of digoxin is now 0.5–0.8 mg/mL.)
29. c
30. d
31. c (Hypokalemia increases the risk of digoxin-induced dysrhythmias.)
32. b, c
33. 6 mL/h (calculates to 5.625 mL/h)
34. Yes, 5 mg falls within the range of 1.75–5.25 for this patient and is safe.

CHAPTER 52

1. Absence
2. Abnormal
3. Slower
4. Faster
5. Ventricular
6. c
7. a
8. b
9. c

10. b
11. a
12. a (In their mildest forms, dysrhythmias have only modest effects on cardiac output. In their most severe forms, however, dysrhythmias can so disable the heart that no blood is pumped at all.)
13. a (Not all the P-waves are able to conduct through the AV node, resulting in a ventricular rate that is not as fast as the atrial rate.)
14. b
15. b (Patients with QT prolongation often present with syncope as torsades de pointes, which is a nonperfusing rhythm.)
16. a
17. d (Atrial fibrillation carries a high risk of stroke.)
18. b
19. b
20. a
21. b (Cinchonism [overdose/toxicity] is characterized by tinnitus [ringing in the ears], headache, nausea, vertigo, and disturbed vision. These symptoms can develop with just one dose.)
22. a
23. b (Warning signs of cardiotoxicity include QRS widening of more than 50%.)
24. a, b, c, e (these are all signs and symptoms of cardiotoxicity.)
25. d (A postvoid residual of >100 mL may necessitate urinary catheterization.)
26. b
27. d (Prolonged vomiting can lead to dehydration and electrolyte disturbances, including hypokalemia. Propafenone can cause PR prolongation; hypokalemia can worsen PR prolongation.)
28. b
29. a
30. a (The most common adverse effects are hypotension and bradydysrhythmias. Hypotension develops in 15% to 20% of patients and may require discontinuation of treatment.)
31. a, c, d
32. a
33. c (Verapamil may produce a decrease in BP below normal levels, which may result in dizziness or symptomatic hypotension.)
34. d
35. c
36. 18.75 mg/dose
37. 30 mL/h

CHAPTER 53

1. Hormones, bile salts
2. Liver
3. Saturated
4. Lipoproteins
5. Affinity for water; repel water
6. 500
7. 150
8. 30; 60
9. c
10. b
11. a (People with very high triglyceride levels are at increased risk for developing pancreatitis.)
12. d (Creatine kinase [CK] elevations occur with rhabdomyolysis; elevated aspartate aminotransferase/alanine aminotransferase [AST/ALT] indicates liver injury.)
13. d (With statins, the risks to the fetus outweigh any potential benefits of treatment.)
14. c (Elevated CK level is an indication of muscle damage. Rhabdomyolysis is the breakdown of muscle tissue that leads to the release of muscle fiber contents into the blood. These substances are harmful to the kidney and often cause kidney damage.)
15. d
16. c
17. a
18. d
19. c
20. b
21. b
22. c
23. c
24. b, e
25. c
26. 3 tablets
27. 1 tablet

CHAPTER 54

1. Oxygen; heart
2. Preload; afterload
3. Diastolic
4. Aspirin
5. c (Anginal pain is precipitated when the oxygen supply to the heart is insufficient to meet oxygen demand. Cardiac oxygen supply is determined by myocardial blood flow.)
6. b
7. d
8. c
9. b (Long-acting formulations of nitroglycerin [patches/sustained release] should be used on an intermittent schedule that allows at least 10–12 drug-free hours a day; usually at night.)
10. a
11. d
12. a (Initial nitroglycerin therapy can produce severe headaches. This response diminishes over the first few weeks of treatment. The headaches can be treated with acetaminophen.)
13. a
14. c (Smoking increases the risk for cardiovascular mortality by 50%. Fortunately, smoking cessation greatly decreases cardiovascular risk.)
15. b
16. c
17. d

18. a, c, e
19. d (Ranolazine is contraindicated in patients with preexisting QT prolongation.)
20. 2 inches
21. 3 mL/h

CHAPTER 55

1. T
2. F
3. T
4. T
5. F
6. T
7. d
8. c (In heparin-treated patients, platelet aggregation is the major remaining defense against hemorrhage. A depressed platelet count means this defense is weakened; hence, heparin must be employed with caution.)
9. a
10. b (In older adults, the use of anticoagulants must outweigh risk of bleeding secondary to falls, decreased renal function, or polypharmacy.)
11. a (Initial response may not be evident until 8–12 hours after first dose; peak effects take several days to develop.)
12. c
13. c
14. d
15. b (Headache or faintness suggest cerebral hemorrhage.)
16. b
17. b, c, d, e
18. d (Spinal hematomas may occur in patients anticoagulated with drugs such as enoxaparin and who receive spinal anesthesia; these hematomas may result in long-term or permanent paralysis.)
19. a, b, c, e
20. c, d
21. b (Most patients do not need to interrupt warfarin for dental procedures [including surgery]; however, it is important that international normalized ratio [INR] be in target range.)
22. d
23. b (Dabigatran dosing has not been determined for patients with an estimated glomerular filtration rate [eGRF]/[CrCl] of <15.)
24. a (12% of patients receiving bivalirudin experience hypotension; patients are advised to change positions slowly to minimize orthostatic hypotension.)
25. a
26. d
27. b
28. c
29. a
30. d (Heparin-induced thrombocytopenia (HIT) is a potentially fatal immune-mediated disorder characterized by reduced platelet counts (thrombocytopenia) and a seemingly paradoxical *increase* in thrombotic events.)
31. b, c, d
32. a, d, e
33. c
34. c (If treatment begins soon after symptoms start, heart attack deaths and heart damage can often be avoided.)
35. b, c, d
36. b, d
37. 5 mL
38. 120 mL/h

CHAPTER 56

1. Myocardial infarction (MI)
2. ST-elevation myocardial infarction (STEMI)
3. Necrosed
4. ST elevation
5. High serum cholesterol; hypertension; smoking; diabetes
6. Atherosclerotic plaque
7. 20
8. Angiotensin II
9. Troponins; creatine kinase
10. Oxygen
11. a, b, d, e
12. a, b
13. b
14. d (Patients with asthma or other similar diseases should not receive β-blockers, including metoprolol. Because of its relative β_1 selectivity, however, metoprolol may be used with caution in patients with asthma who cannot tolerate other treatments. Since β_1 selectivity is not absolute, a β_2-stimulating agent should be administered concomitantly and the lowest possible dose of metoprolol used. In this instance, the nurse should clarify the dose [which totals 200 mg/day] with the provider.)
15. a
16. d (Nitroglycerin should be avoided in patients with tachycardia [heart rate > 100 bpm] due to the increased risk of reflex tachycardia.)
17. d
18. a
19. c
20. 0.8 mL

CHAPTER 57

1. F
2. T
3. F
4. F
5. T
6. F
7. T
8. T
9. b (Trauma can cause profuse hemorrhage in persons with severe hemophilia; bleeding within the skull carries 30% risk of death. Signs of severe head injury include loss of consciousness, confusion, and disorientation.)
10. c
11. a
12. d (Risk of injury is high due to abnormal blood profile/altered clotting factors.)

13. c
14. d
15. b
16. b (Symptoms of anaphylaxis include wheezing, tightness in the throat, shortness of breath, and swelling of the face. The treatment of choice is epinephrine.)
17. a, c
18. c
19. 1125 units of factor VIII for this child
20. 2.25 mL desmopressin will be injected into 50 mL 0.9% normal saline (NS) and infused at 100 mL/h.

CHAPTER 58

1. Proerythroblasts
2. Erythroblasts
3. Reticulocytes
4. Erythropoietin
5. Iron
6. Folic acid
7. Myoglobin
8. 120 days
9. Bowel
10. Hemosiderin
11. Iron binding capacity
12. Ferrous sulfate
13. Antacids
14. a
15. d
16. c
17. b
18. e
19. d (Reticulocytes are immature red blood cells [RBCs]. They normally make up about 1% of RBCs in circulation. A low count suggests the bone marrow is not making enough RBCs.)
20. b (Anemia is common in patients with chronic kidney disease; healthy kidneys produce erythropoietin to help stimulate the bone marrow to make RBCs.)
21. a
22. c, d
23. c
24. d
25. c (In children, iron deficiency can cause developmental problems and impaired cognition.)
26. b
27. a
28. c (Oral iron may impart a dark green or black color to stools.)
29. a (To minimize anaphylactic reactions, intravenous [IV] iron dextran should be administered following a small test dose [25 mg over 5 minutes], and observe the patient for signs and symptoms of anaphylaxis for at least 15 minutes.)
30. d
31. c (Epoetin has been associated with an increase in cardiovascular events. Among these are cardiac arrest, hypertension, heart failure [HF], and thrombotic events, including stroke and myocardial infarction [MI].)
32. b (Approval of the other four forms (iron sucrose, sodium–ferric gluconate complex, ferric pyrophosphate citrate, and ferumoxytol) is limited to treating iron deficiency anemia in patients with chronic kidney disease. However, sodium ferric gluconate complex and ferric pyrophosphate are reserved for those on hemodialysis; the patient in this scenario is not on hemodialysis.)
33. b, d, e (Only rarely is insufficient B_{12} in the diet the cause. Potential causes of poor absorption include (1) regional enteritis, (2) celiac disease (a malabsorption syndrome involving abnormalities in the intestinal villi), and (3) development of antibodies directed against the vitamin B_{12}–intrinsic factor complex.)
34. c (Early manifestations of pernicious anemia include paresthesia of the hands and feet; if deficiency is prolonged, neurologic damage can become permanent.)
35. b (A reduction in deep tendon reflexes may occur as an early manifestation of vitamin B_{12} deficiency.)
36. a, d
37. a (Hematopoietic growth factors have been associated with an increase in cardiovascular events. Erythrocytes incorporate significant amounts of potassium. As large numbers of erythrocytes are produced, potassium levels may fall.)
38. Yes, dose is safe and effective (50 mg in divided doses).
39. 0.2 mL

CHAPTER 59

1. Erythropoietin
2. Cancer
3. Cardiovascular events
4. 1
5. Two
6. Yeast
7. Increase
8. Thrombotic/thromboembolic events
9. a (Epoetin has been associated with an increase in cardiovascular events. Among these are cardiac arrest, hypertension, heart failure [HF], and thrombotic events, including stroke and myocardial infarction [MI].)
10. b
11. d
12. a (Darbepoetin is generally well tolerated; the most common problem is hypertension.)
13. b (In patients receiving chemotherapy, epoetin alfa may be administered three times per week.)
14. c (If endogenous erythropoietin level is >500, epoetin alfa is unlikely to help: Hold the drug, and notify the provider.)
15. c (High levels of uric acid in the blood can cause solid crystals to form within joints. This causes joint inflammation.)
16. c ($240/300 \times 1 = 0.8$; Filgrastim is supplied in single-use vials. Do not reenter vial; discard unused portion.)
17. b
18. b
19. c (Pleural and pericardial effusions have occurred, but only when dosage was massive.)

20. c
21. d (Eltrombopag may cause bone marrow fibrosis, hematologic malignancy, and thrombotic/thromboembolic events and may pose a risk of bleeding; in addition, the drug may cause liver injury. Accordingly, safety is a priority in patients receiving this drug.)
22. b
23. Body surface area (BSA) 1.521; 380.25 mcg = 38 mL/dose
24. 290 mcg; select 300-mcg/0.5-mL prefilled syringe and administer 0.48 mL

CHAPTER 60

1. T
2. T
3. F
4. T
5. F
6. T
7. F
8. T
9. T
10. F
11. F
12. a
13. d (Diabetic gastroparesis affects 20–30% of long-term patients with diabetes; manifestations include nausea, vomiting, delayed gastric emptying, and gastric/intestinal distension.)
14. a, b, d
15. d
16. c (Persons receiving insulin are at risk for hypoglycemia; sweating and confusion/altered level of consciousness are signs of hypoglycemia.)
17. b
18. b
19. a
20. a (Insulin should be refrigerated but not frozen.)
21. d (In addition to regular insulin, only insulin apsart, insulin lispro, and insulin glulisine can be given IV.)
22. c (Because onset is delayed, neutral protamine Hagedorn [NPH] insulin cannot be administered at mealtime to control postprandial hyperglycemia.)
23. a
24. c
25. b
26. b, d, e
27. c (If the swallowing reflex or the gag reflex is suppressed, nothing should be administered by mouth.)
28. d
29. b (Alcohol can inhibit breakdown of lactic acid and can thereby intensify lactic acidosis caused by metformin.)
30. a
31. c
32. b
33. c (Blood levels peak within 1 hour of oral dosing and return to baseline about 4 hours later; administration must always be associated with a meal.)
34. d
35. a
36. c, d
37. d
38. 24 mL/h

CHAPTER 61

1. T
2. F
3. T
4. F
5. F
6. T
7. T
8. F
9. T
10. c (Measurement of serum thyroid-stimulating hormone [TSH] is an important means of evaluation; successful replacement therapy causes elevated TSH levels to fall.)
11. a (By the second trimester, the fetal thyroid gland is fully functional; hence, the fetus can supply its own hormones from then on. Therefore, to help ensure healthy fetal development, maternal hypothyroidism must be diagnosed and treated very early.)
12. a (Thyrotoxic crisis is characterized by profound hyperthermia, severe tachycardia, restlessness, agitation, and tremor. A β-blocker is given to reduce heart rate [HR], and additional measures include sedation, cooling, glucocorticoids, and IV fluids.)
13. c
14. d (Thyrotoxic crisis can occur in patients who develop severe intercurrent illnesses.)
15. a, b, d, e
16. a (Levothyroxine accelerates the degradation of vitamin K–dependent clotting factors; effects of warfarin are enhanced.)
17. b
18. c
19. d (Thionamides can cause neonatal hypothyroidism and goiter. Accordingly, this drug should be avoided during the first trimester.)
20. d (Sore throat and fever may be the earliest indications of agranulocytosis.)
21. b
22. c
23. c (In thyrotoxic crisis, β-blockers are administered to lower HR.)
24. No. At 8–10 mcg/day, safe range is 32.7–40 mcg/day.
25. 1/2 tablet

CHAPTER 62

1. h
2. a
3. e
4. c
5. g
6. d
7. i
8. f

9. b
10. d
11. b (Somatropin is contraindicated in children who are severely obese, as fatalities have occurred.)
12. a (GH is diabetogenic. When used in patients with preexisting diabetes, significant hyperglycemia may result. Glucose levels should be monitored, and insulin dosage should be adjusted accordingly. Blurred vision is a sign of hyperglycemia – the rest are signs of hypoglycemia.)
13. d (A few patients have experienced liver injury; tea-colored urine is a sign of liver injury.)
14. b, c, d (Patients may experience water intoxication at the start of treatment; vasopressin should not be given with creatinine clearance of <50 mL/min; by constricting arteries in the heart, it can cause angina or myocardial infarction [MI].)
15. b
16. b (In a few patients treated with pegvisomant, serum levels of hepatic transaminases rise, indicating liver injury. Monitoring of hepatic function is recommended.)
17. 2 mg/dose
18. 0.08 mL

CHAPTER 63

1. c
2. a
3. b
4. F
5. T
6. T
7. F
8. T
9. F
10. F
11. T
12. T
13. T
14. F
15. a
16. b
17. a (Cushing syndrome is characterized by hyperglycemia and glycosuria, among other symptoms.)
18. d (When aldosterone levels are high, cardiovascular effects are harmful, increasing risk of heart failure [HF] and hypertension.)
19. c
20. b (At times of stress, patients must increase their glucocorticoid dosage. Failure to increase the dosage can be fatal.)
21. d (With fludrocortisone, salt and water may be retained in excess, resulting in the expansion of blood volume. Patients should be monitored for weight gain.)
22. a
23. a (At these doses, ketoconazole can cause significant liver dysfunction.)
24. b, c, d, e
25. 0.5 (1/2) tablet
26. Yes. The safe dose is 24–30 mg. (Body surface area [BSA] is 2 m^2.)

CHAPTER 64

1. d
2. b
3. a
4. e
5. c
6. a
7. a, b, d
8. a, c, d
9. b (Dyspnea while resting is associated with pulmonary embolism.)
10. a, d
11. b
12. d (Selective estrogen receptor modulators [SERMs] can increase the risk of endometrial cancer and thromboembolism.)
13. a (High-dose therapy during the first 4 months of pregnancy has been associated with an increased incidence of birth defects.)
14. a (Estradiol acetate vaginal ring is absorbed in amounts sufficient to cause systemic effects, both beneficial (e.g., suppression of vasomotor symptoms) and adverse (e.g., increased risk for thrombosis).
15. c, e

CHAPTER 65

1. T
2. F
3. F
4. F
5. T
6. T
7. T
8. T
9. F
10. T
11. T
12. F
13. T
14. b (The principal concern with drospirenone is venous thromboembolism, which occurs more often than with other progestins. The thromboembolism can break apart, causing pieces to travel through the bloodstream, resulting in pulmonary embolism.)
15. d
16. c (Drospirenone is a structural analog of spironolactone, a potassium-sparing diuretic that blocks receptors for aldosterone; taken with NSAIDs, there is an increased risk of hyperkalemia.)
17. d
18. b (By increasing levels of clotting factors, oral contraceptives [OCs] can decrease the effectiveness of warfarin; therefore, it is important for patients adhere to blood testing schedules.)
19. a (These signs may be an indication of reduced OC blood levels. The OC should be combined with a second form of birth control.)
20. b (Among females of higher weight, efficacy is reduced.)

21. c (Combination OCs have been associated with an increased risk of venous thromboembolism [VTE], arterial thromboembolism, and pulmonary embolism.)
22. d (OCs may precipitate gallbladder disease in females who already have gallstones or a history of gallbladder disease; right upper quadrant pain is a symptom of gallbladder disease.)
23. a (Hyperkalemia can cause muscle fatigue, weakness, paralysis, arrhythmia, and nausea.)
24. d (If a period is missed while taking monthly-cycle OCs, the possibility of pregnancy should be assessed.)
25. c (OCs can counteract the benefits of insulin and other hypoglycemic agents used in patients with diabetes. Symptoms of hyperglycemia include increased thirst.)
26. d
27. b, c, d
28. c
29. c

CHAPTER 66

1. c
2. a
3. b
4. d
5. F
6. F
7. T
8. F
9. F
10. T
11. T
12. F
13. F
14. F
15. c (Very rarely, clomiphene can cause ovarian hyperstimulation. Symptoms include low abdominal pain, pressure, weight gain, and swelling.)
16. c
17. d
18. b (Of great concern is ovarian enlargement that occurs rapidly and that may be accompanied by ascites, pleural effusion, and considerable pain.)
19. a (Hyperstimulation syndrome following human chorionic gonadotropin [hCG] therapy may provoke rupture of ovarian cysts and resultant bleed into peritoneal cavity.)
20. a
21. b
22. 0.5 (1/2) tablet
23. 2.5 mL in 2 sites (total 5 mL)

CHAPTER 67

1. F
2. F
3. T
4. T
5. F
6. a, b, d, e
7. d (An adverse effect of greatest concern when administering terbutaline is pulmonary edema; shortness of breath and foamy sputum are signs and symptoms of pulmonary edema.)
8. c (There is some concern that nifedipine may compromise uteroplacental blood flow.)
9. c (Risk for adverse effects can be reduced by monitoring magnesium levels, renal function [renal impairment may cause magnesium levels to rise], fluid balance, and deep tendon reflexes.)
10. c
11. a, c, e
12. a (Because it poses a risk of severe hypertension, methylergonovine is considered a second-line drug for controlling postpartum hemorrhage.)
13. a, d, f, g
14. d, e
15. d (The pouch is removed when active labor occurs.)
16. 9 mL/h
17. 2 tabs

CHAPTER 68

1. Follicle-stimulating hormone (FSH); luteinizing hormone (LH)
2. Erythropoietin
3. Liver function
4. Water; sodium (or salt)
5. Irreversible
6. a (Androgens can lower plasma levels of high-density lipoprotein [HDL] cholesterol ["good cholesterol"] and elevate plasma levels of low-density lipoprotein [LDL] cholesterol ["bad cholesterol"]. These actions may increase the risk of atherosclerosis and related cardiovascular events.)
7. c (Edema can result from androgen-induced retention of salt and water. This complication is a concern for patients with heart failure [HF] and for those with a predisposition to developing edema from other causes.)
8. d
9. d
10. b
11. d
12. d
13. b (The 17-α-alkylated androgens can cause cholestatic hepatitis, jaundice, and other liver disorders. Rarely, liver cancer develops. Obtain periodic tests of liver function. Inform patients about signs of liver dysfunction [jaundice, malaise, anorexia, fatigue, nausea], and instruct them to notify the provider if these occur.)
14. c (Androgens can cause cholestatic hepatitis and other disorders of the liver. Since this patient does not report symptoms that are emergent in nature, it is a priority to gather all assessment data [history and physical] plus laboratory data prior to calling the provider.)
15. 0.25 mL
16. 4 pellets

CHAPTER 69

1. F
2. F
3. T
4. F
5. F
6. T
7. F
8. F
9. F
10. T
11. T
12. F
13. F
14. F
15. b, d
16. c (Priapism [painful erection lasting more than 6 hours] may occur with sildenafil use. If erection persists after 4 hours, medical intervention is required to avoid permanent damage to penile tissue.)
17. d (If sildenafil and isosorbide are combined, life-threatening hypotension could result. Therefore, sildenafil is absolutely contraindicated for males taking nitrates.)
18. a (Although sildenafil is generally well tolerated, it can be dangerous for males taking certain vasodilators—specifically, α-adrenergic blockers, nitroglycerin, and other nitrates used for angina pectoris.)
19. d
20. b (Vardenafil can prolong the cardiac QT interval and might therefore pose a risk for serious dysrhythmias.)
21. a
22. a
23. c (Causes of persistent erection [PE] include psychologic factors, genetics, and physiologic variations, as well as alterations in neurotransmitters and receptor sensitivity; while d is correct from a medical perspective, it is unlikely a patient would understand this explanation. Therefore, c is the most correct response by the nurse.)
24. a, b, d
25. a, b, c, e
26. c (Finasteride promotes regression of prostate epithelial tissue, decreasing mechanical obstruction of the urethra.)
27. d (Dutasteride is teratogenic. It can be absorbed through the skin, so pregnant females should not handle the drug.)
28. b (Nonselective α_1 blockers may be dangerous for males with reduced BP.)
29. b (Doxazosin's principal adverse effects are hypotension, fainting, and dizziness.)
30. c

CHAPTER 70

1. T
2. T
3. F
4. T
5. F
6. T
7. T
8. F
9. e
10. f
11. b
12. a
13. c
14. d
15. a, c, d
16. c
17. c
18. a, c
19. a, b, c
20. c
21. b, c, d, e
22. b
23. a, b, e
24. c

CHAPTER 71

1. d
2. c
3. e
4. i
5. b
6. g
7. a
8. f
9. j
10. h
11. c
12. e
13. a
14. d
15. b
16. Gamma-globulins; immunoglobulins
17. B lymphocytes (cells); T lymphocytes (cells)
18. d
19. b (Because of helper T-cell loss, AIDS patients are at high risk of death from opportunistic infections.)
20. c
21. d
22. c
23. c
24. b
25. c

CHAPTER 72

1. f
2. g
3. c
4. d
5. m
6. i
7. e

8. k
9. l
10. b
11. a
12. j
13. h
14. d
15. b (Current antimicrobial therapy and mild acute illness with low-grade fever are not contraindications for vaccines.)
16. c (Rarely, acute encephalopathy may occur with DTaP immunization.)
17. b
18. d, e (Live vaccines can be dangerous in recipients who are immunocompromised because they are unable to mount an effective immune response.)
19. a
20. b, d, e
21. c (Children with severe immunodeficiency should NOT be given MMR. Severe immunodeficiency may result from immunosuppressive drugs [e.g., glucocorticoids, cytotoxic anticancer drugs], certain cancers [e.g., leukemia, lymphoma, generalized malignancy], and advanced HIV infection.)
22. a, c, d
23. c
24. d (Children receiving vaccines should avoid aspirin and other salicylates for 6 weeks, based on the theoretical risk of developing Reye syndrome.)
25. b
26. a, e
27. b, d
28. a (Annual vaccination against influenza is now recommended for all children between 6 months and 18 years, as well as all adults.)
29. d (Rotavirus vaccines may carry a small risk of intussusception, a rare, life-threatening form of bowel obstruction that occurs when the bowel folds in on itself, like a collapsing telescope. Bloody, mucus-like bowel movement, sometimes called a "currant jelly" stool, is a symptom.)
30. b

CHAPTER 73

1. Hypothalamic-pituitary-adrenal axis
2. Azathioprine
3. Toxicity
4. Infection, neoplasm
5. Fat
6. Antacids
7. c (Immunosuppressive drugs inhibit immune responses, which poses increased risk of infection.)
8. d
9. d
10. b
11. a (Renal damage occurs in up to 75% of patients taking cyclosporine. Injury manifests as reduced renal blood flow and reduced glomerular filtration rate.)
12. d (Signs of anaphylaxis include flushing, respiratory distress, hypotension, and tachycardia. If anaphylaxis develops, discontinue the infusion and treat with epinephrine and oxygen.)
13. c, d, e
14. a, b, d
15. b (Grapefruit juice can increase tacrolimus levels, resulting in toxicity.)
16. d (Like tacrolimus, NSAIDs can injure the kidneys. Accordingly, NSAIDs should be avoided.)
17. c
18. a (Owing to the risk of infection, patients taking sirolimus should avoid sources of contagion. In addition, for 12 months after transplant surgery, patients should take medicine to prevent pneumocystis pneumonia.)
19. a
20. b (The full range of glucocorticoid adverse effects can be expected in persons taking prednisone, including osteoporosis with resultant fractures.)
21. b
22. a, c, d
23. c, e
24. b
25. b
26. 2.7 mL
27. 1635 mg

CHAPTER 74

1. T
2. T
3. T
4. F
5. T
6. T
7. F
8. T
9. T
10. F
11. b
12. d
13. a
14. a
15. c
16. d (Antihistamines should be avoided late in the third trimester because newborns are particularly sensitive to the adverse actions of these drugs—in this case, the sedating effects. The normal respiratory rate for a newborn is 30–60 breaths/min.)
17. c
18. d (GI side effects can be minimized by administering antihistamines with food.)
19. 5 mL
20. 0.5 mL; administer over 30 seconds (each 25 mg should be administered over at least 1 minute).

CHAPTER 75

1. 8 days
2. 1 week

3. 2
4. Reye syndrome
5. Vinegar
6. Acetaminophen
7. Acetylcysteine
8. 2000 mg
9. b (Long-term aspirin—even in low doses—can cause life-threatening gastric ulceration, perforation, and bleeding. Coffee ground emesis is a sign of gastrointestinal [GI] bleeding.)
10. d (Stomach pain and bloating may be signs of peptic ulcers.)
11. a
12. b
13. d
14. c (Smoking increases platelet aggregation; caution should be exercised when treating patients who smoke cigarettes with aspirin alone. Smokers may need to take an adenosine diphosphate receptor inhibitor.)
15. a (The aspirin hypersensitivity reaction begins with profuse, watery rhinorrhea and may progress to generalized urticaria, bronchospasm, laryngeal edema, and shock. Maintaining a patient's airway is the highest priority.)
16. c
17. d
18. b
19. a (The principal risks to pregnant females are [1] anemia [from GI blood loss], and [2] postpartum hemorrhage. A uterus that has not contracted down well [boggy] is the main cause of postpartum hemorrhage.)
20. b (Because of its sodium content, sodium salicylate should be avoided in patients with heart failure.)
21. c
22. c
23. b (Celecoxib contains a sulfur molecule and can precipitate an allergic reaction in patients allergic to sulfonamides.)
24. b (Celecoxib can impair renal function, thereby posing a risk to patients with hypertension, edema, heart failure, or kidney disease. A daily weight increase is a marker of fluid accumulation.)
25. c (There is strong evidence that COX-2 inhibitors increase the risk of myocardial infarction [MI], stroke, and other serious cardiovascular events.)
26. b (Overdose with acetaminophen can cause severe liver injury and death.)
27. b (Acetaminophen use has also been associated with SJS, acute generalized exanthematous pustulosis (AGEP), and toxic epidermal necrolysis (TEN). SJS and TEN are characterized by painful rash, blistering of the skin and mucous membranes, and detachment of the epidermis. These are considered medical emergencies because they can result in death.)
28. a (Use of aspirin in children under 18 is associated with Reye syndrome; characteristic symptoms are encephalopathy and fatty liver degeneration.)
29. 200 mL/h
30. 1.5 mL/dose

CHAPTER 76

1. b
2. c
3. e
4. d
5. a
6. c (Because of their mineralocorticoid activity, glucocorticoids can cause sodium and water retention and potassium loss.)
7. d (By suppressing host defenses [immune responses and phagocytic activity of neutrophils and macrophages], glucocorticoids can increase susceptibility to infection.)
8. b (Glucocorticoids can suppress growth in children.)
9. a, c, e (Nasal influenza, MMR, and varicella vaccines are live attenuated vaccines. Glucocorticoids can decrease antibody response and increase risk of infection for live virus vaccines.)
10. b (Glucocorticoids can cause potassium loss; risk of hypokalemia can be reduced by consuming potassium-rich foods [e.g., potatoes, bananas, and citrus fruits.]
11. c
12. a
13. a (Symptoms of glucocorticoid withdrawal include hypotension, hypoglycemia, myalgia, arthralgia, and fatigue.)
14. a, d, e (Signs of digoxin toxicity include confusion, fast and irregular pulse, loss of appetite, nausea, vomiting, diarrhea, and visual changes.)
15. 0.75 mL
16. Yes. Safe dose is up to 11.25 mg/day or 5.625 mg/dose.

CHAPTER 77

1. c
2. e
3. a
4. b
5. d
6. b, c, d
7. c (When symptoms flare, patients may be given 10–20 mg/day until symptoms are controlled, followed by gradual drug withdrawal over 5–7 days.)
8. a
9. d
10. c (Methotrexate can cause fetal death and congenital abnormalities, and therefore is contraindicated during pregnancy.)
11. a
12. a
13. d (Retinal damage, which is rare, is the most serious toxicity. Retinopathy may be irreversible and can produce blindness.)
14. b (Because disease-modifying antirheumatic drugs [DMARDs] suppress immune function, they all pose a risk for serious infections.)
15. c
16. d (Varicella is a live attenuated vaccine. DMARDs and tumor necrosis factor [TNF] antagonists may increase

the risk of acquiring or transmitting infection following immunization with a live virus. Pediatric patients should be current on vaccinations before therapy starts.)
17. c (Infliximab may pose a risk of heart failure. Exercise caution in patients with existing heart failure and monitor them closely for disease progression.)
18. b (Induration of 5 mm is considered positive for people whose immune system is suppressed. Adalimumab is indicated for people who have not responded to one or more DMARDs [immunosuppressive drugs].)
19. d
20. a (Rituximab can cause severe infusion-related hypersensitivity reactions. The immediate reaction and its sequelae include hypotension, bronchospasm, angioedema, hypoxia, pulmonary infiltrates, myocardial infarction, and cardiogenic shock.)
21. b, d (Tocilizumab can reduce neutrophil counts. Patients should discontinue the drug if absolute neutrophil count [ANC] falls below 500/mm^3. Serious adverse effects include GI perforation, particularly in those with preexisting diverticulitis.)
22. b, e
23. No. The safe dose is 20 mg.
24. 0.6 mL

CHAPTER 78

1. F
2. T
3. T
4. F
5. T
6. T
7. a (Acetaminophen may help control pain but not inflammation. Nonsteroidal antiinflammatory drugs [NSAIDs] control inflammation.)
8. a
9. b (The most serious toxicity is a rare but potentially fatal hypersensitivity syndrome, characterized by rash, fever, eosinophilia, and dysfunction of the liver and kidneys. To prevent renal injury, fluid intake should be sufficient to maintain a urine flow of at least 2 L/day.)
10. c
11. c (Allopurinol can inhibit hepatic drug-metabolizing enzymes, thereby delaying the inactivation of other drugs. This interaction is of particular concern for patients taking warfarin, whose dosage should be reduced.)
12. b
13. a (During premarketing trials, pegloticase triggered anaphylaxis in 6.5% of patients. Symptoms include wheezing, perioral or lingual edema, hemodynamic instability, and rash. Also during premarketing trials, *infusion reactions* were seen in 26% to 41% of patients. Symptoms include urticaria, dyspnea, chest discomfort, erythema, and pruritus.)
14. b
15. 1 1/2 tablets per dose
16. 125 mL/h

CHAPTER 79

1. Parathyroid hormone; vitamin D; calcitonin
2. Hypercalcemia
3. Clot
4. Lethargy; depression
5. Tetany, convulsions
6. Increases
7. Whole grains (or bran); spinach (or rhubarb, Swiss chard, beets)
8. Vitamin D
9. Bisphosphonates and thyroid hormone
10. a (preservation of calcium levels in blood takes priority over preservation of calcium in bone. Therefore, if serum calcium is low, calcium will be resorbed from bone and transferred to the blood, even if resorption compromises the structural integrity of bone.)
11. a
12. c
13. b (For severe hypercalcemia, initial therapy consists of replacing lost fluid with intravenous [IV] saline.)
14. d (Hypocalcemia increases neuromuscular excitability. As a result, tetany, convulsions, and spasm of the pharynx and other muscles may occur.)
15. a (Blood levels of calcium are tightly controlled by three processes: absorption of calcium from the GI tract, excretion by the kidneys, and resorption and deposition in bone.)
16. b
17. d
18. b, e
19. d
20. d (Parenteral calcium may cause severe bradycardia in patients taking digoxin.)
21. b, c, e
22. a, c (Reactions that occur in the liver produce the major transport form of vitamin D. A later reaction in the kidney produces the fully active form.)
23. d
24. c, e
25. a (Esophagitis, sometimes resulting in ulceration, is the most serious adverse effect of alendronate. The cause of injury is prolonged contact with the esophageal mucosa, which can occur if alendronate fails to pass completely through the esophagus, as would be the case in dysphagia.)
26. b
27. b
28. c, d
29. a (Poor oral hygiene is a risk factor for osteonecrosis of the jaw [ONJ].)
30. c
31. b
32. d (Raloxifene increases the risk of thromboembolic events. Because inactivity promotes deep vein thrombosis [DVT], patients should discontinue raloxifene at least 72 hours before prolonged immobilization and should not resume the drug until full mobility has been restored.)
33. d (The potential for fetal harm from taking raloxifene outweighs any possible benefits of use during pregnancy.)

34. b
35. c
36. b (Denosumab increases the risk of serious infections; patients who develop signs of severe infection should seek immediate medical attention. Flank pain and fever may indicate UTI or infection of the abdomen.)
37. b, c, d, e
38. d (Hypocalcemia is a concern with cinacalcet administration—numbness and tingling in the perioral area, fingers, and toes are symptoms of hypocalcemia.)
39. b
40. 2.5–10 minutes
41. 1.7 mL
42. 2 tablets (180lbs/2.2 = 81.81 kg × 10 mg = 818.1 mg. Round down to 800 mg, which is 2 tabs.)

CHAPTER 80

1. k
2. e
3. j
4. d
5. i
6. a
7. h
8. c
9. g
10. b
11. f
12. c (Symptoms of asthma result from a combination of inflammation and bronchoconstriction. Accordingly, treatment must address both components.)
13. c
14. a
15. d
16. d (Although inhaled glucocorticoids may promote bone loss—at least in premenopausal females—the amount of loss is much lower than the amount caused by oral glucocorticoids.)
17. c = 1, b = 2, a = 3, d = 4, f = 5, e = 6
18. a (The selectivity of the β_2-adrenergic agonists is only relative, not absolute. Accordingly, these drugs are likely to produce some activation of β_1 receptors in the heart. If dosage is excessive, stimulation of cardiac β_1 receptors can cause angina pectoris and tachydysrhythmias.)
19. d (Following withdrawal of oral glucocorticoids [or transfer to inhaled glucocorticoids], several months are required for recovery of adrenocortical function. Throughout this time, all patients—including those switched to inhaled glucocorticoids—must be given supplemental oral or IV glucocorticoids at times of severe stress. Failure to do so can prove fatal.)
20. b
21. c (β_2-Adrenergic agonists are likely to produce some activation of β_1 receptors in the heart. Stimulation of β_1 receptors can cause tachydysrhythmias, leading to fainting.)
22. a
23. b
24. d
25. a
26. b
27. c (Benefits are much less than those of intranasal glucocorticoids. Cromolyn reduces symptoms by suppressing the release of histamine and other inflammatory mediators from mast cells.)
28. d (Smoking either tobacco or marijuana accelerates metabolism and decreases the half-life.)
29. b
30. c
31. d (Important sources of asthma-associated allergens include warm-blooded pets. To the extent possible, exposure to these factors should be eliminated or reduced.)
32. 4 mL/dose
33. 1.2 mL at 2 subcutaneous sites (total 2.4 mL)

CHAPTER 81

1. c
2. g
3. a
4. f
5. d
6. b
7. h
8. e
9. e
10. b
11. h
12. g
13. c
14. a
15. d
16. f
17. a
18. b, d, e
19. b
20. c (Although rare, systemic effects are possible. Of greatest concern are adrenal suppression and slowing of linear growth in children.)
21. b (If nasal congestion is present, a topical decongestant should be used [if prescribed] before glucocorticoid administration.)
22. c
23. a
24. d
25. b (By activating α_1-adrenergic receptors on systemic blood vessels, sympathomimetics can cause widespread vasoconstriction; for individuals with cardiovascular disorders—hypertension, coronary artery disease, cardiac dysrhythmias, cerebrovascular disease—widespread vasoconstriction can be hazardous.)
26. b
27. b
28. b
29. d
30. b (If benzonatate is sucked or chewed, rather than swallowed, the drug can cause laryngospasm, bronchospasm, and circulatory collapse.)

31. a, b
32. 2 capsules
33. 8 capsules

CHAPTER 82

1. h
2. a
3. e
4. g
5. b
6. f
7. c
8. d
9. T
10. F
11. T
12. F
13. T
14. F
15. T
16. T
17. F
18. c (Smoking delays ulcer healing and increases the risk of recurrence.)
19. d
20. b
21. c
22. a (Bismuth can impart a harmless black coloration to the tongue and stool. Patients should be forewarned. However, stool discoloration may confound interpretation of gastric bleeding. Therefore, an abdominal assessment is a priority.)
23. a (No antibiotic is effective alone when treating *Helicobacter pylori.* If drugs are used alone, risk of developing resistance is increased.)
24. b
25. b, d, e
26. c
27. a, b, e
28. a
29. d (PPIs have been associated with a dose-related increase in the risk of infection with *Clostridium difficile*, a bacterium that can cause severe diarrhea. Patients experiencing diarrhea while taking omeprazole or other PPIs should report immediately to their health care provider for testing. To avoid transmitting the disease from one patient to another, or to other healthcare providers, handwashing is the most important thing a nurse can do. Patients with C. diff are placed on contact precautions, no isolation.)
30. b, c (Omeprazole and other PPIs increase the risk for community-acquired and hospital-acquired pneumonia. Possible causes include alteration of upper GI flora (because of reduced gastric acidity.)
31. b, c, d
32. b (Sucralfate may impede the absorption of some drugs, including phenytoin, theophylline, digoxin, warfarin, and fluoroquinolone antibiotics (e.g., ciprofloxacin, norfloxacin; INR should be 2.5 for mechanical valve replacemnt.)
33. d (Misoprostol during pregnancy has caused partial or complete expulsion of the developing fetus.)
34. 10 mL
35. 16–17 drops per 15 seconds

CHAPTER 83

1. c
2. d
3. a
4. b
5. d
6. c (Rome criteria determine constipation more by stool consistency [degree of hardness] than by how often bowel movements occur.)
7. a
8. a
9. d
10. b (Bulk-forming laxatives should be administered with a full glass of water or juice to prevent esophageal obstruction.)
11. c
12. d
13. a (Lactulose can enhance intestinal excretion of ammonia. This property has been exploited to lower blood ammonia content in patients with portal hypertension and hepatic encephalopathy secondary to chronic liver disease. Normal ammonia levels range from 15 to 110 mcg/dL [this number may vary depending upon lab].)
14. b (In patients with renal impairment, magnesium can accumulate to toxic levels.)
15. d
16. b (Laxatives should be used with caution during pregnancy, as GI stimulants can induce labor.)
17. d
18. a (Easy bruising and mucosal bleeding can occur when medications interfere with vitamin K absorption.)
19. b
20. 30 mL
21. 1 capsule

CHAPTER 84

1. Medulla oblongata
2. Reflexive (or reflex)
3. Chemoreceptor trigger zone
4. Vagus
5. Before (or prior to) chemotherapy
6. Serotonin (or 5-HT3)
7. Dexamethasone
8. Doxylamine; vitamin B_6
9. Prolong
10. Irritable bowel syndrome
11. b (A patient with prolonged vomiting and diarrhea will show a decrease in sodium and potassium [electrolytes] and an elevated blood urea nitrogen [BUN].)
12. a

13. b, d, e (Side effects of prochlorperazine include hypotension, sedation, and respiratory depression.)
14. d (Patients should be advised to report local burning or pain immediately when receiving promethazine IV. Extravasation of IV promethazine can cause abscess formation, tissue necrosis, and gangrene that require amputation. Therefore, the priority action is to stop the IV infusion.)
15. c
16. c (Cannabinoids can cause tachycardia and hypotension. Normal blood pressure [BP] is less than 120/80 mm Hg. Symptoms of hypotension are not typically present unless BP is less than 90/60 mm Hg. Tachycardia is a resting heart rate greater than 100 bpm. Therefore, the priority for this patient is a pulse increase.)
17. b
18. c
19. c
20. a
21. d (Management of diarrhea is directed at diagnosis and treatment of underlying cause, replacement of lost water and salts, relief of cramping, and reducing passage of unformed stools. Infectious diarrhea is usually self-limiting and does not require antidiarrheals.)
22. b (Users should be aware that the drug may blacken stools and the tongue.)
23. b
24. c
25. b, f
26. c
27. a, b
28. b
29. d (Tuberculosis and opportunistic infections are of particular concern in patients receiving infliximab. Therefore, a productive cough would be a priority nursing concern.)
30. d
31. b
32. c (Drug is approved for decreasing oral mucositis in patients receiving high-dose chemotherapy for hematologic malignancy.)
33. a
34. Yes. The recommended dose calculates to 5.2 mg, so a 5-mg capsule is safe and effective.
35. 377 mg

CHAPTER 85

1. d
2. a
3. b
4. e
5. c
6. b
7. a
8. d, e
9. a (Vitamin A intoxication affects multiple organ systems, especially the liver.)
10. b, d, e
11. a (High doses of vitamin E can inhibit platelet aggregation.)
12. c
13. a (Derivatives of vitamin A have been used for dermatological disorders, including acne; vitamin A can cause birth defects, liver injury, and bone-related disorders.)
14. b
15. a (There is evidence that high-dose vitamin E may actually increase the risk for heart failure, cancer progression, and all-cause mortality.)
16. d
17. b, c, e
18. c (Research has failed to show any benefit for vitamin C therapy for patients with advanced cancer.)
19. 1 1/2 tablets
20. 0.25 mL

CHAPTER 86

1. b
2. a
3. d
4. c
5. T
6. T
7. F
8. T
9. F
10. T
11. T
12. b
13. d
14. d
15. c (By reducing fat absorption, orlistat can reduce absorption of fat-soluble vitamins [vitamins A, D, E, and K]. Vitamin K deficiency can intensify the effects of warfarin, an anticoagulant. In patients taking warfarin, anticoagulant effects should be monitored closely.)
16. a
17. a, c, d, e
18. 2 capsules (120 mg)
19. 0.5 (1/2) tablet

CHAPTER 87

1. c
2. g
3. a
4. e
5. d
6. h
7. b
8. f
9. c
10. g
11. a
12. h

13. d
14. f
15. b
16. e
17. F
18. T
19. F
20. T
21. T
22. T
23. F
24. T
25. a
26. c (Rather than wait for implementation of Current Good Manufacturing Practices [CGMPs], four private organizations—the US Pharmacopeia [USP], ConsumerLab, the Natural Products Association, and NSF International—have already begun testing dietary supplements for quality. A "seal of approval" is given to products that meet their standards, which are very similar to the CGMPs described previously. The USP standards are enforceable by the FDA.)
27. a (Herbal products and other dietary supplements can interact with conventional drugs, sometimes with significant harmful results. The principal concerns are increased toxicity and decreased therapeutic effects. Clinicians and consumers should be alert to these possibilities.)
28. a, b, e
29. b
30. c
31. a, b, c
32. a (The patient is not acute; continue to gather assessment data [the first step in the nursing process] to have all data necessary when contacting the provider.)
33. c
34. d (Symptoms of hypoglycemia include pounding heart, sweating, chills, and clamminess.)
35. d (There is concern that ginkgo may promote seizures. Accordingly, the herb should be avoided by patients at risk for seizures, including those taking drugs that can lower the seizure threshold, including antipsychotics, antidepressants, cholinesterase inhibitors, decongestants, first-generation antihistamines, and systemic glucocorticoids.)
36. a
37. a (St. John wort is known to interact adversely with many drugs—and the list continues to grow. Three mechanisms are involved: induction of cytochrome P450 enzymes, induction of P-glycoprotein, and intensification of serotonin effects.)
38. c
39. b (Ma Huang contains ephedrine, a compound that can elevate blood pressure and stimulate the heart and CNS.)

CHAPTER 88

1. T
2. F
3. T
4. F
5. T
6. T
7. F
8. F
9. T
10. T
11. F
12. T
13. F
14. T
15. F
16. T
17. F
18. T
19. d (The first rule of antimicrobial therapy is to *match the drug with the bug*. If treatment is begun in the absence of a definitive diagnosis, positive identification should be established as soon as possible so as to permit adjustment of the regimen to better conform with the drug sensitivity of the infecting organism.)
20. c
21. a
22. b, c, d, e
23. c (As a rule, patients with a history of allergy to penicillin should not receive it again. The exception is treatment of a life-threatening infection for which no suitable alternative is available. For emergency treatment, people typically receive epinephrine; antihistamines and corticosteroids may also be ordered.)
24. b (Tetracycline should be avoided during pregnancy due to risk of permanent bone/teeth discoloration and enamel hypoplasia, as well as possible risk of spontaneous abortion.)
25. d
26. c
27. a, c, d, e
28. a

CHAPTER 89

1. F
2. T
3. F
4. T
5. F
6. F
7. T
8. T
9. T
10. F
11. T
12. F
13. T
14. a (All patients who are candidates for penicillin therapy should be asked if they have penicillin allergy.)
15. c
16. b
17. d

18. c (Anaphylaxis [laryngeal edema, bronchoconstriction, severe hypotension] is an immediate hypersensitivity reaction, mediated by immunoglobulin E [IgE]. Anaphylactic reactions occur more frequently with penicillins than with any other drugs.)
19. a (Whenever a penicillin is used, keep the patient under observation for at least 30 minutes following administration.)
20. c
21. a, e
22. c (Neurotoxicity (seizures, confusion, hallucinations) if blood levels of penicillin G are too high.)
23. c
24. No. Dose is 500 mg/day. 7.5 kg × 20 mg = 150 mg/day; 7.55 kg × 40 mg = 300 mg/day.
25. 200 mL/h

CHAPTER 90

1. β-Lactamases
2. Positive
3. Methicillin-resistant *Staphylococcus aureus* (MRSA)
4. Increased
5. Negative
6. Ceftaroline
7. Good
8. c (In patients with renal insufficiency, dosages of most cephalosporins must be reduced [to prevent accumulation to toxic levels].)
9. c (Ceftriaxone can cause bleeding tendencies.)
10. b (Hypersensitivity reactions are the most frequent adverse events. Maculopapular rash that develops several days after the onset of treatment is most common. Prior to any other action, since a rash is not a severe reaction requiring administration of epinephrine, the assessment must be completed to have all relevant information available for the provider.)
11. b
12. a
13. c (Because of structural similarities between penicillin and cephalosporins, a few patients allergic to one type of drug may experience cross-reactivity with the other. For patients with mild penicillin allergy, cephalosporins can be used with minimal concern. However, because of the potential for fatal anaphylaxis, cephalosporins should not be given to patients with a history of severe reactions to penicillin.)
14. a
15. a
16. c
17. a (Drug may cause elevation in liver enzymes (alanine aminotransferase [ALT], aspartate aminotransferase [AST], alkaline phosphatase [Alk Phos], and lactate dehydrogenase [LDH].)
18. c (Imipenem can reduce blood levels of valproate, a drug used to control seizures. Breakthrough seizures have occurred. The patient is a safety risk due to the possibility of seizures.)
19. d
20. a
21. d
22. No. 750 mg is higher than the 10 mg/kg recommended for persons with normal renal function.
23. 254 mg. Yes, this is a safe dose.

CHAPTER 91

1. T
2. T
3. T
4. F
5. F
6. T
7. F
8. F
9. T
10. F
11. b, c, e
12. d (Tetracyclines may exacerbate renal impairment in patients with preexisting kidney disease.)
13. a
14. c
15. c
16. d (Treatment with tetracyclines may result in superinfection of the bowel with staphylococci or with *Clostridium difficile*, producing severe diarrhea that can be life-threatening. Patients should notify provider if significant diarrhea occurs.)
17. a
18. a, c, d
19. c
20. a, b, c
21. d
22. c
23. c
24. c (Drugs that decrease bowel motility [e.g., opioids and anticholinergics] may worsen symptoms and should not be used in persons with *C. difficile*–associated disease [CDAD].)
25. d
26. c (Linezolid can cause reversible myelosuppression, manifesting as anemia, leukopenia, thrombocytopenia, or even pancytopenia. Complete blood counts should be done weekly.)
27. a
28. c
29. a
30. 4 mL
31. 125 mg

CHAPTER 92

1. Bactericidal
2. Cerebrospinal fluid (CSF)
3. Kidneys
4. Narrow
5. Negative
6. Hours

7. Concentration dependent
8. Enzymes
9. Anaerobes
10. a, c, f
11. a
12. a (Patients on aminoglycoside therapy should be monitored for ototoxicity. The first sign of impending vestibular damage is headache, which may last for 1 or 2 days. A complete assessment must be performed prior to notifying the provider for them to determine whether the headache is related to tobramycin. Therefore, assessment is the priority action.)
13. d (Caution must be exercised when combining gentamicin with other nephrotoxic or ototoxic drugs.)
14. c (Aminoglycosides can inhibit neuromuscular transmission, causing flaccid paralysis and potentially fatal respiratory depression. Most episodes of neuromuscular blockade have occurred following intraperitoneal or intrapleural instillation of aminoglycosides. However, neuromuscular blockade has also occurred with intravenous [IV], intramuscular [IM], and oral dosing.)
15. b
16. d (Comparing the estimated glomerular filtration rate [eGFR] to the dosing recommendations provided in the package insert or IV drug book, in concert with trough drug level, will enable the nurse to determine if the dosing is appropriate.)
17. c
18. b (Peak gentamicin levels should range between 4 and 10 mcg/mL for traditional dosing or between 16 and 24 mcg/mL for once-daily dosing; trough should not exceed 2 cg/mL.)
19. a (In patients with normal renal function, half-lives of the aminoglycosides range from 2 to 3 hours. However, because elimination is almost exclusively renal, half-lives increase dramatically in patients with renal impairment. Accordingly, to avoid serious toxicity, dosage must be reduced or the dosing interval increased in patients with kidney disease.)
20. c (Aminoglycosides can intensify neuromuscular blockade induced by pancuronium or other skeletal muscle relaxants. If used with these agents, caution must be exercised to avoid respiratory arrest.)
21. 100–170 mg every 8 hours. However, according to table 92.1, the total daily dosing for adults is 3-5 mg/kg. Administering 170 mg every 8 hours would exceed this total daily dose.
22. No. The correct dosing for amikacin is 7.5 mg/kg every 12 hours. This would be 487.5 mg every 12 hours.

CHAPTER 93

1. F
2. T
3. T
4. F
5. F
6. T
7. F
8. T
9. F
10. T
11. T
12. d (Symptoms of Stevens-Johnson syndrome include blisters and sores on the skin and on mucus membranes of the mouth, combined with fever, malaise, and toxemia.)
13. b (To minimize the risk of renal damage, adults should maintain a daily urine output of 1200 mL. This can be accomplished by consuming 8–10 glasses of water each day. Because the solubility of sulfonamides is highest at elevated pH, alkalinization of the urine can further decrease the chances of crystalluria.)
14. c (In addition to hemolytic anemia, sulfonamides can cause agranulocytosis, leukopenia, thrombocytopenia, and, very rarely, aplastic anemia; in hemolytic anemia, the hemoglobin is decreased, the mean corpuscular volume [MCV] remains in normal range, and LDH and reticulocyte count are elevated.)
15. a
16. b
17. a
18. c (Local application of mafenide is frequently painful.)
19. c
20. b (People with hyperkalemia may report symptoms such as muscle weakness, tiredness, tingling sensations, or nausea.)
21. a
22. c
23. a
24. d
25. 160 mg each dose (20 mL); keep in mind, dosing is based on trimethoprim (TMP).

CHAPTER 94

1. c
2. f
3. b
4. a
5. e
6. d
7. b
8. b (Prevention of repeat UTIs in females includes wiping front to back.)
9. a, b, c, d
10. d (If treatment is to succeed, the identity and drug sensitivity of the causative organism must be determined. To do so, urine for microbiologic testing should be obtained before giving any antibiotics.)
11. c

12. b (Acute reactions induced by nitrofurantoin manifest as dyspnea, chest pain, chills, fever, cough, and alveolar infiltrates.)
13. a
14. a, b, c, e
15. c (Nitrofurantoin has caused severe liver injury, manifesting as hepatitis, cholestatic jaundice, and hepatic necrosis. Deaths have occurred. To reduce risk, patients should undergo periodic tests of liver function. Those who develop liver injury should discontinue nitrofurantoin immediately and never use it again.)
16. a
17. 2 capsules
18. 0.5 (1/2) tablet

CHAPTER 95

1. T
2. F
3. F
4. F
5. T
6. F
7. F
8. T
9. F
10. T
11. T
12. b, c, d
13. d
14. b
15. d (Isoniazid can cause hepatocellular injury and multilobular necrosis. Patients should be informed about signs of hepatitis [anorexia, malaise, fatigue, nausea, yellowing of the skin or eyes] and instructed to notify the provider immediately if these develop.)
16. b
17. a, c, e
18. c
19. b
20. a
21. c (Rifampin is a powerful inducer of hepatic isoenzymes. It can hasten the metabolism of many drugs, reducing their effectiveness. The dosage of warfarin may need to be increased. Changes in mental status may be a sign of a stroke.)
22. b
23. a, b, d (The eighth cranial nerve is the vestibulocochlear nerve that is responsible for hearing, balance, and body position sense. Problems with the nerve may result in deafness, nystagmus, tinnitus, dizziness, vertigo, and vomiting. Second-line aminoglycosides may damage the eighth nerve.)
24. b (Ethambutol can produce dose-related optic neuritis, resulting in blurred vision, constriction of the visual field, and disturbance of color discrimination.)
25. a
26. c
27. c (Bedaquiline can cause QT prolongation, which places the patient at risk for dangerous ventricular dysrhythmias.)
28. 507 mL divided by 3 = 169 mL/h
29. Yes. Safe dose range is 400–800 mg/day = 200–400 mg/dose.

CHAPTER 96

1. Tendon
2. *Neisseria gonorrhoeae*
3. *Clostridiodes difficile*
4. Phototoxicity (or severe sunburn)
5. Broad
6. a (If treatment is to succeed and drug resistance reduced, the identity and drug sensitivity of the causative organism must be determined.)
7. d (Ciprofloxacin can induce a variety of mild adverse effects, including GI reactions [nausea, vomiting, diarrhea, abdominal pain]; vomiting and diarrhea put the child at increased risk of electrolyte imbalance.)
8. a, d, e
9. d (Candida infections [thrush] of the pharynx may develop during treatment. Symptoms of thrush include pain when swallowing.)
10. c (Absorption of ciprofloxacin can be reduced by aluminum/magnesium-containing antacids, iron salts, and calcium supplements. These agents should be administered 6 hours before or 2 hours after ciprofloxacin. Because of these timing issues, the provider should be contacted for additional orders concerning the supplements.)
11. c (Ciprofloxacin can increase plasma levels of theophylline. Tachycardia is a symptom of theophylline toxicity.)
12. d
13. b (Moxifloxacin should be used with great caution in patients with hypokalemia; symptoms of hypokalemia include weakness, fatigue, muscle cramps, and constipation.)
14. b (Avoid this drug in patients with hypokalemia or preexisting QT prolongation and in those taking prodysrhythmic drugs.)
15. c
16. c
17. a
18. a
19. a, b, c
20. b, c, e (Please note: Option d is not approved for diarrhea accompanied by fever.)
21. 494 mg is the recommended dose. This is safe.
22. Yes, it is safe. 1.2 g is the recommended dose.

CHAPTER 97

1. Mycosis
2. Nonopportunistic
3. Systemic mycoses; superficial mycoses
4. T

5. T
6. T
7. T
8. F
9. T
10. T
11. F
12. T
13. b
14. d
15. c
16. a
17. c, d, e
18. c
19. b
20. a (Amphotericin is toxic to cells of the kidney. Renal impairment occurs in practically all patients.)
21. a (Amphotericin can cause bone marrow suppression.)
22. a
23. c
24. c
25. b (Itraconazole has negative inotropic actions and should not be used in patients with heart failure or a history of heart failure or other indications of ventricular dysfunction, as it can cause a transient decrease in ventricular ejection fraction.)
26. d
27. c
28. b (Treatment with fluconazole has been associated with Stevens-Johnson syndrome. Fever, along with mucocutaneous lesions, is an early symptom of Stevens-Johnson syndrome.)
29. d
30. b (Patients taking ketoconazole may develop potentially fatal hepatic necrosis. Signs and symptoms include jaundice, ascites, right upper quadrant tenderness, nausea, and vomiting.)
31. a
32. c
33. d
34. a, b, d
35. c
36. 86 or 87 mL/h; total volume is 130 mL over 90 minutes.
37. 12.5 mg; yes, 12 mg is safe.

CHAPTER 98

1. T
2. F
3. T
4. T
5. T
6. F
7. T
8. T
9. F
10. F
11. F
12. T
13. d
14. c
15. a (Intravenous acyclovir is generally well tolerated. The most common reactions are phlebitis and inflammation at the infusion site.)
16. c (Reversible nephrotoxicity, indicated by elevations in serum creatinine and blood urea nitrogen, occurs in some patients. The risk of renal injury is increased by dehydration and use of other nephrotoxic drugs. Dry mucous membranes are indicative of dehydration. To avoid nephrotoxicity, hydrating the patient is priority.)
17. a (For herpes simplex genitalis, valacyclovir is indicated for treatment of initial and recurrent episodes for immunocompetent patients; however, for suppressive therapy, this drug is approved for management in immunocompetent and HIV-infected adults with a CD4+ cell count of at least 100 cells/mm^3.)
18. a
19. b
20. d
21. c (Valganciclovir is presumed to pose the same risks for mutagenesis, aspermatogenesis, and carcinogenesis as ganciclovir. Ganciclovir may present a hazard for nurses who administer this drug. NIOSH requires special handling of drugs identified as hazardous.)
22. c (Foscarnet frequently causes electrolyte and mineral imbalance. Signs of hypocalcemia include numbness, tingling, and muscle cramps progressing to spasm.)
23. c
24. a
25. a (Patients treated with these drugs have developed lactic acidosis. If lactic acidosis develops, these drugs should be discontinued. A sign of lactic acidosis is deep, rapid breathing.)
26. a
27. a, d, e
28. c
29. d
30. a, b
31. 200 mg every 8 hours
32. 3800 mg each dose (40 × 95); 158 mL in each dose (3800/24=158.33 or 158.)

CHAPTER 99

1. e
2. b
3. a
4. f
5. h
6. d
7. g
8. c
9. c
10. a
11. Single episode: Extended multiple response

Cognitive skill: Recognize cues.

Military Time: 0830 Received patient from emergency department. Patient is HIV-1+. Admit to unit with pneumocystis pneumonia (PCP) infection. Most recent CD4 count (1 month ago) was 200 cells/mm^3, and their HIV viral load was 10,000 copies/mL. Patient is taking Biktarvy 1 tab orally (PO) daily at 0700 hrs. Alert and oriented x 4. Responds to questions appropriately. Cleanly dressed. Patient states they feel worn out. Lungs with diminished breath sounds throughout, dry cough. Becomes short of breath with activity. Heart with regular rate and rhythm. Skin cool and dry; patient is pale. No edema. Blood pressure 142/88, respirations 18, heart rate 95, temperature 102.5°F. Oxygen saturation 92% on room air. Patient is 5'8" and weighs 150 pounds. Orders received for trimethoprim-sulfamethoxazole 340 mg IV every 8 hours for 21 days. Discussed therapy with patient including drug dosing, actions, and side effects. All patient questions answered.	Which laboratory tests should the nurse monitor during drug therapy? **Select all that apply.** a. Aspartate aminotransferase (AST) b. Alanine aminotransferase (ALT) c. Blood urea nitrogen (BUN) d. Complete blood count e. Creatinine f. Lipid profile g. Prothrombin time (PT) h. Total bilirubin

Answer: c, d, e

Rationale: Trimethoprim-sulfamethoxazole has been associated with kidney failure and elevated BUN and creatinine, as well as hemolytic anemia in patients with glucose-6-phosphate dehydrogenase (G6PD) deficiency, agranulocytosis, thrombocytopenia, and aplastic anemia. Complete blood count (CBC) should be monitored. AST, ALT, lipid profile, PT, and total bilirubin do not require monitoring during therapy.

12. d
13. b (Rilpivirine can cause depression. Instruct patients to contact the provider immediately if they start feeling sad, hopeless, or suicidal.)
14. c (CNS symptoms occur in over 50% of patients and include dizziness, insomnia, impaired consciousness, drowsiness, vivid dreams, and nightmares.)
15. d, e, f (The most common adverse effect is rash; for most patients, the rash is benign. However, if the patient experiences severe rash or rash associated with fever, blistering, oral lesions, conjunctivitis, muscle pain, or joint pain, nevirapine should be withdrawn because these symptoms may indicate development of erythema multiforme or Stevens-Johnson syndrome.)
16. c
17. d
18. d (Use of protease inhibitors [PIs] has been associated with redistribution of body fat, sometimes referred to as *lipodystrophy syndrome* or *pseudo-Cushing syndrome*. Fat accumulates in the abdomen ["protease paunch"], in the breasts of males and females, and between the shoulder blades ["buffalo hump"]. Fat is lost from the face, arms, buttocks, and legs. Leg and arm veins become prominent.)
19. a
20. a, b, c, d
21. d (The major adverse effect of indinavir is nephrolithiasis.)
22. a, b, d
23. d (Enfuvirtide has been associated with pneumonia. Cough, shortness of breath, and fever are symptoms of pneumonia.)
24. a
25. b
26. a
27. a, b
28. c
29. c
30. 30 mL
31. 40 mg

CHAPTER 100

1. T
2. T
3. F
4. T
5. F
6. T
7. a
8. d (About half of the infants born to females with cervical *Chlamydia trachomatis* acquire the infection during delivery, putting them at risk for pneumonia.)
9. a
10. c
11. b

12. c (Among preadolescent children, the most common cause of gonococcal infection is sexual abuse. Vaginal, anorectal, and pharyngeal infections are most common.)
13. a
14. b
15. d (Neonatal gonococcal infection is acquired through contact with infected cervical exudates during delivery. Infection can be limited to the eyes, or it may be disseminated. Gonococcal neonatal ophthalmia is a serious infection. The initial symptom is conjunctivitis.)
16. b
17. d
18. a
19. c
20. b
21. 40 mg every 6 hours; 160 mg total per day.
22. 100 mL/h

CHAPTER 101

1. e
2. b
3. c
4. d
5. f
6. a
7. g
8. F
9. F
10. T
11. T
12. F
13. T
14. F
15. T
16. F
17. a, b, d
18. a
19. b
20. a (Isopropanol promotes local vasodilation and can thereby increase bleeding from needle punctures and incisions.)
21. a, b
22. b
23. b
24. a (Because benzalkonium chloride is inactivated by soap, all soap must be removed by rinsing with water and 70% alcohol prior to benzalkonium chloride application.)
25. b
26. c, d, e

CHAPTER 102

1. T
2. T
3. F
4. T
5. F
6. T
7. T
8. T
9. F
10. b (Infestation is associated with chronic blood loss and progressive anemia. Pale skin may be an indication of anemia.)
11. d
12. c
13. b, c, d, g
14. c (Relatively low doses of mebendazole are embryotoxic and teratogenic in animal models. Pregnant females should avoid this drug, especially during the first trimester.)
15. a
16. a
17. d (Indirect effects of diethylcarbamazine, occurring secondary to death of the parasites, can be more serious. These include rashes, intense itching, encephalitis, fever, tachycardia, lymphadenitis, leukocytosis, and proteinuria.)
18. 5 tablets
19. Yes. Safe dosage ranges from 375 to 750 mg × 1.

CHAPTER 103

1. Young
2. *Anopheles* mosquito
3. Hepatocytes (or liver cells)
4. Erythrocytes
5. Vivax
6. Relapse
7. Black water fever
8. c
9. b
10. c
11. c
12. b (*Plasmodium falciparum* can destroy up to 60% of circulating red blood cells [RBCs]; the hemoglobin released from these cells causes the urine to darken, giving rise to the term "black water fever.")
13. a (Falciparum malaria can produce serious complications, including pulmonary edema.)
14. a (Symptoms of hypoglycemia include sweating, chills, and clamminess.)
15. d
16. a (The most serious and frequent effect from primaquine is hemolysis, which can develop in patients with glucose-6-phosphate dehydrogenase [G6PD] deficiency. During primaquine therapy, the urine should be monitored [darkening indicates the presence of hemoglobin].)
17. c (Quinine has quinidine-like effects on the heart and must be used cautiously in patients with atrial fibrillation. By enhancing atrioventricular conduction, quinine can increase passage of atrial impulses to the ventricles, thereby causing a dangerous increase in ventricular rate.)
18. b
19. a

20. a (When proguanil is used alone, the most common side effects are oral ulceration, GI effects, and headache. In addition, the drug may cause hair loss, urticaria, hematuria, thrombocytopenia, and scaling of the soles and palms. Bleeding gums are a symptom of thrombocytopenia.)
21. c (Patients taking mefloquine who develop psychiatric symptoms [hallucinations, depression, suicidal ideation] should discontinue the drug immediately and contact their provider.)
22. c
23. a, b, d
24. 18 mL (165 lb = 75 kg; 75 kg × 2.4 mg/kg = 180 mg/10 mg/mL = 18 mL.)
25. 166 (or 167) mg every 8 hours

CHAPTER 104

1. b
2. d
3. a
4. c
5. c (Cryptosporidiosis is characterized by diarrhea, abdominal cramps, anorexia, low-grade fever, nausea, and vomiting. For immunocompromised individuals, the disease can be prolonged and life-threatening, with diarrhea volume up to 20 L/day. For this person on prednisone for chronic illness, fluid volume deficit would be a priority, as they are immunocompromised and could potentially have life-threatening diarrhea.)
6. d
7. a
8. c
9. a
10. a, b, e
11. b
12. 6 mg (2 tablet). 65 pounds = 29.5 kg; 29.5 kg × 0.2 mg (200 mcg)/kg = 5.9 mg or 6 mg = 2 tablets.

CHAPTER 105

1. P
2. S
3. S
4. B
5. P
6. S
7. B
8. B
9. P
10. B
11. b
12. a, c, d
13. b
14. c
15. 2 oz

CHAPTER 106

1. 27%
2. Drug therapy
3. Prostate
4. Surgery
5. Immunotherapy
6. Cytotoxic
7. Division
8. d
9. b, d
10. a
11. c
12. a
13. b
14. a (Normal red blood cell [RBC] range is greater than 4.5×10^6/mL. Symptoms of anemia include fatigue, sore or aching muscles, weakness, and slowed reflexes and responses.)
15. c
16. a
17. b (Caution should be exercised when performing procedures that might promote bleeding.)
18. c (The major concern with hyperuricemia is injury to the kidneys secondary to deposition of uric acid crystals in renal tubules.)
19. b (Certain anticancer drugs are highly chemically reactive and can cause severe local injury if they make direct contact with tissues.)

CHAPTER 107

1. T
2. F
3. T
4. F
5. T
6. T
7. F
8. F
9. T
10. F
11. d (To prevent bleeding secondarily to thrombocytopenia, use soft toothbrush and electric razor and eat a high-fiber diet.)
12. a (Bone marrow suppression [neutropenia, thrombocytopenia] is the usual dose-limiting toxicity for patients receiving cytotoxic drugs.)
13. b, c
14. a
15. b
16. d
17. c (Other adverse effects of cisplatin include ototoxicity, which manifests as tinnitus and high-frequency hearing loss.)
18. b
19. d
20. c (High doses can directly injure the kidneys. To promote drug excretion, and thereby minimize renal damage, the urine should be alkalinized and adequate hydration maintained.)
21. b (It should be noted that leucovorin rescue is potentially dangerous: failure to administer leucovorin in the right dose at the right time can be fatal.)

22. a (One of the dose-limiting toxicities associated with methotrexate therapy is pulmonary infiltrates and fibrosis.)
23. c
24. a, d, e (Cytarabine syndrome: fever, aches, bone pain, rash and conjunctivitis may occur 6-12 hours post-administration.)
25. a
26. d (Bone marrow suppression [neutropenia, thrombocytopenia, anemia] is the principal dose-limiting toxicity. Petechiae often occur in the setting of thrombocytopenia.)
27. d
28. d
29. c (The major dose-limiting toxicity is injury to the lungs. Injury manifests initially as pneumonitis.)
30. a (Alopecia develops in about 20% of patients receiving vincristine. For adolescents, hair loss secondary to chemotherapy can be devastating; nurses must assist the adolescent to find ways to cope with this problem.)
31. b (Severe hypersensitivity reactions [hypotension, dyspnea, angioedema, urticaria] have occurred during infusion of paclitaxel.)
32. c (Severe hypersensitivity can occur with docetaxel infusion. Manifestations include hypotension, bronchospasm, and generalized rash or erythema.)
33. d (Diarrhea, seen in 47% of patients receiving cabazitaxel, can be severe. Deaths resulting from electrolyte imbalance have occurred.)
34. 300 mcg
35. Body surface area (BSA) is 2.25 m^2. 2.25 × 550 = 1237.5 mg

CHAPTER 108

1. F
2. T
3. T
4. F
5. F
6. F
7. d (Perhaps the biggest concern with tamoxifen is endometrial cancer. Tamoxifen acts as an estrogen agonist at receptors in the uterus, causing proliferation of endometrial tissue.)
8. b
9. a (Because of its estrogen agonist actions, tamoxifen poses a small risk of thromboembolic events, including deep vein thrombosis, pulmonary embolism, and stroke.)
10. c
11. d (Toremifene administration increases the risk of thrombosis.)
12. a, d, e
13. a (The principal concern with trastuzumab is cardiotoxicity, manifesting as ventricular dysfunction and congestive heart failure.)
14. d
15. a, d
16. c
17. d
18. b (One of the presenting signs of hypercalcemia is weakness.)
19. c
20. d
21. c (Nilutamide can cause hepatotoxicity and interstitial pneumonitis.)
22. a, e
23. a, c
24. a (One of the major adverse effects of these drugs is neutropenia. A normal absolute neutrophil count [ANC] ranges from 1500/mm^3 to 8000/mm^3.)
25. d
26. b
27. a (Fluid retention occurs in 52–68% of patients taking imatinib and may lead to pleural effusion, pericardial effusion, pulmonary edema, or ascites.)
28. d
29. b (Sunitinib frequently causes thrombocytopenia.)
30. c (Rapid and massive death of tumor cells can lead to TLS, characterized by acute renal failure, hyperkalemia, hypocalcemia, hyperuricemia, or hyperphosphatemia)
31. a (Rituximab can cause severe infusion-related hypersensitivity reactions. Prominent symptoms are hypotension, bronchospasm, and angioedema.)
32. c
33. a (Bevacizumab can cause life-threatening side effects, including gastrointestinal [GI] perforation, hemorrhage, and thromboembolism.)
34. d
35. a
36. a
37. c (Practically all patients experience significant toxicity with aldesleukin. The drug must be administered in a hospital with intensive care unit [ICU] and a cardiopulmonary/ICU specialist available. One of the most often seen effects is pulmonary congestion and dyspnea.)
38. c
39. c
40. d (In patients taking interferon alfa-2b, neuropsychiatric effects—especially depression—are a serious concern, owing to a risk of death by suicide. Therefore, preventing injury is the priority.)
41. Yes. The patient's body surface area (BSA) = 2 m^2. 2 × 400 mg = 800 mg.

CHAPTER 109

1. c
2. m
3. f
4. d
5. a
6. n
7. e

8. g
9. i
10. j
11. k
12. l
13. b
14. h
15. Central
16. Drusen
17. Dry; wet
18. Anemia
19. b (Since primary open-angle glaucoma [POAG] has no symptoms [until significant and irreversible optic nerve injury has occurred], regular testing for early POAG is important among individuals at high risk. With early detection and treatment, blindness can usually be prevented.)
20. d (Angle-closure glaucoma develops suddenly and is extremely painful. In the absence of treatment, irreversible loss of vision occurs in 1–2 days.)
21. a, e
22. a
23. c
24. b
25. a, d
26. c
27. c, e (By relaxing the iris sphincter, anticholinergic drugs can induce closure of the filtration angle. In persons who have narrow angles to begin with, topical anticholinergic drugs can be absorbed in sufficient amounts to produce systemic toxicity, including tachycardia.)
28. c
29. d (The biggest concern is endophthalmitis, an inflammation inside the eye caused by bacterial, viral, or fungal infection. Patients who experience symptoms [e.g., redness, light sensitivity, pain] should seek immediate medical attention.)
30. a
31. b
32. 0.05 mL
33. 2.5 mL

CHAPTER 110

1. Epidermis
2. Stratum germinativum or basal layer
3. Keratin
4. Corneum
5. Melanin
6. Dermis
7. Sebum
8. Fat
9. f
10. e
11. g
12. d
13. a
14. b
15. c
16. a
17. d (Assessment is the first step in the nursing process. To describe what the skin looks like when contacting the provider, the nurse must assess first.)
18. a (Salicylic acid is readily absorbed through the skin, so systemic toxicity [salicylism] can result when large amounts are used for a prolonged period. Symptoms of salicylism include tinnitus.)
19. b
20. a (Some formulations of benzoyl peroxide contain sulfites, which can cause potentially serious allergic reactions. The incidence of reactions is highest in patients with asthma.)
21. a
22. a, c, e
23. a, b, c
24. a
25. b
26. a
27. d
28. b
29. d
30. c
31. d
32. a (Sunscreens alone cannot completely protect against sun damage. Accordingly, to further reduce risk, sunglasses, protective clothing, and a wide-brimmed hat should be worn. In addition, avoid sun exposure in the middle of the day, especially between 10:00 a.m. and 4:00 p.m. If you must be outside at these times, try to stay in the shade as much as possible. These all work together to reduce chronic exposure of the skin to sunlight.)
33. c
34. a
35. b (Podophyllin is teratogenic and must not be used during pregnancy.)
36. b
37. 83 mL/h
38. 1 mL

CHAPTER 111

1. Auricle; pinna
2. External ear
3. Eardrum; inner
4. Eustachian tube
5. Semicircular canals
6. F
7. T
8. F
9. T
10. F
11. c
12. d
13. a
14. d
15. a, b, d

16. d
17. d
18. 0.8 mL
19. 15 mL

CHAPTER 112

1. b
2. e
3. d
4. b
5. b
6. b, c, f
7. b
8. b (Supportive care is the most important element in managing acute poisoning. Support is based on the clinical status and requires no knowledge specific to the poison involved. Maintenance of respiration and circulation are primary concerns.)
9. b, e
10. a
11. d
12. c
13. b (Whole-bowel irrigation should not be used in patients with bloody vomitus.)
14. d
15. a (The principal disadvantage of hemoperfusion is loss of platelets.)
16. a
17. b (Rapid IV infusion may cause hypotension, tachycardia, erythema, and urticaria.)
18. c
19. d
20. a
21. d
22. c (Bone marrow suppression can result in leukopenia, agranulocytosis, and aplastic anemia, all of which can be fatal.)
23. c
24. a
25. 840 mg; 0.84 mL; 200 mL/h
26. 333 mL/h

CHAPTER 113

1. T
2. T
3. F
4. T
5. T
6. T
7. T
8. T
9. F
10. d (Initial symptoms of anthrax include fever, cough, malaise, and weakness. They may be relatively mild.)
11. a
12. d
13. a (The correct dosage of streptomycin is 10 mg/kg twice a day for 7 to 10 days.)
14. d (Pneumonic plague is acquired by inhaling aerosolized *Yersinia pestis*; aerosolized particles require airborne precautions.)
15. b
16. b
17. a
18. a (Accordingly, people who have these conditions [pregnancy] should not be vaccinated—unless, of course, they have been exposed to the smallpox virus, in which case the risk for infection would far outweigh the risk of the vaccine.)
19. a (Supportive care, which may be needed for several months, includes mechanical assistance of ventilation; hence, effective breathing is the highest nursing priority.)
20. c (Prussian blue can bind with potassium and other electrolytes. Some patients have developed hypokalemia. To reduce risk, serum electrolytes should be monitored closely. Exercise caution in patients with cardiac dysrhythmias [which are sensitive to hypokalemia] or preexisting electrolyte imbalance. Therefore, patients on digoxin should be monitored closely.)
21. c
22. c
23. 1/2 tablet
24. Yes, the dose is safe and effective; 300 mg is 14 mg/kg for a child under 12 (calculates out to 299.09 mg).